Kay Lawson

Progress in Pathology

Volume 7

Progress in Pathology reviews many aspects of pathology, describing issues of everyday diagnostic relevance and the mechanisms underlying some of these processes. Each volume in the series reviews a wide range of topics and recent advances in pathology of relevance to daily practice, keeping consultants, trainees, laboratory staff and researchers abreast of developments as well as providing candidates for the MRCPath and other examinations with answers to some of the questions they will encounter.

Highly illustrated in full colour, topics covered in this volume include:

Immunohistochemistry as a diagnostic aid in gynaecological pathology, Drug induced liver injury, Childhood lymphoma, Immune responses to tumors, Post-mortem imaging, Understanding the Human Tissue Act 2004 and much more.

Volume 7 of Progress in Pathology will be an essential addition to the shelves and laboratory benches of every practising pathologist.

Nigel Kirkham is Consultant Histopathologist in the Department of Cellular Pathology at the Royal Victoria Infirmary, Newcastle upon Tyne, UK.

Neil A. Shepherd is Consultant Histopathologist at Gloucestershire Royal Hospital, Gloucester, UK.

D1337914

Progress in Pathology

Volume 7

Edited by

Nigel Kirkham, MD FRCPath

Consultant Histopathologist
Royal Victoria Infirmary
Newcastle upon Tyne, UK

Neil A. Shepherd, DM FRCPath

Consultant Histopathologist &
Visiting Professor of Pathology
Gloucestershire Royal Hospital
Gloucester, UK

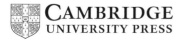
CAMBRIDGE
UNIVERSITY PRESS

CAMBRIDGE UNIVERSITY PRESS

Cambridge, New York, Melbourne, Madrid, Cape Town, Singapore, São Paulo

Cambridge University Press
The Edinburgh Building, Cambridge CB2 2RU, UK

Published in the United States of America by Cambridge University Press, New York

www.cambridge.org
Information on this title: www.cambridge.org/9780521694599

First published 2007

Printed in the United Kingdom at the University Press, Cambridge

A catalogue record for this publication is available from the British Library

ISBN-13 978-0-521-69459-9 hardback
ISBN-10 0-521-69459-0 hardback

Contents

Contributors

Editors

Dr Nigel Kirkham
Consultant Histopathologist
Department of Cellular Pathology
Royal Victoria Infirmary
Newcastle upon Tyne, UK

Professor Neil A. Shepherd
Consultant Histopathologist
Gloucestershire Royal Hospital
Gloucester, UK

Contributors

Dr Adrian C. Bateman
Consultant Pathologist
Department of Cellular Pathology
Southampton General Hospital
Southampton, UK

Dr Clare Craig
Clinical Academic Training Fellow
Department of Histopathology
Royal Free and University College
Medical School
London, UK

Dr Susan E. Davies
Consultant Pathologist
Department of Histopathology
Addenbrooke's Hospital
Cambridge University Hospitals
NHS Foundation Trust
Cambridge, UK

Dr Jayne L. Dennis
Centre for Oncology and
Applied Pharmacology
Cancer Research UK Beatson
Laboratories
University of Glasgow
Glasgow, UK

Dr Victoria Elliot
Specialist Registrar in Histopathology
Department of Cellular Pathology
Southampton General Hospital
Southampton, UK

Professor T. R. Jeffry Evans
Centre for Oncology and
Applied Pharmacology
Cancer Research UK Beatson
Laboratories
University of Glasgow
Glasgow, UK

Dr Jyoti Gupta
Consultant Histopathologist
Preston Hall Hospital
Maidstone
Kent, UK

Dr Linda M. Harrison
Clinical Scientist
Department of Pathology
Royal Lancaster Infirmary
Lancaster, UK

Dr Siân E. Hughes
Consultant Pathologist
Honorary Senior Lecturer
Department of Histopathology
Royal Free and University College
Medical School
London, UK

Dr Richard Jones
Specialist Registrar in Histopathology
Hammersmith Hospitals NHS Trust
Charing Cross Hospital
London, UK

Dr Keith P. McCarthy
Consultant Pathologist
Department of Histopathology
Cheltenham General Hospital
Gloucestershire, UK

Professor W. Glenn McCluggage
Consultant Gynaecological Pathologist
Department of Pathology
Royal Group of Hospitals Trust
Belfast
Northern Ireland

Dr Sanjiv Manek
Consultant Gynaecological Pathologist
John Radcliffe Hospital
Oxford, UK

Professor James A. Morris
Consultant Pathologist
Department of Pathology
Royal Lancaster Infirmary
Lancaster, UK

Dr Karin A. Oien
CR-UK Clinician Scientist
and Hon. Consultant Pathologist
Centre for Oncology and Applied
Pharmacology
Cancer Research UK Beatson
Laboratories
University of Glasgow and University
Department of Pathology
Glasgow Royal Infirmary, UK

Dr Susan F. D. Robinson
Consultant Neuropathologist
Institute of Neurological Sciences
Southern General Hospital
Glasgow, UK

Dr Elizabeth J. Soilleux
Consultant Pathologist
John Radcliffe Hospital
Oxford, UK

Dr William Stewart
Specialist Registrar in Neuropathology
Honorary Clinical Teacher
Department of Neuropathology
Institute of Neurological Sciences
Southern General Hospital
Glasgow, UK

Dr Bryan F. Warren
Consultant Gastrointestinal Pathologist
John Radcliffe Hospital
Oxford, UK

Preface

In the years that have passed since the publication of the last volume of *Progress in Pathology* have seen many developments and changes in the practice of Pathology. The basis of our work in the diagnosis and understanding of disease processes remains much the same as ever but, as our society becomes more developed and more demanding of its healthcare workers, the challenges that we face grow beyond the basic task of diagnosis, to considerations of the place of the specialty of Pathology within that complex animal, the multidisciplinary team in the hospital, as well as more widely in society itself.

Some of these developments are reflected in the range of chapters to be found within these covers. The selection in this volume extends from basic science and issues in neuropathology and lymphoma, through the effects of drugs in causing, as well as treating, disease in the liver, to consideration of why small children come to die suddenly, and what may be found in the hearts of some adults who also come to autopsy after unexpected deaths. We also include contributions on the developing role of the pathologist as part of the multidisciplinary team and on the legislation that has been enacted in England as a reaction to some of the negative publicity that has impinged upon the specialty in recent years.

This review of the state of Pathology will, we hope, give you, our readers, an opportunity to develop your knowledge as well as to reflect upon some of the ways in which our work is changing, whether preparing for professional examinations or as part of continuing professional development. Once again we cannot disagree with the old adage that you cannot 'stand in the way of Progress'. We trust that you will find much of interest here.

The observant amongst you will have noticed that this, the 7th volume of *Progress*, sees us with, apparently, new publishers. In fact our new publishers, Cambridge University Press, have bought out our former publishers Greenwich Medical Media. We look forward to working with Cambridge for many editions to come.

N.K. and N.A.S
Newcastle upon Tyne and Gloucester
January 2007

1

The microbiological investigation of sudden unexpected death in infancy

James A. Morris and Linda M. Harrison

INTRODUCTION

Sudden unexpected death in infancy (SUDI) is simply defined as the death of an infant that is sudden and is unexpected. If a detailed post-mortem examination fails to reveal an adequate explanation for death then the term 'sudden infant death syndrome' (SIDS) is used. If the autopsy does not reveal an explanation for death, but there are suspicious features, the term 'unascertained' is often applied. The difference between SIDS, which legal authorities will regard as natural disease, and unascertained is, therefore, related to the level of suspicion. The latter term can cause distress to parents and lead to unnecessary inquests. It should be used sparingly. In strict logic, of course, the difference between 'I don't know' (SIDS) and 'I don't know' (unascertained) is unascertained and unascertainable.

The age distribution of SUDI and SIDS is the most consistent and characteristic feature of sudden infant death. The risk of SUDI and SIDS is low in the first few days of life, the risk then rises to a peak at two to three months, followed by a rapid fall so that the condition is uncommon after six months and rare after twelve months (Fig. 1.1). This risk profile is approximately reciprocal to infant serum IgG levels, and therefore sudden death occurs when infants have least protection against common bacteria and common bacterial toxins. For this reason it is important that careful microbiological investigation is carried out in all sudden infant deaths.

There are published protocols for the microbiological investigation of these cases, with which we broadly concur [1], [2]. Certain aspects of the investigation, however, are more important than others and the time when specimens are obtained is crucial. In this chapter we intend to concentrate on aspects of the investigation, giving background information as to why the tests are needed and placing emphasis on practical procedures as well as discussing the difficult task of interpreting the results obtained.

Progress in Pathology Volume 7, ed. Nigel Kirkham and Neil Shepherd. Published by Cambridge University Press. © Cambridge University Press 2007.

James A. Morris and Linda M. Harrison

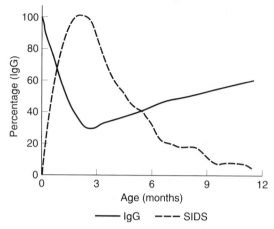

Fig. 1.1 Serum IgG levels in infancy expressed as a percentage of the adult level. The age distribution of SIDS is for cases in England and Wales between 1993 and 1995 (1311 cases).

CEREBROSPINAL FLUID

The diagnosis of meningitis in life depends on the examination of cerebrospinal fluid (CSF). In a suspected case of meningitis, CSF is obtained using an aseptic technique to avoid contamination by bacteria from the skin surface. The specimen is examined promptly; a white cell count and differential cell count are performed; protein, glucose and, in some laboratories, lactate levels are determined. The specimen is then examined for bacteria using Gram stain and bacterial culture. Part of the specimen is sent to a specialised laboratory for viral culture and some saved in case other specialised techniques are required, such as nucleic acid amplification or immunoassay to identify specific organisms.

We suggest that exactly the same approach should be used in cases of SUDI. The problem is, however, to obtain the specimen sufficiently soon after death for the investigation to be useful.

WHITE CELL COUNT

Normal CSF contains no more than four mononuclear cells per cubic mm and no polymorphs [3]. Inflammation of the meninges (meningitis) leads to protein and white cell exudation so that the white cell count rises. The rise is predominantly lymphocytic in viral infection, while polymorphs predominate in bacterial infection. A major problem of interpretation of post-mortem CSF, however, is that the mononuclear cell count rises after death in the absence of inflammation. Thus Platt *et al.* [4] found CSF counts ranged between 37 and 3250 cells per cubic mm (mean = 647 per cubic mm) in 26 cases of SIDS, in which there was no evidence of meningitis. The post-mortem intervals were stated as 2 to 28 hours. In adult autopsies the CSF pleocytosis was less marked, with a mean of 28 white cells per cubic mm (mean post-mortem interval 15 hours). In SIDS cases the typeable cells were mononuclear and consisted of 60 to 70% lymphocytes and

Table 1.1 Normal CSF protein ranges in infancy	
Term	
neonate	0.2–1.7 g/l
1–30 days	0.2–1.5 g/l
30–90 days	0.2–1 g/l
3–6 months	0.15–0.3 g/l
6 months–10 years	0.15–0.3 g/l

20 to 40% macrophages. The authors did not record the presence of polymorphs. When the post-mortem interval exceeded 12 hours the cells became vacuolated and could not be identified. The CSF cell count rises with the duration of the post-mortem interval, but the rate of rise is decreased if the body is stored at 4 °C as opposed to 20 °C [3].

The mononuclear cells in the CSF are apparently derived from the lining cells of the arachnoid membranes. In the absence of inflammation polymorphs should not cross the blood–brain barrier and therefore, if polymorphs are seen, they are, in theory, an absolute indicator of inflammation. This seems to be borne out in practice as neither of the above publications [3], [4] record the presence of polymorphs in the absence of meningitis. In order to gain maximum information, therefore, a differential cell count should be performed on post-mortem CSF samples, but they would have to be obtained within a few hours of death for this to be useful. The distinction between polymorphs and mononuclear cells in samples showing degenerative changes can be difficult, and modern staining techniques, using a range of specific antisera, on cytocentrifuge preparations should be deployed (a useful research project for someone).

PROTEIN

Fishman [3] gives normal ranges for CSF protein in infancy (Table 1.1)

The blood–brain barrier is maintained in health so that the protein concentration in plasma is much higher than in CSF (i.e. 200-fold difference in adults). Meningeal inflammation, however, leads to increased permeability of meningeal vessels, and proteins leak into the CSF. The blood–brain barrier was first described in autopsy studies conducted in the nineteenth century [5]. Ehrlich and his students injected aniline dyes intravenously, the dyes became attached to albumin in blood. At autopsy it was found that the tissues were stained blue but not the CSF, which remained clear, nor the brain. Thus with rapid death and a short post-mortem interval there is no leakage of protein into the CSF in experimental animals.

There are relatively few studies of CSF protein changes in humans following death and no large systematic studies in infants [6]–[9]. The study by Mangin et al. [7] demonstrates a good correlation between the clinical history and the CSF protein concentration when the samples were obtained within 24 hours of death. If death was rapid, such as in cases of homicide, the CSF protein was within the normal range. If the process of dying was prolonged and associated with inflammation and cytokine release, as in patients in intensive care, the CSF protein was raised. In the study conducted by Osuna *et al.* [9], in comparison, all the CSF protein values were raised and bore little relation to the premorbid condition. In this study, however, the samples were obtained after a mean interval of 48 hours. Thus it appears that the CSF protein estimation can be useful but only if obtained soon after death. This is another area in which more research is required.

CSF GLUCOSE AND LACTATE LEVELS

Polymorphs are anaerobic cells, when activated they metabolise glucose and cause a fall in pH and a rise in lactate levels. Thus bacterial infection is associated with a fall in CSF glucose and a rise in CSF lactate. The same changes, however, can follow death in the absence of infection and therefore these analyses are of limited value in post-mortem samples.

PRACTICAL CONSIDERATIONS

The usual practice of taking a CSF sample 24, 48 or even 72 hours after death results in loss of information. In most cases of sudden death the infants are taken urgently to A&E departments and a consultant paediatrician attends to supervise resuscitation and to decide when to desist. The consultant paediatrician should be empowered by the coroner to commence the investigation by obtaining samples for microbiology, including CSF. The sample should then be sent to the laboratory and treated urgently, as for a case of suspected meningitis in life. There is no point in getting the specimen early and then allowing it to deteriorate over several hours. The sample should be taken with full aseptic precautions to reduce the possibility of bacterial contamination. The result of the analysis will then be ready prior to the autopsy. The pathologist should also take a sample when the autopsy is undertaken, preferably by cisternal puncture (after careful cleaning of the skin with alcohol wipes) so as to obtain sufficient fluid in case further studies are required (see below). Paediatricians are skilled at taking clean samples but pathologists are better at getting large volumes of fluid.

HISTOPATHOLOGICAL CORRELATION

There is a school of thought that meningitis can be diagnosed on the basis of histological examination alone, and that therefore counting white cells in the CSF and measuring the protein level is unnecessary. In my opinion this view is misguided for the following reasons:

1. Histological examination of the meninges is 100% specific for meningitis, i.e., by definition, those without meningitis will not show lymphocytic and polymorph infiltration of the meninges. Since no biological test is both 100% sensitive and 100% specific it follows that histological examination cannot identify every case of meningitis (sensitivity is the percentage of individuals with meningitis who show diagnostic histological features of meningitis).

2. In viewing a section of meninges on microscopy we would expect to see at least one polymorph per high power field in a case of meningitis. The mean diameter of a high power field is 0.5 mm and the section thickness is 0.005 mm. Thus one polymorph per high power field is equivalent to 800 polymorphs per cubic mm of tissue. Eighty polymorphs per cubic mm of CSF is more than enough for a diagnosis of meningitis, but the equivalent (one polymorph per 10 high power fields) is not enough. Thus, simple calculations indicate that in the early stages of meningitis examination of the CSF will allow a diagnosis to be made before diagnostic changes are seen in tissue sections. The CSF white cell count is a more sensitive indicator than histology.

3. Sonnabend *et al.* [10] conducted a very careful microbiological study of 70 cases of SUDI. They found evidence of overwhelming infection in eleven. They comment that 'the post-mortem cultures were of diagnostic value, providing the sole means of identifying the cause of death in 8 (11%) of the 70 infants, in whom the presence of an infection could be established only after repeated and extensive histological investigations'. Thus, initial histological investigations were negative but further sections revealed foci of inflammation. This principle applies generally, in the earliest stages of infection the changes may be focal and missed with standard samples.

Sadler [11] reviewed 95 infant deaths examined according to a detailed protocol in which the autopsy was conducted between 2.5 and 53 hours (mean 11 hours, median 5 hours) after death. The author records 'ten (16%) of the apparent cot deaths were explained on the sole basis of unexpected positive microbiological findings, mostly meningococcal or pneumococcal meningitis and/or septicaemia'. Thus, infection, particularly meningitis, can be missed if reliance is placed on histology alone.

INTERPRETATION OF POSITIVE MICROBIOLOGICAL CULTURES

The interpretation of positive microbiological cultures from blood or CSF is fraught with problems[12]. In theory, positive cultures can be due to:

1. Bacteria invading the blood and tissues in life. This is usually associated with inflammation and in the absence of another explanation it is assumed that the bacteria cause or contribute to death.
2. Bacteria entering the blood in the agonal phase or during attempts at resuscitation.
3. Bacterial growth after death followed by tissue invasion. This is reduced but not eliminated by storage of the body at 4 °C.
4. Contamination of the samples, when they are obtained, by surface organisms. This can also be reduced, but not eliminated, by careful technique.

The following is a useful working rule:

A. A pure growth of a pathogen in the CSF in association with inflammation is regarded as the likely cause of death.
B. A pure growth of a pathogen without evidence of inflammation is regarded as a possible cause of death.

C. Other results, such as a mixed growth of organisms in the absence of inflammation, are more likely to be a consequence of mechanisms 2, 3 or 4.

If the specimen is obtained soon after death using a good technique, the chance of false positives due to mechanisms 3 and 4 is reduced.

VIROLOGY

A specimen of CSF should be sent for virological studies. This also applies to blood, upper and lower respiratory secretions and bowel contents. The interpretation of the results is even more difficult than with bacteria. Infants will encounter a number of viruses in the first year of life, and therefore their presence does not necessarily imply significant disease. Isolation of a virus, together with evidence of inflammation at an appropriate site, should be regarded as a possible explanation for death. Isolation of a virus without other evidence of disease leaves the case unexplained.

TOXICOLOGY

The idea that common bacterial toxins could have a role in the pathogenesis of SUDI and SIDS [13] has been strengthened by the discovery that over 50% of SIDS cases have detectable staphylococcal pyrogenic enterotoxins in brain and other tissues [14]. These toxins (toxic shock syndrome toxin (TSST)), and staphylococcal enterotoxins A, B and C) are only produced by staphylococci when the temperature is raised to between 37 and 40 °C. Thus, the presence of these toxins in tissues indicates production in life rather than after death. These results need to be confirmed, but there is a good case for measuring staphylococcal toxins in CSF in every case of SUDI and SIDS.

RESEARCH POINTS

1. The concept that a post-mortem mononuclear cell pleocytosis in the CSF has no pathological significance is open to challenge. The CSF post-mortem cell counts in SIDS are much higher than in adults and there is a possibility that meningitis is being missed. Enumeration of cell sub-types using antisera against the wide range of cluster differentiation antigens (CD) now recognised should aid in distinguishing blood—borne mononuclear cells from the lining cells of the arachnoid membranes.
2. Proteomics is replacing genomics as the vanguard of biological science [15]. Proteins in fluids, such as CSF, can be separated by two-dimensional electrophoresis and then analysed by mass spectroscopy, and their amino acid sequence determined. This entire process can be automated, and in the future it will be possible to recognise foreign proteins, such as bacterial toxins, and products of inflammation. This is big science, rather than the small-scale science we are accustomed to in pathology, but it should be brought to bear on the problem of SUDI.

Table 1.2 Causes of bacteraemia and meningitis in infancy

Under 1 month old	1–3 months old	Over 3 months old
Group B streptococcus	Streptococcus pneumonia	Streptococcus pneumoniae
Enterobacteriaceae	Group B streptococcus	Haemophilus influenzae
Listeria monocytogenes	Neisseria meningitidis	Neisseria meningitidis
Streptococcus pneumonia	Salmonella spp.	Salmonella spp.
Haemophilus influenzae	Haemophilus influenzae	
Staphylococcus aureus	Listeria monocytogenes	
Neisseria meningitidis		
Salmonella spp.		

This table is adapted from Brook [16]

BLOOD CULTURE

A blood culture should also be taken prior to the autopsy and as soon after death as possible. The specimen should be obtained by the consultant paediatrician who attends in A&E. The subsequent assessment of any bacterial growth must take into account the four possible routes of bacterial access noted in the previous section: invasion prior to death, invasion during the agonal phase or as part of resuscitation, post-mortem growth, or contamination. But if the specimen is obtained soon after death using a careful aseptic technique, the possibility of post-mortem growth and contamination is greatly reduced.

Table 1.2 lists the organisms that cause bacteraemia and meningitis in infants [16]. If one of these organisms is isolated in pure growth, then it is a likely explanation for death. If the culture produces a mixed growth of skin commensals then contamination should be suspected. A mixed growth of organisms from the gut or respiratory tract points towards an agonal ingress of bacteria. None of these rules, however, is absolute.

Correlation of the microbiological findings with histology can aid interpretation. If there is evidence of inflammation on serosal surfaces or in the liver or lung, then this increases the likelihood of genuine infection. The absence of inflammation, however, as in meningitis, does not exclude infection.

Table 1.3 shows the results of positive blood cultures obtained in Lancaster, UK from all age groups for one year ($n = 371$). Positive cultures judged to be a result of contamination are excluded. *Escherichia coli* and *Staphylococcus aureus* together account for 40% of serious infections in all age groups except infants aged 1 month to 12 months. This is in spite of the fact that colonisation of the upper airways by *S. aureus* is maximal in the first few months of life [17] and infant serum IgG levels reach their lowest levels at two to three months of age. Brook states [16] 'Most young children who develop bacteraemia are immunologically intact. The process is initiated by nasopharyngeal colonisation and followed by bacterial invasion of the blood and rare systemic dissemination. Both colonisation and bacteraemia are often associated with a preceding viral respiratory tract infection'. It appears that *S. aureus* bacteraemia and meningitis is not observed at the very time one would expect it to be most common.

Table 1.3 Clinically significant blood culture isolates in one year from Royal Lancaster Infirmary, UK ($n = 371$)

Organism	Percentage
Escherichia coli	24.5
Staphylococcus aureus	15.9
Streptococcus pneumoniae	9.2
Klebsiella pneumoniae	5.7
Enterococcus faecalis	4.0
Proteus mirabilis	2.9
Group B streptococci	2.9
Pseudomonas aeruginosa	2.4
Group A streptococci	2.4
Serratia marcescens	1.8
Enterococcus faecium	1.8
Candida albicans	1.8
Other organisms	24.7

The absence of significant *S. aureus* infection in infancy is also at variance with the finding of staphylococcal toxins in the brain of over 50% of SIDS cases [14]. Is it that staphylococcal toxaemia kills before bacteraemia occurs? Is it that termination of bacteraemia by polymorphs leads to toxin release and sudden death? Or is it that the microbiological investigation of SUDI is too cursory, and disseminated staphylococcal infection is missed or ignored?

A specimen of blood should also be obtained at autopsy for possible virological, toxicological or genetic analyses. It is best to clean the skin with alcohol wipes, then cut down to a vein with a new scalpel blade and obtain blood by venepuncture. The specimen of blood should be separated and stored.

SPLENIC CULTURE

A specimen of spleen can be obtained at autopsy for bacterial culture, and this is a useful adjunct to blood culture. The specimen should be obtained immediately the abdomen is opened. One approach is to push a swab into the spleen. A second is to cut off a small piece using a clean knife and send it for microbiology. The piece is subsequently placed in boiling water to sterilise the surface, and then splenic tissue from the centre is used for culture.

RESEARCH POINT

E. coli and *S. aureus* are common causes of bacteraemia except in infants between one and twelve months of age. Either these organisms do not cause bacteraemia in this age group, or they do, but the infection progresses rapidly to death and is missed. The observation that staphylococcal enterotoxins and *E. coli* endotoxin can interact synergistically to cause death in experimental models [18] is pertinent to answering these questions. Nucleic acid amplification techniques (polymerase chain reaction) need to be used on blood and CSF specimens from cases of SUDI to see if the bacteria have been present, even if they cannot be grown. If blood can be obtained soon after death, then endotoxin measurements may also be useful [19].

UPPER RESPIRATORY TRACT

The nasopharyngeal bacterial flora of SIDS infants is different from that in healthy live infants matched for age, gender and season [20]. A study conducted in the 1980s, when most infants slept prone, revealed increased carriage of staphylococci, streptococci and Gram negative bacilli in infants at autopsy [20]. Although the possibility of Post-mortem change cannot be discounted as an explanation for the difference, a similar pattern is found in the early morning in infants suffering from a viral upper respiratory infection who have slept prone in the night [17]. Enterobacteriaceae, such as *E. coli* and *Klebsiella* spp., are rarely found in healthy infants, occur in less than 3% of those with clinical upper respiratory tract infections (URTI) who sleep supine, but are commonly found in the early morning in those with URTI who sleep prone, and were found in up to 45% of SIDS cases in the 1980s [17], [20].

S. aureus is found in approximately 50% of normal healthy infants in the first three months of life. The carriage rate thereafter gradually falls to 30% by 6 months of age. *Streptococcus pneumoniae*, by comparison, occurs in 5% in the first month of life and then gradually rises to 30% by 6 months. *Haemophilus influenzae* is rarely found in the first month but then rises to 10% at 6 months. Enterobacteriaceae remain under 3% throughout the first six months of life [17]. Streptococci are commonly found but group A haemolytic streptococci are rare. Other pathogens, such as meningococci and *Bordetella pertussis* are also rare.

In SUDI a pernasal swab should be taken as soon after death as possible, once again this is best obtained in A&E rather than waiting till the autopsy is undertaken. A full analysis of the nasopharyngeal flora requires examination using a wide range of culture media. In practice, most laboratories will concentrate on the identification of possible pathogens, but this should include *S. aureus* and at least partial identification of the enterobacteriaceae.

If *S. aureus* is isolated, the organism should be sent for genetic analysis to see if it produces any of the pyrogenic enterotoxins such as toxic shock syndrome toxin (TSST) and the staphylococcal enterotoxins A, B, C or D. These toxins are superantigens, their production is switched on when the temperature rises above 37 °C. They cause a polyclonal proliferation of T-lymphocytes, leading to an outpouring of cytokines, and this in turn can cause profound shock as in the toxic shock syndrome. These toxins have been found in the brain tissue of over 50% of SIDS cases, as noted above [14] and, therefore, are leading contenders for a causative role in SIDS.

In my opinion, if a toxigenic *S. aureus* is isolated, then the CSF and blood should be analysed for the respective toxin using an antibody probe. This test is not routinely available but can be performed. A positive result would point strongly to a mechanism of death based on toxic shock.

A pernasal swab, passed through the nose to touch the posterior nasopharyngeal wall, is the best method of sampling the flora of the upper respiratory tract. A throat swab is less useful overall but may give a higher isolation rate for pathogenic streptococci. Thus, either a pernasal swab alone or a pernasal swab plus a throat swab should be obtained, but not a throat swab alone.

LOWER RESPIRATORY TRACT

Microbiological investigation of the lower respiratory tract depends on samples obtained at autopsy. If the autopsy cannot be undertaken immediately the body should be stored at 4 °C. The samples should be obtained as soon as the chest is opened and before the abdomen is opened. A clean scalpel blade should be used to obtain a sample of lung, and swabs should be passed down the trachea and into the bronchi as soon as the chest contents are removed. The specimens obtained can be used for both bacteriology and virology. If, during the subsequent dissection of the lungs, a focal area of consolidation is noted, a further sample should be obtained for bacteriology, but the chance of contamination will inevitably be increased.

The results of bacterial culture must be interpreted with care. In life the upper airways have a resident bacterial flora but the lower airways do not, and therefore the presence of bacteria in the lower respiratory tract is of significance. The problem, however, is that the lower airways may be contaminated from the upper airways during attempts at resuscitation. This is where careful analysis of the flora of the upper airways can help. If the mixture of organisms in the upper and lower airways is the same, then contamination is the more likely explanation. But if there is a pure growth of a pathogen in the lower respiratory tract and a mixed growth in the upper respiratory tract, a genuine infection is more likely. Furthermore, if the same organism is found elsewhere, e.g. in the blood or CSF, then infection is clearly the most likely explanation.

Correlation of bacteriology and histology is an important, but a vexed, problem. If there is histological evidence of pneumonia and a pathogen is isolated, then the diagnosis is clear. The difficulty arises when the bacteriological findings point to infection and histology is negative. The process of inflammation is defined by the histological appearance and histology is 100% specific; therefore, it cannot be 100% sensitive or we would be denying the essential uncertainty and variability that underlies biology and pathology. Thus, there will be false negatives and cases of genuine infection will be missed if we regard histology as the gold standard. This is particularly important in SUDI, as recent evidence suggests that infants can go from being apparently well to death in under 20 minutes [21]. This does not give time for the classical signs of inflammation to arise.

THE GASTROINTESTINAL TRACT

The microbial flora of the gastrointestinal tract are much more complex than those of the respiratory tract. In fact, there are close to ten times more bacterial cells in the gut than there are human cells in the body. The number of different species far exceeds those found in the respiratory system, and many, perhaps most, cannot be grown using conventional techniques. It is, therefore, not possible to analyse the gastrointestinal flora in the way that the respiratory tract flora can be assessed.

If bacteria and bacterial toxins have a role in the pathogenesis of SUDI then the numerical superiority of the gut flora makes it a prime candidate for the site of origin of the infection. The seasonality of SUDI, however, with an increased risk in the winter months, points more to the respiratory tract. Furthermore, epidemiological evidence indicates that breast feeding is not protective, which would be a surprising finding if the gut flora were important in pathogenesis.

Thus, there are theoretical as well as practical reasons for concentrating on the respiratory tract rather than the gastrointestinal tract in attempting to elucidate the cause of SUDI. There is nothing to gain from any attempt to analyse the gut flora in detail, but it is possible to look for specific pathogens such as salmonella, shigella and campylobacter organisms. In addition tests can be done for verotoxin-producing *E. coli* and toxigenic clostridia [10]. This is particularly useful if any of these organisms are isolated from the blood or CSF, or if any lesions of the bowel are found at autopsy.

VIROLOGY

In the CESDI SUDI study [2], viruses were isolated from 4.5% of nasopharyngeal aspirates (5 of 112 cases), 4.2% of lung tissue (11 of 264 cases) and 18% of gastrointestinal samples (bowel contents) (43 of 237 cases). There were six cases in which virology confirmed the main cause of death, and one in which the virology confirmed a probable contributory cause. This is from a total of 450 autopsies. The cases included myocarditis (Coxsackie B2 in nasopharyngeal aspirate and gut), transverse myelitis (Coxsackie B1 in gut contents) and neonatal HSV infection (HSV1 in gut).

Polio viruses was isolated in 22 cases, rotavirus in 5, adenovirus in 4, echovirus in 4, coxsackie virus in 3 and enterovirus not specified in 2. These isolates were not associated with significant clinical illness or pathology.

The message is that virological studies are of only limited value, and the results must be interpreted in conjunction with the clinical picture and the pathological findings.

CONCLUSION

The microbiological investigation of SUDI requires specimens of CSF, blood, upper respiratory tract secretions, lower respiratory tract tissue and bowel contents for both bacteriological and virological studies.

A specimen of CSF should be obtained within a few hours of death and processed urgently, as for the investigation of meningitis in life. Examination should include a white cell count, a differential cell count, a protein estimation and bacterial culture.

A blood culture should be obtained within a few hours of death. Techniques based on nucleic acid amplification (PCR) and antigen immuno-recognition should be developed and used to seek evidence of infection by S. aureus and E. coli.

A pernasal swab should also be obtained within a few hours of death and examined for pathogens including S. aureus and enterobacteriaceae. If S. aureus is isolated, the toxigenic profile should be determined and the toxins measured in CSF and blood.

Tissue and swabs from the lower respiratory tract should be obtained, and the results of culture carefully compared with histology and with the upper respiratory tract flora. Histology aids diagnosis but cannot be regarded as the gold standard for infection.

Examination of bowel contents should be undertaken but provides only limited information.

The results of virology need to be interpreted in the light of clinical and pathological findings.

The investigation of SUDI in the twenty-first century must be taken beyond the concept that morphological assessment of tissues two to three days after death is sufficient, and is a gold standard against which other investigations are to be measured. Specimens must be obtained soon after death, examined urgently and the full range of modern techniques employed. Evidence of bacteraemia should be sought by culture and by antigen and genomic analysis. Evidence of bacterial toxaemia should be sought using antibody probes, and in the future by the emerging techniques of proteomics. Morphological analysis would also benefit from the wider use of immunohistological methods to type inflammatory cells and distinguish normal from the earliest stages of inflammation.

SUDI poses an intellectual challenge to pathology. There are big scientific questions to address: the acquisition of protective immunity to the microbial flora, the role of bacteraemia and bacterial toxaemia in switching on or off physiological systems, the specification of those systems by genes, and the effect of deleterious genetic mutations on physiological function. The science of genomics and proteomics will provide answers to these questions, but only if pathologists learn to take the correct samples at the correct time.

REFERENCES

1. Royal College of Pathologists. Guidelines for Postmortem Examination after Sudden Unexpected Death in Infancy. (RCP, London, 1993).
2. Berry J, Allibone E, McKeever P, Moore I, Wright C, Fleming P. The Pathology Study: the contribution of ancillary tests to the investigation of unexpected infant death. In *Sudden Unexpected Deaths in Infancy: the CESDI SUDI Studies*, Fleming P *et al.* eds (The Stationery Office, London, 2000) pp. 97–112.
3. Fishman RA. *Cerebrospinal Fluid in Diseases of the Nervous System*. (London, W B Saunders, 1980).
4. Platt MS, McClure S, Clarke R, Spitz WU, Cox W. Postmortem cerebrospinal fluid pleocytosis. *Am J Forens Med Pathol* 1989; **10**: 209–12.

5. Ehrlich P. Das Sauerstoffbedurfhis des Organismus. Eine Farbenanalytische Studie. (Berlin, A Hirschfeld, 1885).
6. Wyler D, Marty W, Bar W. Correlation between the post-mortem cell content of cerebrospinal fluid and time of death. *Int J Legal Med* 1994; **106**: 194–9.
7. Mangin P, Lugnier AA, Chaumont AJ, Offner M, Grucker M. Forensic significance of postmortem estimation of the blood cerebrospinal fluid barrier permeability. *Forens Sci Int* 1983; **22**: 143–9.
8. Coe JI. Postmortem chemistry update: emphasis on forensic application. *Am J Forens Med Path* 1993; **14**: 91–117.
9. Osuna E, Perez-Carceles MD, Luna A, Pounder DJ. Efficacy of cerebro-spinal fluid biochemistry in the diagnosis of brain insult. *Forens Sci Int* 1992; **52**: 193–8.
10. Sonnabend OAR, Sonnabend WFF, Krech U, Molz G, Sigrist T. Continuous microbiological and pathological study of 70 sudden and unexpected infant deaths. *Lancet* 1985; **i**: 237–41.
11. Sadler DW. The value of a thorough protocol in the investigation of sudden infant deaths. *J Clin Pathol* 1998; **51**: 689–94.
12. Morris JA, Harrison LM, Partridge SM. Postmortem bacteriology: a re-evaluation. *J Clin Pathol* 2006; **59**: 1–9.
13. Morris JA. The common bacterial toxin hypothesis of sudden infant death syndrome. *FEMS Immunol Med Microbiol* 1999; **25**: 11–17.
14. Zorgani A, Essery SD, Al Madani O *et al*. Detection of pyrogenic toxins of *Stapylococcus aureus* in sudden infant death syndrome. *FEMS Immunol Med Microbiol* 1999; **25**: 103–8.
15. Banks RE, Dunn MJ, Hochstrasser DF *et al*. Proteomics: new perspectives, new biomedical opportunities. *Lancet* 2000; **356**: 1749–56.
16. Brook I. Unexplained fever in young children: how to manage severe bacterial infection. *Br Med J* 2003; **327**: 1094–7.
17. Harrison LM, Morris JA, Telford DR, Brown SM, Jones K. The nasopharyngeal bacterial flora in infancy: effects of age, season, viral upper respiratory tract infection and sleeping position. *FEMS Immunol Med Micobiol* 1999; **25**: 19–28.
18. Sayers NM, Drucker DB, Morris JA, Telford DR. Lethal synergy between toxins of staphylococci and enterobacteria: implication for sudden infant death syndrome. *J Clin Pathol* 1996; **49**: 365–8.
19. Sayers NM, Crawley BA, Humphries K *et al*. Effect of time post mortem on the concentration of endotoxin in rat organs: implications for sudden infant death syndrome. *FEMS Immunol Med Microbiol* 1999; **25**: 125–30.
20. Telford DR, Morris JA, Hughes P *et al*. The nasopharyngeal bacterial flora in the sudden infant death syndrome. *J Infect* 1989; **18**: 125–30.
21. Meny RG, Carroll MD, Carbone MT, Kelly DH. Cardiorespiratory recordings from infants dying suddenly and unexpectedly at home. *Pediatrics* 1994; **93**: 44–8.

2

An overview of childhood lymphomas

Jyoti Gupta and Keith P. McCarthy

INTRODUCTION

Lymphomas encompass a diverse group of neoplasms that arise from the clonal proliferation of lymphoid precursor cells. They are triggered by a series of genetic events that may be related to genetic predispositions, viral and other environmental factors, or may simply be accidental genetic rearrangements.

Lymphomas are the third most common cancer in children in the UK, behind acute leukaemias and brain tumours. They account for approximately 11–13% of all childhood malignancies with an annual incidence of 13.2 per million children [1]–[4]. The age-specific incidence rates and clinical features of paediatric lymphomas in white children in the USA correspond to those in Europe [5]. In equatorial Africa, 50% of all childhood cancers are due to lymphomas, because of the high incidence of Burkitt's lymphoma.

Paediatric lymphomas can be classified into Hodgkin's lymphoma (HL) and non-Hodgkin's lymphoma (NHL). The main subtypes are defined in the REAL classification [6], but the more recent WHO classification updates and expands this [7]. NHLs represent 60–70% of all childhood lymphomas in developed countries [2], [8], affecting children mainly between 7 and 10 years of age. The male-to-female ratio recorded in a Dutch study was 2.5 [5]. There is, however, an increased incidence in children with inherited or acquired immunodeficiencies [9], [10]. HL represents the remaining 30–40% of childhood lymphomas. Their incidence increases steadily throughout life and studies show a male-to-female ratio of 2.7 [5].

Unlike adult NHLs, which are often low-to-intermediate grade, the paediatric NHLs are frequently high-grade lymphomas and are clinically aggressive. However, low-grade tumours of both B- and T-cells do occur rarely in children [11]. Childhood NHLs are also more likely to present as extranodal disease in comparison to adults, where they tend to present as peripheral lymphadenopathy. A leukaemic phase is also more common in children, particularly in lymphoblastic lymphoma.

15

Progress in Pathology Volume 7, ed. Nigel Kirkham and Neil Shepherd. Published by Cambridge University Press. © Cambridge University Press 2007.

The subtypes of NHL in children are predominantly of three main types, Burkitt's and atypical Burkitt's lymphomas (together accounting for about 35–50% of cases), lymphoblastic lymphoma (about 30–40%) and large cell lymphoma (15–25%). Individually, anaplastic large cell lymphomas are reported as the most common NHLs in children, in some studies accounting for even 25% of paediatric lymphomas [12]. Other subtypes of NHL are rare in children [3], [13] and in particular follicular lymphoma is very rare.

These groups are distinguished from one another by their clinical presentation, histological appearance, immunophenotype and cytogenetic profile.

Burkitt's lymphoma is a B-cell neoplasm. The WHO recognises three subtypes, including endemic BL, non-endemic (sporadic) BL and immunodeficiency associated BL [7]. The Revised European–American Lymphoma classification originally provisionally included a lymphoma subtype – 'Burkitt-like Lymphoma' – that was essentially defined as a variant of diffuse large B-cell lymphoma with features resembling Burkitt's lymphoma [6]. The new WHO classification of haematolymphoid diseases has dropped the term 'Burkitt-like lymphoma', replacing it with 'atypical Burkitt's lymphoma'; this is defined as a variant of Burkitt's lymphoma [7]. The difference between Burkitt's and atypical Burkitt's is based on subtle morphologic differences, but they do not appear to have different aetiology or clinical behaviour, and their diagnostic reproducibility is open to serious question. For these reasons, it must be questioned whether atypical Burkitt's lymphoma is a real entity.

Lymphoblastic lymphomas are derived from precursor B- or T-cells and are commonly associated with a leukaemic manifestation. Histologically, they are indistinguishable from ALL (acute lymphoblastic leukaemia), since they derive from precursor B- or T-cells that are analogous to the blasts seen in ALL. Although ALL predominantly involves B-cells, 80% of the lymphomas are of T-cell origin and only 20% are of B-cell origin [14]. The number of blasts in the bone marrow and presence or absence of mediastinal or nodal disease is used to distinguish lymphoblastic lymphoma from ALL. If more than 25% of blasts are present in the bone marrow, this implies ALL.

Large cell lymphomas can be of B-cell, T-cell, or intermediate (null) origin. They include diffuse large B-cell lymphomas, peripheral T-cell lymphomas (subtype; large cell) and anaplastic large cell lymphoma (T- and null-cell type). In general, B-cell lineage LCLs have centroblastic or immunoblastic morphological features, lack CD30 expression, affect older patients and involve less-advanced disease. In contrast, T-cell lineage LCLs in children usually express CD30 and are often of the anaplastic LCL subtype.

Other subtypes of NHL have been described in children, but are rare. For instance, although follicular lymphomas are one of the most common lymphomas in adults, they are rarely found in children and they tend to present extranodally [15].

Hodgkin's lymphoma represents 30–40% of childhood lymphomas. As with adult HL, they can be divided into classic HL (nodular sclerosis, mixed cellularity, lymphocyte depletion, lymphocyte rich) and nodular lymphocyte predominant. The histologic subtype does not influence survival [16].

Prompt diagnosis and staging of paediatric lymphomas is important due to the rapid growth of lymphomas. In addition to pathological typing and staging, various clinical investigations are required before commencing treatment. These include blood count, electrolytes, liver function tests, chest X-ray and possibly CT scan of the chest, abdominal and pelvic ultrasound (US) or CT scan, bone scan, bone marrow biopsy and occasionally spinal fluid analysis.

As with other malignancies, the two groups of genes involved in the pathogenesis of malignant transformation are proto-oncogenes and tumour suppressor genes.

In paediatric NHL, the mechanism by which oncogenes are activated usually involves genetic translocations that correlate with cell lineage. Recent data have suggested that the role of tumour suppression genes and its inactivation may be associated with the loss of the multitumour suppressor (MTS1) gene, in the pathogenesis of certain lymphoblastic lymphomas [2].

In paediatric Hodgkin's disease, there is now evidence to suggest that its pathogenesis may be due to deregulated cytokine production [2], [17].

BURKITT'S LYMPHOMA

Burkitt's lymphoma (BL) was previously referred to as small, non-cleaved cell, Burkitt's lymphoma according to the Working Formulation and Kiel classification.

CLINICAL FEATURES

BL was first recognised as the endemic form presenting as tumours in the jaws of children [18]. It occurs endemically in Africa and parts of New Guinea, but is seen sporadically elsewhere in the world. The sporadic form is the predominant type in USA and Europe. Whereas the endemic form affects children ranging in age from 3 to 15 years, the sporadic form affects older children and young adults [12]. The male:female ratio is approximately 2–3:1, such that in the American Burkitt Lymphoma Registry, the incidence of BL was 1.4 per million in white males compared to only 0.4 per million for white females during 1973–1981 [19].

BL is associated predominantly with extranodal disease, but occasionally can present as leukaemic, and is then synonymous with ALL L3 [6], [20].

The endemic form is strongly associated with the Epstein–Barr virus (EBV) and can be found in up to 95% cases, but EBV is seen in only 20% of sporadic cases and 30–40% of HIV-positive cases. It still remains unclear how EBV contributes to the pathogenesis of Burkitt's lymphoma. However, a high antibody titer to EBV antigen is associated with a better prognosis [21]. They often show a dramatic response to chemotherapy, but spontaneous remission rarely occurs [22]. BL can also be found less frequently in ovaries, retroperitoneum, bones, salivary glands, thyroid and breast.

The sporadic cases usually present as intra-abdominal tumours. The commonest presentation is as a right iliac fossa mass and not infrequently a right hemi-colectomy is performed, usually because of intussusception or bleeding; needless to say, such surgery is not curative. Such cases are assumed to arise from Peyers patches in the ileo-caecal region or possibly from mesenteric nodes.

Rarely, there may be other intra-abdominal presentations, possibly because of involvement of kidney, liver or spleen. Sporadic BL may also present as CNS disease or in Waldeyer's ring, or even in the jaw [23], [24]. In sporadic cases, Burkitt's lymphoma may occur in AIDS patients and other cases of immunosuppression. The clinical course is aggressive, but as with the endemic form, cures can be achieved with chemotherapy. However, occasionally relapses may occur in the CNS.

PATHOLOGICAL FEATURES

Usually, the normal architecture, whether it be of intestinal wall or lymph node, is completely effaced by monomorphic population of cohesive, medium-sized lymphocytes admixed with macrophages containing apoptotic debris, which give a 'starry sky' appearance. Although the growth pattern is usually diffuse, occasionally a more follicular arrangement of cells is seen (due to follicular colonisation), and this rare pattern should be borne in mind should a nodular lymphoma present in childhood.

The neoplastic cells have large round–oval nuclei, often angulated, containing dense, clumped chromatin, which obscures the nucleoli (usually 2–5) and abundant basophilic cytoplasm that may contain characteristic cytoplasmic vacuoles; however, it is important to remember that these may also seen in other lymphoma subtypes, particularly when cells are degenerate. Characteristically, there is a high proliferation fraction of very nearly 100%; this is an extremely important diagnostic feature, since no other lymphoma has such a high proliferation rate (except possibly atypical Burkitt's lymphoma, see below). The neoplastic cells often appear to infiltrate around nerves, muscles and other structures, thereby compressing them rather than destroying them [25].

The morphological features of sporadic and endemic types of Burkitt's lymphoma are indistinguishable.

DIFFERENTIAL DIAGNOSIS

This includes other types of high-grade lymphomas such as B- and T-lymphoblastic lymphoma and the small-cell variant of diffuse large B-cell lymphoma. Poorly fixed BL may well lose its characteristic cytological and morphological features (such as the 'starry sky' pattern, and the monotonous appearance). Under these circumstances, the high proliferation index may help to distinguish BL from diffuse large B-cell lymphoma (DLBCL) (which generally has a lower percentage of cells in cycle), although atypical BL/Burkitt-like lymphoma will remain a problem. Another useful diagnostic feature is the demonstration of cytoplasmic vacuoles. Although these are best demonstrated in cytological preparations, they may be seen at the edge of sections, where cells are tending to separate in areas of relatively good preservation.

Should BL grow in an apparent follicular or nodular pattern (due to follicular colonisation), there may be superficial resemblance to follicle centre cell lymphomas, and this may be strengthened by the positivity for CD10. High-power examination should reveal, at least in areas, the characteristic cytology of the cells.

True lymphoblastic lymphomas are Terminal deoxynucleotide Transferase (TdT) positive whereas BL is always negative. However TdT is a technically difficult antibody and care should be taken in interpreting a negative result. If the lymph node is well fixed, then the morphological characteristics should enable distinction from BL.

IMMUNOHISTOCHEMISTRY

The immunophenotype of the BL cell is essentially that of a peripheral B cell, although CD10 is also often present, suggesting derivation from germinal centre cells. Neoplastic cells express monoclonal surface IgM, pan B-cell markers (CD19, CD20, CD22 and CD79a) and CD10. They are CD5 and CD23 negative. Ki67/MIB-1 is a useful marker in the differentiation of BL from other high-grade lymphoma subtypes due to the characteristically extremely high proliferation index (see above). As might be assumed, the tumour cells are TdT negative, allowing their distinction from true lymphoblastic lymphoma. The tumour cells may be positive for Epstein−Barr virus (EBV) associated antigens such as LMP-1 and may, similarly, be positive on in-situ hybridisation for EBERs.

GENETICS

Almost all cases, from whatever the subtype, show a chromosomal translocation involving the C-MYC gene on chromosome 8, which appears to be the critical event in the pathogenesis of Burkitt's lymphoma [2]. The most common abnormality [t (8:14)(q24;q32)] results in the translocation of C-MYC into the heavy chain (IgH) gene locus. The IgH gene locus is actively transcribing in B-cells and the translocation means that C-MYC comes under the influence of the IgH gene promotor, with consequent constitutive expression of C-MYC protein. C-MYC protein is a powerful cell-proliferation protein.

Variant chromosome translocations include the t(2;8)(q11;q24) and t(8;22) (q24:q11), in which the C-MYC gene is translocated, in an exactly analogous manner to the t(8;14), in the actively transcribing immunoglobulin kappa light chain gene and the immunoglobulin lambda light chain gene.

As will be obvious from the foregoing discussion, BL invariably shows rearrangements of the IgH and IgL gene loci. It may also show promiscuous rearrangements of T-cell receptor genes, especially of the T-cell receptor gamma chain genes. Such rearrangements are usually only partial and rarely complete.

ATYPICAL BURKITT'S LYMPHOMA/BURKITT-LIKE LYMPHOMA

Although both the REAL classification and new WHO classification consider that there is a subtype of high-grade lymphoma with features intermediate between DLBCL and BL, they vary in their positions as to its nature. The REAL system implies that it is more closely akin to DLBCL, the WHO considers it to be a variant of BL. From a clinical point of view, it is treated as BL.

There is considerable controversy concerning this entity, not least because published studies indicate that its reproducibility is poor [26]. Indeed, it seems not unlikely that both atypical Burkitt's lymphoma and Burkitt-like lymphoma are actually both the same thing — poorly fixed or poorly processed BL — since it is well recognised amongst experienced haematolymphoid pathologists that these factors may have a significant effect on several aspects of cytomorphology, including cell size and nuclear appearance. However, the information that is presented below is predicated on the assumption that such an entity has an objective existence.

CLINICAL FEATURES

It occurs more commonly in adults than children, and may also be seen in patients with immunosuppression. Cases are said more frequently to involve lymph nodes rather than extranodal sites, in contrast to BL [27]. Some studies have shown an apparent reduced long-term survival in Burkitt-like lymphoma, compared to Burkitt's, particularly in adults [24], [28].

PATHOLOGICAL FEATURES

Atypical Burkitt's lymphoma shows subtle morphological differences from Burkitt's lymphoma, the main one being that cases exhibit increased cellular pleomorphism. The cells are of intermediate size (possibly slightly larger than typical Burkitt's lymphoma cells) and have round—oval nuclei (with more irregularity of nuclear shape than in BL). The chromatin is more clumped and nucleoli may be prominent, but fewer in number compared to Burkitt's lymphoma. A 'starry sky' appearance is sometimes present, but is less often seen than in BL. Cases have a high proliferation index, as judged by MIB-1 or Ki-67 staining, approaching that of BL. Atypical cells may be present in the peripheral blood, again similar to BL.

DIFFERENTIAL DIAGNOSIS

Not surprisingly, given the difficulties described above, the main differential diagnoses are BL and DLBCL. The difficulties of the situation are highlighted in Figs. 2.1 and 2.2; these two pictures are from the same section of a case of Burkitt's lymphoma. The morphology of the cells in Fig. 2.1 is characteristic of Burkitt's lymphoma, yet the morphology of those in Fig. 2.2 more closely resembles DLBCL. This illustrates the effects of fixation and other factors and explains why distinguishing BL, DLBCL and the 'intermediate' entities of Burkitt-like or atypical BL can be all but impossible.

True lymphoblastic lymphoma, especially in small or poorly-fixed samples, may also present in the differential diagnosis. Staining for TdT (only positive in true lymphoblastic lymphomas) will be of use.

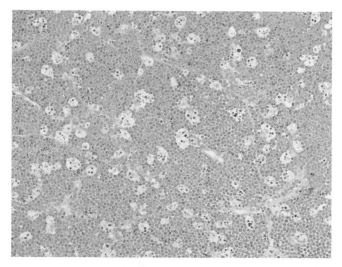

Fig. 2.1 Burkitt's lymphoma, showing a monomorphic population of lymphocytes admixed with macrophages containing apoptic debris giving a 'starry sky' appearance. (H&E, magnification × 20.)

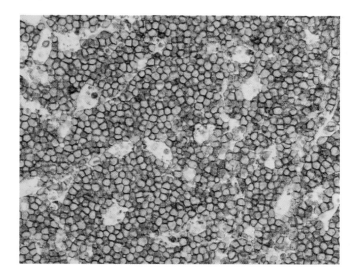

Fig. 2.2 Burkitt's lymphoma (CD20, magnification × 40.)

IMMUNOHISTOCHEMISTRY

The differentiation between BL, DLBCL and atypical BL/Burkitt-like lymphoma cannot be resolved with certainty by immunohistochemistry and cytogenetics. Like BL and DLBCL, these entities exhibit a mature B-cell phenotype, showing positivity for Pan B markers (e.g. CD19, CD20, CD22, CD79a). They are CD5−, and are usually CD10+. They may show evidence of surface immunoglobulin (IgM or IgG), but are always negative for TdT. There are no published data concerning the percentage of cases showing bcl-2 positivity.

As has already been mentioned, accurate estimation of the percentage of cells in cycle may allow a pragmatic distinction between DLBCL and atypical BL/ Burkitt-like lymphoma. The diagnosis of atypical BL/Burkitt-like lymphoma should not be made if the proliferation index is less than 98%.

GENETICS

As would be expected of a mature B-cell lymphoma, this entity shows both IgH and IgL gene rearrangements, as detected by both restriction enzyme analysis and polymerase chain reaction. C-MYC rearrangements are reportedly less common than in BL, but this can be attributed to the heterogeneity of lymphoma subtypes included under this heading – cases of DLBCL may well not have such a translocation.

Bcl-2 gene rearrangements have been reported in 30% of patients [6]; this contrasts with BL (where no such rearrangements occur) but again may well represent a subset of DLBCL included in this category.

DIFFUSE LARGE B-CELL LYMPHOMA

This was previously referred to as centroblastic, B-immunoblastic or B-large cell anaplastic under the Kiel classification. However, there was no convincing evidence for the validity of the distinction between centroblastic and immunoblastic lymphomas and they were therefore combined. Under the working formulation, they were classified as diffuse large-cell lymphomas. Under the REAL classification, this category includes all high grade B-cell lymphomas other than distinct clinicopathological entities such as Burkitt's lymphomas. The new WHO classification similarly makes no distinction between large B-cell lymphomas containing centroblasts, immunoblasts or a mix thereof, but it does separate out primary mediastinal large B-cell lymphoma.

CLINICAL FEATURES

This is a heterogeneous entity that may affect all age groups. It often presents as a rapidly growing, localised mass. In children, large B-cell lymphomas primarily affect lymph nodes or mediastinum, but can also affect spleen and extranodal sites, including gastrointestinal tract, mediastinum, skin, bone, soft tissue and rarely the CNS. It must be remembered that DLBCL may arise in the caecum, and so a diagnosis of BL cannot be made automatically when a child presents with a right iliac fossa mass.

Primary mediastinal (thymic) sclerosing B-cell lymphoma (recognised as a rare subtype of large B-cell lymphoma in the REAL system, but as a distinct clinicopathological entity in the revised WHO system) presents as an anterior or superior mediastinal mass. It may present with airway compromise, superior vena caval syndrome or other local disease. It has mainly been described in young women. It is thought to arise from thymic B-cells [29].

In adults a proportion of cases will represent transformation of pre-existing low grade B-cell lymphomas or rarely from nodular lymphocyte-predominant Hodgkin's disease. Clearly, in the paediatric age group, such a situation is extremely unlikely, with the great majority of cases representing de novo high-grade disease.

They have an aggressive course, but remission can be achieved with combination chemotherapy.

PATHOLOGICAL FEATURES

The main characteristic feature of this histologically diverse group is a diffuse pattern of growth effacing the lymph node architecture. Some cases have a high mitotic count and occasionally a 'starry sky' appearance; such a growth pattern should not be taken as evidence of BL, but is merely evidence of a high mitotic (and therefore apoptotic) rate. The neoplastic cells are large with nuclei even larger than tissue macrophage nuclei (Fig. 2.3); this comparison is of use in the distinction from BL, where the nuclei are smaller than, or the same size as, the interspersed macrophages. They have prominent nucleoli and a moderate amount of variably basophilic cytoplasm (Fig. 2.4).

Cases of DLBCL show marked cytological variation, with several distinct subpopulations of cells. Centroblasts are intermediate to large cells that may show a cerebriform or polylobulated nuclei with several, relatively inconspicuous nucleoli distributed around the nuclear membrane. Immunoblasts are larger cells with large nuclei, characterised by a prominent nuclear membrane. They have open chromatin, a single, large central eosinophilic nucleolus and variable amounts of cytoplasm. Plasmacytoid cells are round with eccentrically placed nuclei, prominent central nucleoli, peripherally condensed chromatin and occasionally a pale perinuclear hof.

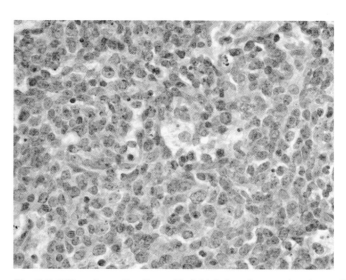

Fig. 2.3 Diffuse large B-cell non-Hodgkin's lymphoma, showing a diffuse population of neoplastic cells with large nuclei. (H&E, magnification × 60.)

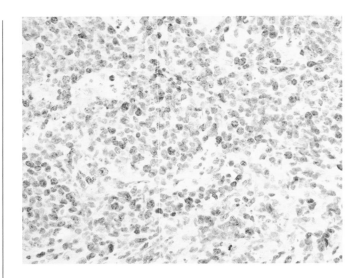

Fig. 2.4 Diffuse large B-cell non-Hodgkin's lymphoma (Ki67, magnification × 40.)

Prominence of one of these subpopulations does not change the diagnosis, which is still one of DLBCL. Another point to remember is that some cases, even in childhood, may show a marked over-predominance of mature or activated T-cells — so-called 'T-cell rich B-cell lymphoma'. This is not a distinct subtype of lymphoma and should not be proffered as a diagnosis. Another point to bear in mind is that other non-neoplastic cells, including reactive plasma cells, small B-cells, macrophages and eosinophils, may be present in excess, leading to a resemblance to peripheral T-cell lymphomas. Sometimes necrosis is a prominent feature.

Occasionally, bizarre giant cells may be seen. These may closely resemble Reed–Sternberg cells. It may be that bizarre or anaplastic morphology is prominent, leading to a resemblance to anaplastic large-cell lymphoma.

Mediastinal B-cell lymphoma often shows a characteristic pattern of fibrosis, with a 'compartmentalising' pattern, producing small packets of tumour cells surrounded by strands of sclerosis.

DIFFERENTIAL DIAGNOSIS

Although there may be a morphological similarity with various types of tumour (including poorly differentiated carcinoma, anaplastic myeloma, malignant melanoma and Merkel cell tumour), basic immunohistochemistry should exclude these. Anaplastic large-cell lymphoma may be a problem if there is anaplastic morphology, but it is now generally accepted that the B-cell variant of anaplastic large-cell lymphoma does not exist. Thus positivity for any pan-B-cell markers precludes this diagnosis, even if there is positivity for ALK-1 and/or CD30.

If there is prominence of reactive inflammatory cells, the appearance may resemble peripheral T-cell lymphoma. Here, careful examination of the results of immunohistochemistry is essential, so that the precise immunophenotype of the cytologically atypical cells can be discerned.

The main problem in the differential diagnosis is with BL and atypical BL/Burkitt-like lymphoma. This problem has already been addressed in detail, but points that should be considered are the proliferation index, the presence of bcl-2 positivity, the absence of CD10 positivity (although DLBCL may be positive, BL is always positive) and the presence of intracytoplasmic vacuoles.

IMMUNOHISTOCHEMISTRY

This entity demonstrates a mature B-cell immunophenotype, with neoplastic cells expressing pan-B-cell markers (CD19, CD20, CD22 and CD79a). Most at CD45+ (leukocytes common antigen), but some lymphomas with immunoblastic features may not express CD45. CD44 expression has been shown to be a strong prognostic predictor in localised large B-cell lymphoma [30]. They may or may not express CD5 and CD10. TdT is always negative.

They show immunoglobulin light chain restriction, with variable expression of surface and cytoplasmic immunoglobulin. A small percentage of cases express CD30, but CD15 positivity is rare.

Thymic B-cell lymphoma also has a mature B-cell phenotype, but usually does not express immunoglobulin. It is more likely to express CD30 than other types of DLBCL.

GENETICS

In 25% of cases, there is t(14;18)(q32;q23) chromosomal translocation [12]. This translocation inserts the entire BCL-2 gene on chromosome 18 into the actively transcribing IgH locus on chromosome 14. This results in the constitutive expression of BCL-2, and anti-apoptotic gene. It is the characteristic abnormality of low-grade follicle centre cell lymphoma, and has been taken as evidence of transformation from a pre-existing low-grade lymphoma. There is evidence to suggest that the presence of the translocation may be an important prognostic factor, indicating poorer response to therapy [31].

In 30−40% of cases there is a cytogenetic abnormality involving the BCL-6/LAZ3 gene on chromosome 3q27 [6]. Rearrangement of the C-MYC gene is uncommon, but can occur in association with other genetic rearrangements [31]. The most common variant is the t(8;14)(q23;q35), and thus the presence of this abnormality cannot be taken as evidence that it is BL.

PRECURSOR B-LYMPHOBLASTIC LEUKAEMIA/ LYMPHOMA

These were previously referred to as malignant lymphoma, lymphoblastic B-cell type (Kiel classification) and malignant lymphoma lymphoblastic (convoluted cell, non-convoluted cell) under the Working Formulation.

B-cell lymphoblastic lymphomas are less common than T-cell derived ones and they have a high propensity for marrow and CNS infiltration. They are the most common NHL subtype associated with a leukaemic manifestation.

CLINICAL FEATURES

They usually occur in children with peak incidence between 2 and 10 years with a 75% long-term survival. However, adults have a poorer prognosis with only a 20% long-term survival [12]. Lymphoblastic neoplasms of B-cell type usually present as a leukaemia with bone marrow and blood involvement, but can occur as localised solid tumours, usually in lymph nodes as intra-abdominal masses. Lymphomatous deposits may present peripherally, usually below the diaphragm, or with primary bone or skin disease; the latter have more mature phenotype. In contrast, T-cell-type lymphoblastic lymphomas often present as mediastinal masses.

Should relapse occur, it may occur in the CNS and other sites, such as the testis, a consideration that is important when considering treatment and prophylaxis options.

It is an aggressive disease, but is frequently curable with aggressive chemotherapy. Poor prognostic factors include age less than 1 year or more than 10 years, male sex, CNS disease and a high white cell count at presentation.

PATHOLOGICAL FEATURES

If arising in a lymph node, there is usually diffuse or partial replacement of normal architecture by a monotonous infiltrate of non-cohesive, but closely packed, uniform, medium-sized lymphoblasts. The tumour cells characteristically grow in an interfollicular growth pattern, a useful feature in establishing the diagnosis. The neoplastic cells contain large round or convoluted nuclei with a fine chromatin pattern and inconspicuous nucleoli. There is scanty cytoplasm, varying from pale to slightly basophilic in colour. Morphologically, the neoplastic cells are indistinguishable from those seen in ALL [32].

Mitotic figures are abundant and necrosis may be extensive; if this is the case, it may preclude a tissue diagnosis [8].

DIFFERENTIAL DIAGNOSIS

T-lymphoblastic lymphoma and B-lymphoblastic lymphoma may closely resemble each other, especially if the fixation is less than optimal. However in T-lymphoblastic lymphoma, cells are less uniform and nuclei show more tendency towards convolution. Immunohistochemistry is needed, however, to make a reliable distinction.

Myeloblastic lesions (presenting as soft tissue masses – chloroma) can resemble this entity, as it can mimic many lesions. However, the presence of maturing myeloid cells and scattered immature eosinophils may help in arousing suspicions. Once again, immunohistochemistry should allow a definite distinction, with the tumour cells showing positivity for MT1, CD11c and negativity for TdT.

In the paediatric age range, there are a number of small round cell tumours of childhood, such as Ewing's sarcoma, peripheral neuro-ectodermal tumours and neuroblastoma, that may closely resemble lymphoblastic lymphoma. Immunohistochemical staining should exclude these.

Subclassification is by cell lineage and stage differentiation. These include mature B-ALL, common B-ALL, pre-B-ALL and pre-pre-B-ALL [12], [33].

IMMUNOHISTOCHEMISTRY

True lymphoblastic lymphomas of B-cell phenotype express early B-cell markers (CD19, CD22, CD79a) but may not express CD20 if the phenotype is relatively immature. They also show variable positivity for CD10 and may be positive for CD34, CD13 and CD33. Although they may express cytoplasmic immunoglobulin, they are negative for surface immunoglobulin. TdT is usually positive, although it is technically difficult and is lost in the more mature lesions.

GENETICS

There are no consistent characteristic cytogenetic abnormalities found in true lymphoblastic lymphomas of B-cell phenotype. For the purpose of prognostication, various broad groupings of abnormality are recognised, including hypodiploid, pseudodiploid, hyperdiploid (whether less than 51 chromosomes, or 51 or more), and the presence of specific abnormalities.

The t(1;19)(q23;p13) translocation results in an expressed fusion gene between E2A (encoding a transcription factor) and the PBX gene, a homeobox gene. Its presence indicates poor response to some treatment regimens.

The t(9;22)(q34;q11) translocation (the Philadelphia chromosome) occurs in only 5% of cases in children, but is an important independent prognostic marker [34].

T-CELL LYMPHOMAS

Non-Hodgkin's lymphomas of T-cell phenotype occurring in the paediatric age range are almost universally of true lymphoblastic subtype [35]. It must be noted, however, that peripheral T-cell lymphoma, although rare, does occur and this should always be borne in mind when considering the diagnosis of a T-cell lymphoma in children [36]. Another point for consideration is that anaplastic large cell lymphoma (ALCL) frequently marks with CD3, thus apparently exhibiting a T-cell phenotype (indeed it is believed to be derived from cytotoxic T-cells [37], although for the purposes of classification, prognosis and treatment, it is considered as a separate entity. It is thus important to exclude this possibility by always undertaking staining for CD30, ALK-1 and EMA, since the 'small-celled' variant of ALCL may be a morphological mimic of T-cell lymphoma [37].

T-CELL LYMPHOBLASTIC LYMPHOMA (TLL)

CLINICAL FEATURES

This is by far the most common subtype of T-cell phenotype NHL occurring in the paediatric age range. Although representing only approximately 30% of all childhood NHL [38], it constitutes 98% of all T-NHL. The male-to-female ratio is approximately 7 to 3 [35]. The presentation is usually one of leukaemia accompanied by a mass. In about two thirds there is an anterior mediastinal mass and/or a pleural effusion, but a quarter have peripheral — usually cervical — lymphadenopathy (possibly with an as yet undetected mediastinal mass) [39]. Unusual sites of presentation include the mastoid cavity, an infra-orbital mass and ovary [40], [41].

TLL occurs in older children, with only 15% occurring in those under 5 years of age. Interestingly, although almost universally a highly aggressive lesion, in 1999 a case of clinically indolent TLL was reported [42].

PATHOLOGICAL FEATURES

At low power, TLL presents a relatively uniform appearance with a diffuse, monotonous growth pattern. Although a 'starry-sky' appearance (due to the presence of tingible-body macrophages) may be present, this is not usually as prominent as is seen in Burkitt's lymphoma [43]. Nodal disease frequently shows extracapsular extension, together with paracortical infiltration, possibly with sparing of germinal centres [43], [44]. The majority of cells are approximately 1.5—2 times a lymphocyte diameter and have a high nucleocytoplasmic ratio, with only a thin rim of cytoplasm (Fig. 2.5). The nuclear chromatin is either

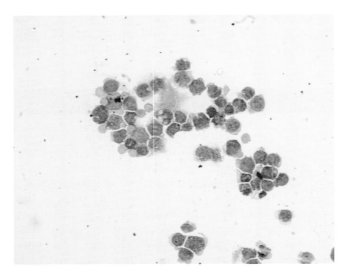

Fig. 2.5 Fine needle aspiration cytology of lymph node showing T-lymphoblastic lymphoma consisting of large cells with a high N:C ratio and thin rim of cytoplasm. (Giemsa, magnification × 60.)

dispersed or only very finely condensed. There are a variable number of incon-spicuous nucleoli [44]. Not infrequently, there are subpopulations of cells with somewhat differing cytological features, including slightly larger, more obviously blastic cells with larger nucleoli, and cells resembling mature small lymphocytes [40]. The mitotic rate and apoptotic rate are high, although not as high as is seen in Burkitt's lymphoma [7]. There is no known clinical signif-icance in the division, based on nuclear morphology, into 'convoluted' and 'non-convoluted' subtypes [45].

The cytoplasmic vacuolation seen in cytological preparations is less conspic-uous than is seen in Burkitt's lymphoma, and the condensation of the chromatin is more obvious [46]. The nucleoli are seen as chromocentres and nuclear outline is more obviously convoluted.

IMMUNOHISTOCHEMISTRY

TdT is expressed in almost 100% of cases and is extremely useful in confirming the diagnosis, although there can be technical difficulties in using it [47]. TLL also expresses T-lineage markers (CD2, CD3, CD5 and CD7) and may co-express CD4 and CD8 [40]. It is also positive with CD1a. Approximately 50–60% of cases express CD10 [48] and rarely cases may be positive for CD79a; this does not signify bi-lineage differentiation [7]. Positivity for CD1a, CD4 and CD8 appears to correlate with normal T-lymphoblast ontogeny [49], although there is some dispute concerning the correlation of the stage of differentiation with clinical behaviour [35], [50].

Rare cases may exhibit true bi-lineage differentiation with expression of myeloid markers such as CD13 and CD33 [40], although it should be noted that myeloblastic lesions may express T-cell antigens [35]. A case of TLL arising nine months after the diagnosis of acute myeloblastic leukaemia has been reported [51].

There are various case reports of an association with viruses and TLL [52], [53], although the biological relevance of these instances is not clear.

GENETICS

There is no known recurrent cytogenetic abnormality that defines TLL. In one third of cases there are cytogenetic abnormalities involving either the T-cell receptor beta chain locus at 7q35, the T-cell receptor gamma chain locus at 7p14, or the T-cell receptor alpha/delta receptor loci at 14q11 [54], [55]. It is hypothesised that these aberrations result in the inappropriate activation of cellular oncogenes, a situation that parallels the activation of BCL-2 by its trans-location into the immunoglobulin heavy chain locus in follicle centre cell lymphoma [56]. In the great majority of cases, the precise nature of the onco-genes being thus activated is at present unknown, although cases have been reported that involve MYC, HOX-11, RBTN-1 and RBTN-2 [57].

In approximately one third of cases of TLL there is a deletion of 9p, resulting in loss of the tumour suppressor gene CDKN2a; the product of this gene inhibits cyclin-dependent kinase-4 [57]. The locus 1p32 is the site of the TAL-1 gene (also known as SCL or TCL-5). A deletion of this locus is present in 25% of cases (although it is only karyotypically visible in only 5% of cases) [58]. TAL-1 encodes a transcription factor containing a basic helix-loop-helix motif and it appears to be fundamental in haematopoietic stem cell development [59]. It binds as a heterodimer to the E2A and HEB/HTF4 gene products, although details suggest a complex picture in which the TAL-1 gene product can act as both an activator and repressor of transcription [60]. Overexpression of TAL-1 is the most common molecular abnormality found in T-cell leukaemia [61].

Although rearrangement of the T-cell receptor chain loci can be used as a diagnostic tool, it should be remembered that such rearrangements, especially of the gamma chain, are seen also in myeloid lesions as well as in B-lineage lesions [62]–[65].

OTHER T-LINEAGE NHL

As stated above, it should be remembered that not all T-lineage lymphomas in this age group are TLL [36]. In the past three years, there has been one case of peripheral T-cell lymphoma (PTCL) presenting to the UKCCSG Review Panel. This presented as a mass in the forearm of an eight-year-old boy and had the morphological growth pattern of angio-immunoblastic lymphadenopathy.

MEDIASTINAL MASSES

The majority of cases of mediastinal mass in children are due to TLL, but other lymphoid and non-lymphoid causes of such a lesion must be excluded. Not only Hodgkin's disease but also anaplastic large cell lymphoma and sclerosing B-cell lymphoma (even in childhood) may present with a such a mass. Non-lymphoid causes include thymoma and germ cell tumour.

ANAPLASTIC LARGE CELL LYMPHOMA

CLINICAL FEATURES

Anaplastic large cell lymphoma (ALCL) is the third most common childhood lymphoma, accounting for approximately one fifth of cases of paediatric NHL in the UK. There is a striking male preponderance, with a male-to-female ratio of approximately 7 to 1 [66]. It may present as a nodal disease, but it must be remembered that it is often extranodal in presentation, especially affecting skin, soft tissues, lung and bone marrow; synchronous nodal and extranodal disease is considered to represent high-risk disease [66]. Because of this, disease at presentation is late stage (III or IV) and often associated with B symptoms. Bone marrow involvement occurs in about 30% of cases [67].

There are several subtypes of ALCL. The 'common' or 'classical' subtype occurs with highest frequency and was the first to be recognised [68]. Of diagnostic importance are the 'small cell' and the 'lymphohistiocytic' variants, since these appear mistaken for peripheral T-cell lymphoma [69]. Other subtypes include the 'sarcomatoid' variant (which has a spindle-celled morphology and which may therefore be mistaken for a soft tissue tumour), the 'giant cell' variant and the 'Hodgkin-like' variant [69], [70].

It is now generally accepted that ALCL and HL are different disease entities [71]. That said, some cases may present features that present diagnostic difficulties. Originally it was conceived that truly intermediate forms did exist, but this view is now discounted [72]. The generally accepted view now is that 'Hodgkin-like' cases (possibly with classical Hodgkin and Reed–Sternberg cells, a nodular growth pattern and capsular thickening) should be considered Hodgkin-like ALCL only if they express ALK-1 protein (see below), and HL if this stain is negative [73].

Mixed forms are not uncommon and are of significance since one pattern may predominate in relapse [74].

ALCL was originally defined by its positivity for the CD30. It is a cell surface protein that belongs to the tumour necrosis factor–nerve growth factor receptor family [75], is an antigen normally found on activated lymphoid cells (both B and T) and sometimes CD30 on activated macrophages [69]. Its overexpression may be seen not only in lymphomas but also in germ cell tumours, and this must be taken into consideration if the presentation or morphology is unusual [76]. Its function remains unknown [77].

Although the usual differential diagnosis of ALCL is Hodgkin's lymphoma (CD30 was first characterised in classical HL) other lymphomas and lympho-proliferative disorders may be CD30 positive [69]. Diffuse large B-cell lymphoma (especially mediastinal B-cell lymphoma) may be CD30 positive, but this does not mean that a designation of ALCL of B-lineage is appropriate, even if the lesion shows extreme cellular pleomorphism. The general view is that ALCL of B-cell lineage does not exist; but there is a caveat. It was originally thought that those rare cases of DLBCL that stain positively with the ALK-1 antibody (the characteristic marker of ALCL, see below) were not expressing the fusion gene product that is characteristic of ALCL, but the full-length, normal ALK protein [78]. However, it is now recognised that they may well be expressing a particular fusion gene product of the t(2;17) translocation, involving the clathrin heavy chain gene. This does not usually occur in the paediatric age range.

CD30 positivity may also occur in cells that morphologically resemble ALCL cells in certain lymphohistiocytic proliferations of the skin, including regressing atypical histiocytosis and lymphomatoid papulosis [79]. These are usually negative both for ALK-1 and EMA (both characteristically positive in ALCL) and should not therefore be considered as isolated skin deposits of ALCL [69], unless there is obvious lymph node or other site involvement. The distinction is important, since isolated lymphohistiocytic proliferations of the skin are self-limiting and may be cured by local surgery, whereas skin and lymph node involvement by ALCL requires chemotherapy [80].

PATHOLOGICAL FEATURES

The cell that characterises ALCL is the 'Hallmark cell' (Fig. 2.6). This is approximately equivalent in size to a macrophage, mononuclear and has a characteristic nuclear shape variously described as 'reniform', 'horse-shoe' or 'grooved'. These are seen in all variants of ALCL and should be identified for the diagnosis

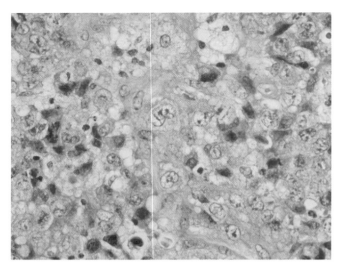

Fig. 2.6 Anaplastic large cell lymphoma, showing a hallmark cell. (H&E, magnification × 60.)

to be made. ALCL may show great nuclear pleomorphism and may even contain cells that are morphologically and immunophenotypically indistinguishable from Hodgkin and Reed–Sternberg cells; this must be remembered when considering the differential diagnosis from HL. However, ALCL, somewhat paradoxically, may show little or no nuclear pleomorphism and may even, in the small-cell variant, consist predominantly of cells relatively small in size.

The chromatin is usually coarsely clumped and may be condensed on the nuclear membrane. Nucleoli are usually prominent and may be multiple. There is usually a moderate amount of eosinophilic cytoplasm. If fixation and staining conditions are optimal, one may be able to appreciate intensification of eosinophilia within the region of the Golgi complex.

These cells may be seen growing in cohesive sheets within paracortical areas (hence the confusion in earlier days with metastatic carcinoma), but a characteristic feature is an intra-sinusoidal growth pattern, an important point of distinction from HL. Another feature of the growth pattern, more frequently associated with the small-cell and lymphohistiocytic variants, is a tendency for perivascular growth.

In the small-cell variant, the characteristic Hallmark cells may be in a minority, most of the atypical cells being small-to-intermediate in size, with insignificant nucleoli and markedly irregular, possible cerebriform, nuclear outline [81]. The cytoplasm is scanty. In the lymphohistiocytic variant, there is predominance of histiocytes, both epithelioid and non-epithelioid, and atypical cells may be hard to find [82], [83]. As in the small-cell variant, these tend to be smaller, although Hallmark cells may be found. It is often difficult to distinguish between the lymphohistiocytic and small-cell variants, raising the possibility that they are, in fact, biologically related.

The giant-cell type is recognised by the fact that the majority of cells are extremely large and multinucleate, often with bizarre morphological features [29], [68]. In the sarcomatoid variant the atypical cells have a spindle-celled morphology and there may be a myxoid stroma [70]. Other variants include the neutrophil-rich variant [84] and the Hodgkin-like variant (in which there may be capsular thickening and banded sclerosis) [69]. This last variant is of interest not only because it highlights the diagnostic difficulties that may be encountered in ALCL, but also because it suggests a possible relationship between the two entities [71]. It is now generally accepted that morphologically at least there are cases of overlap between the two diseases, although use of immunohistochemistry for ALK-1 and PAX-5 (the former characteristic of ALCL, the latter of HL) usually allows distinction [69]. Some authorities believe that this subtype does not exist as a separate entity and that most such cases are in reality HL [85].

IMMUNOHISTOCHEMISTRY

ALCL and its variants are characteristically positive for CD30 [57] (Fig. 2.7). The staining pattern is usually accentuated on the cell membrane, although positive staining of the Golgi complex may impart a 'dot-like' positivity [69]. Epithelial membrane antigen (EMA) is positive in approximately 50% of cases, again staining the cell membrane and Golgi complex [86]. CD45 is positive in only 50% of cases, another fact that contributed to the early confusion with metastatic carcinoma [69].

ALK-1 and ALK-C are monoclonal antibodies against ALK protein and are most commonly used [57], [87]. Polyclonal ALK antibodies may give false positive results and are best avoided. ALK-1 stains not only the NPM-ALK fusion protein that results from the most common cytogenetic marker of ALCL, the t(2;5)(p23;p35), but also against its variants [69]. There is variation in the staining pattern depending on which cytogenetic abnormality is present. The most common pattern (associated with t(2;5)(p23;p35)) is cytoplasmic, nuclear and nucleolar. The second most common pattern is predominantly cytoplasmic

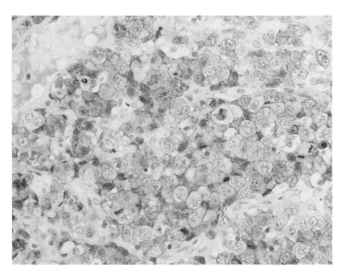

Fig. 2.7 Anaplastic large cell lymphoma. (CD30, magnification × 60.)

and cytoplasmic membrane staining and is associated with the t(1;2)(q25;p23) abnormality.

Interestingly, in the small cell variant, the more characteristic cytoplasmic and nuclear staining may be seen in the scattered Hallmark cells, whereas in the small atypical cells there may be predominant nuclear staining [88].

ALK staining (Fig. 2.8) is not only important diagnostically but also prognostically, since there is considerable evidence to suggest that the 5-year survival rate of 75% in ALK-positive cases is halved in ALK-negative cases [66]. In children, ALK-positive ALCL is the norm, although rare cases of ALK-negative ALCL do occur.

Childhood ALCL is thought to be a proferation of cytotoxic T-cells, and as such may exhibit either a T-cell phenotype or a null cell phenotype [57], [69]. Tumour cells may express any or all of a variety of T-cell markers, but the variability means that it is not recommended to attempt to assign phenotype using only one or two antibodies. Even in those cases that are consistently negative it may prove possible to assign a T-cell phenotype by finding positivity for either granzyme B, perforin or TIA-1 (although this last is not particularly specific). These are characteristic markers of cytotoxic T-cells [89], [90]. Rare cases may express CD56, suggesting a natural killer cell phenotype [89]. Stains for Epstein—Barr virus (such as LMP-1) are almost always negative [90].

As has been remarked above, it is now widely held that ALCL of B-cell phenotype does not exist, and great care should be taken before consideration of this diagnosis.

GENETICS

The t(2;5)(p23;q35) translocation is found in approximately 75% of cases [79]. This results in fusion of the ALK gene on chromosome 2p23 with the NPM

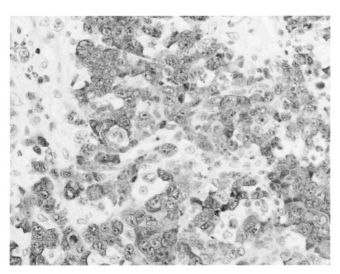

Fig. 2.8 Anaplastic large cell lymphoma showing nuclear, nucleolar and cytoplasmic staining with ALK-1. (ALK-1, magnification × 60.)

(nucleophosmin) gene on chromosome 5q35 [91]. NPM codes for an ubiquitously expressed intranuclear protein. It is a phosphoprotein that binds RNA and transports ribonucleoproteins between the nucleolus and the cytoplasm and is normally located in the nucleolus [91]. ALK, a member of the insulin receptor family that is normally located in the cell membrane, is a tyrosine kinase [93]. Its normal role appears to be in nervous system development, and it is not normally expressed in haematopoietic cells [94]. The translocation results in the expression of a fusion protein that is both in frame and functional [79]. This protein retains the cytoplasmic kinase domain of ALK fused to the 5′ end of the NPM gene [95]. It is a constitutively active kinase under the action of the strong NPM promoter [96]. The fusion protein loses the nuclear localisation signal of wild-type NPM but it is still capable of dimerisation [79]. Homodimerisation results in cytoplasmic localisation, heterodimerisation (with wild-type ALK) in nuclear and nucleolar localisation; it is the homodimers that are thought to be oncogenic [97].

There are several variants of this cytogenetic abnormality, all involving the ALK gene on chromosome 2p23. The second most common, found in approximately 15% of cases, is the t(1;2)(q25;p23), which produces a fusion protein of ALK and tropomysin 3 [98]. Because this fusion protein has no nuclear localisation signal, staining is exclusively cytoplasmic [79].

Five percent of cases have an inversion of chromosome 2, inv(2)(p23;q35), that results in a fusion protein of ALK and ATIC-2, a gene that codes for an enzyme involved in purine nucleotide synthesis [98]. This, too, is restricted to the cytoplasm [79]. In addition, several other cytogenetic abnormalities, all involving 2p23, have been described in cases of ALCL [69], [99].

T-cell receptor gene rearrangements can be found in 90% of cases using either PCR or Southern blotting techniques [69]. Rearrangements of the immunoglobulin genes are not found.

HODGKIN'S LYMPHOMA

In the UK, there are approximately 120 new cases of Hodgkin's lymphoma (HL) per year in the paediatric age range. The currently accepted classifications are the REAL and the Revised WHO systems [57]. The main change in classification in recent years has been the recognition that there are two distinct disease entities encompassed by the term Hodgkin's lymphoma – namely classical Hodgkin's lymphoma (CHL) and nodular lymphocyte predominant Hodgkin's lymphoma (NLPHL) [57], [100], [101]. These two entities will be considered separately, the main part of the discussion concerning CHL, since in children NLPHL is less common.

CLASSICAL HODGKIN'S LYMPHOMA

CLINICAL FEATURES

In children, HL is slightly less common than NHL (ratio about 4:5) and CHL accounts for approximately 85–90% of all cases of HL. Of these, 70% occur in males, only 10% in children under 5, and only 25% occur in those under 10. By far the most common site of presentation is in a lymph node, often a cervical lymph node. Nearly 10% present purely as mediastinal mass.

In CHL the Hodgkin and Reed—Sternberg cells are derived from follicle centre cells that have participated in the primary immune response, but have not completed the normal process of somatic hypermutation in the germinal centre [102]. Somatic hypermutation is the mechanism of affinity maturation whereby the specificity and strength of binding of B-cells to antigen is increased, thus allowing a more targeted secondary immune response [103]. In CHL, there are an abnormally high number of somatic hypermutations, many of which lead to non-functional rearranged immunoglobulin heavy chain genes [69]. The transforming event seems to arise within the environs of the germinal centre itself [104], [105]. There is also evidence of mutations in the IκBα gene, therefore possibly suggesting that a fundamental pathogenetic mechanism in HL is abnormality of the nuclear factor κB signalling pathway [106]. This is an interesting observation in the light of the characteristic inflammatory response of HL [102].

PATHOLOGICAL FEATURES

The Reed—Sternberg cell is the characteristic abnormal cell in CHL. This has traditionally been described as binucleate or multinucleate, but it is now known to be a single bilobed or multilobed nucleus. It is usually some 10—15 times larger than the small lymphocyte and characteristically has a single, centrally placed and exceedingly prominent nucleolus. The chromatin is cleared, with some condensation on the inner nuclear membrane. There is usually a small-to-moderate amount of amphophilic cytoplasm. The Hodgkin cell is the mononuclear variant, which, although highly suggestive of HL, cannot be taken alone as diagnostic of the condition [107]. A diagnostic aid is the presence of so-called 'mummified' cells; these cells are degenerate variants of Hodgkin and Reed—Sternberg cells [57]. They are smaller than Hodgkin or Reed—Sternberg cells with hyperchromatic nuclei, smudged chromatin, insignificant nucleoli and eosinophilc cytoplasm. They tend to stand out at low power.

The growth pattern of HL tends to be a paracortical disease, growing around follicles, which, in early disease, may show quite marked hyperplasia. It does not usually involve sinuses, in contradistinction to ALCL [57].

The Hodgkin and Reed—Sternberg cells are seen against a cellular background that defines the subtype. Thus the histological picture of lymphocyte-rich HL is one of a few atypical cells in a large number of small lymphocytes and histiocytes. The presence of numerous, often highly atypical and pleomorphic, Hodgkin's and Reed—Sternberg cells with relatively few surrounding reactive cells is the characteristic appearance of lymphocyte-depleted HL. Mixed cellularity HL contains atypical cells in moderate numbers set in a background of small lymphocytes, eosinophils, histiocytes and plasma cells [57], [107].

All of the preceeding discussion assumes that the features of nodular sclerosis are not present. Nodular sclerosing HL (Fig. 2.9) is diagnosed when two out of the three of the following are present: banded sclerosis, capsular thickening or Lacunar cells [57], [107]. Lacunar cells are another variant of Hodgkin and Reed—Sternberg cells in which the atypical cell appears to be placed within a 'lacuna' or clear space (Fig. 2.10). They may not have all of the normal morphological characteristics of Reed–Sternberg cells, but stain appropriately. It has been suggested that they are an artefact due to tissue retraction because of the fibrosis, although their presence in cases of so-called 'cellular phase' of nodular sclerosing HL (where there is no established banded sclerosis) suggests otherwise [108]. It should also be noted that the sclerosis in this type of HL must be in the form of thick, acellular and eosinophilic bands, and diffuse, ill-defined sclerosis should not be regarded as indicating nodular sclerosing HL [35], [71].

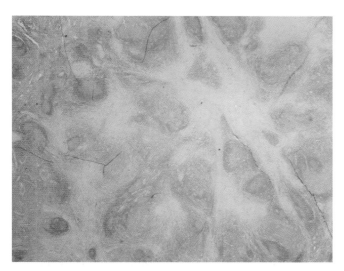

Fig. 2.9 Classical Hodgkin's lymphoma, nodular sclerosing variant, showing fibrous collagen bands dividing the lymph node into nodules. (H&E, magnification × 2.)

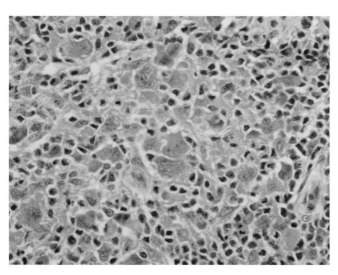

Fig. 2.10 Classical Hodgkin's lymphoma, nodular sclerosing variant, showing lacunar cells. (H&E, magnification × 60.)

If the features of nodular sclerosis are present, the cellularity of the residual lymphoid tissue is not relevant in subcategorisation, but some authorities consider that an attempt should be made to grade the disease [109]. Grade 1 disease has fewer and/or less-pleomorphic atypical cells than grade 2. The clinical usefulness of grading is, however, still debated [110]–[112]. One study has suggested that cellular-phase nodular sclerosing HD may have a worse prognosis [113].

Immunohistochemistry

Hodgkin and Reed—Sternberg cells are almost always positive for CD30 (Fig. 2.11) and a negative result must throw considerable doubt on the diagnosis [71]. It should also be noted that CD30 is not unique to HL and is, of course, positive in ALCL and also in high grade B-NHL, and non-lymphoid tumours, such as germ cell tumours, may also be positive [57], [114]. CD30 belongs to the tumour necrosis factor receptor superfamily [77]. Its function is largely unknown although its activation (by binding with its ligand) is thought to result in pleiotropic effects including cell proliferation and apoptosis [115].

Curiously, considering its lymphoid origin, CHL is consistently negative for CD45, and CD15 positivity is found in approximately 80% of HL; this can be a useful marker, since NHL is rarely positive [116]. Approximately 40% of HL cases are positive with the pan-B-cell marker, CD20, but CHL is not usually positive with CD79a. Rarely, T-cell markers such as CD3 may be positive, but if this is the case, one should question whether the case is really ALCL [57].

CHL shows positivity for Epstein—Barr virus in a varying proportion of cases, depending on subtype. Overall, approximately 50% of cases in Europe and the United States are positive [116], [117]. The pattern of protein expression indicates type-2 latent infection, so that there is positivity for anitbodies against latent

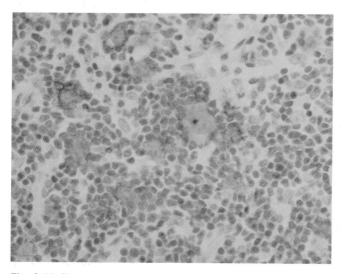

Fig. 2.11 Classical Hodgkin's lymphoma, nodular sclerosing variant showing CD30 expression. (CD30, magnification × 60.)

membrane protein 1 and EBNA1 [116]. A far more sensitive method of detecting EBV infection is in-situ hybridisation for EBERs (small RNA molecules found in the latent state) [117].

Useful in the distinction between HL and ALCL are the facts that Alk-1 is never positive and EMA very rarely so, in CHL [57]. Variable expression of T-cell markers, such as CD2 and granzyme B, may occur [102].

GENETICS

There are no recurrent, consistent characteristic karyotypic abnormalities in CHL, although the lack of t(14;18) and t(2;5) translocations may help in the distinction of HL from B-NHL and ALCL respectively [118]. It is interesting to note that there are frequent, apparently random, abnormalities involving 14q [116]. Also, the finding of marked variability of karyotypes between cells from the same case indicates that genomic instability is a characteristic of HL [118]. Specialised molecular biological techniques have demonstrated a relatively high frequency of amplification and gain of chromosomal material in various distinct regions [119].

Overall, karyotyping demonstrates aneuploidy and hypertetraploidy in both Hodgkin and Reed–Sternberg cells in most cases of HL [57].

It is now recognised that the majority of cases of HL have rearranged immunoglobulin chain genes [116], [120], [121]. Original studies failed to demonstrate this because of technical limitations. The use of single-cell amplification techniques has allowed the separation of Hodgkin's and Reed–Sternberg cells from the surrounding reactive infiltrate, thereby increasing the signal-to-noise ratio. Those cases expressing B-cell antigens are reported to be more likely to have such rearrangments [121]. These findings are in keeping with their postulated B-cell origin. There are, however, a small number of cases in which rearranged T-cell receptor chain genes in the absence of rearranged immunoglobulin chain genes have been found [122].

NODULAR LYMPHOCYTE PREDOMINANT HODGKIN'S LYMPHOMA

CLINICAL FEATURES

In children nodular lymphocyte predominant Hodgkin's lymphoma (NLPHL) is a relatively uncommon tumour type, comprising approximately 10–15% of cases of HL. It is considered to be a relatively indolent lesion, often presenting as stage 1 disease, characteristically as an enlarged node or nodal mass high in the neck or axilla [35], [57]. Because of this, it is often amenable to local radiotherapy. There is a small risk of transformation to high-grade B-cell NHL, which occurs in about 5% of cases [123]. Case reports of transformation to T-cell lymphoma presumably represent instances of coincidental second malignancy [124]. NLPHL may uncommonly present at other sites, such as inguinal nodes and mediastinum.

The male-to-female ratio is approximately 3:1 and, unlike CHL, the age distribution is unimodal with a peak in the 4th decade [102]. Late presentation has a relatively poor prognosis [125].

The original Lukes and Butler classification of HL recognised two variants of lymphocyte predominant Hodgkin's lymphoma − not only a nodular form (also called 'nodular paragranuloma') but also a diffuse form [108]. It is now widely accepted that cases of the diffuse variant are either non-Hodgkin's lymphoma (often so-called 'T-cell rich B-cell lymphoma') or are what would now be termed 'lymphocyte-rich CHL' [57].

NLPHL has an ill-defined relationship with a condition known as 'progressive transformation of germinal centres'. In this condition there is clinical lymph node enlargement without systemic symptoms. Histologically, there is follicular enlargement with germinal centres appearing disrupted, expanded and infiltrated by small lymphocytes [35]. These lymphocytes are CD5+ B-cells derived from the mantle zone. Progressive transformation may occur without relationship to NLPHL, but it may precede NLPHL, may occur synchronously or may occur subsequently. [126], [127].

It is now accepted that, like CHL, NLPHL is derived from follicle centre cells, although in the case of NLPHL the evidence suggests that there is more B-cell differentiation than in CHL [57].

PATHOLOGICAL FEATURES

Nodal architecture is complete or partly effaced by a vaguely nodular lymphoid proliferation. This does not resemble normal follicular architecture and the nodularity may be exceedingly difficult to discern, in contrast to follicle centre cell lymphoma. IHC with pan-B- and pan-T-cell markers may accentuate the nodularity [57], [116].

The proliferation consists large of mature and polyclonal small lymphocytes, together with a variable number of histiocytes, possibly forming small granulomata or congeries, and a small number of L&H or 'popcorn' cells (Fig. 2.12). These cells have nuclei that are 3−4 times the size of a small lymphocyte, and in which the chromatin is cleared and condensed on the nuclear membrane. These nuclei are often bilobated or multilobated [35]. They characteristically have small nucleoli that are less prominent than those seen CHL. They are often multiple and less eosinophilic, again in contrast to Reed−Sternberg cells. The other components of CHL − eosinophils, plasma cells and neutrophils − are absent in NLPHL.

IMMUNOHISTOCHEMISTRY

'Popcorn' cells do not express CD15 or CD30, and this finding may be of use in the distinction between NLPHL and classical HL. Moreover, L&H cells characteristically express CD45 and CD79a, again a distinct difference from CHL. They are also far more frequently positive with other B-cell markers such as CD19, CD20 and CD22 [116]. They also stain with BCL-6 and between 40% and 50% stain positively with EMA [116], [128].

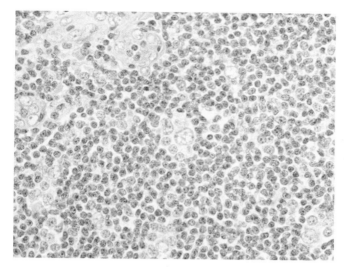

Fig. 2.12 Nodular lymphocyte predominant Hodgkin's lymphoma, showing popcorn cells. (H&E, magnification × 60.)

The surrounding small lymphocytes are a mixture of CD20+ B-cells and CD3+ T-cells, with more B-cells being found in the nodular areas. One useful diagnostic feature is that the L&H cells within the nodules may be surrounded by a ring of CD3+, CD57+ T-cells, a phenomenon not seen in CHL [129], [130]. Staining for follicular dendritic cells (e.g. CD21) highlights large networks within the nodules and is evidence that the nodules are in fact broken up and expanded follicles [116].

GENETICS

Single-cell PCR demonstrates that L&H cells show rearrangement of the immunoglobulin heavy and light chain genes [131]. Sequencing of rearranged immunoglobulin heavy chain genes has shown that the cells are undergoing somatic hypermutation (as with CHL) to an extent greater than is normally seen in follicle centre cells [132]. The resulting genes are functional, thus explaining the evidence of B-cell differentiation, and why, in contrast to CHL, hypermutation continued after the transforming event. They also appear to have been positively selected by antigen [102].

There are no known recurrent cytogenetic abnormalities occurring in NLPHL with any great frequency [116].

REFERENCES

1. Behrman RE, Kliegman RM, Jenson HB. *Nelson Textbook of Paediatrics.* 16th edn. (W.B. Saunders, London, 2000).
2. Goldsby RE, Carroll WL. The moleular biology of paediatric lymphomas. *J Paed Haem Onc* 1998; **20**: 282–96.

3. Sandlund JT, Downing JR, Crist WM. Non-Hodgkin's lymphoma in childhood. *N Eng J Med* 1996; **334**: 1238–48.

4. Stiller CA, Allen MB, Eatock EM. Childhood cancer in Britain: the National Registry of Childhood Tumours and incidence rates 1978–1987. *Eur J Cancer* 1995; **31A**: 2028–34.

5. Coeberg JW, Van der Does-Van den Berg A, Kamps WA *et al.* Malignant lymphomas in children in The Netherlands in the period 1973–1985: incidence in relation to leukaemia: a report from the Dutch Childhood Leukaemia Study Group. *Med Paed Oncol* 1991; **19**: 169–74.

6. Chan JKC, Banks PM, Clearly ML *et al.* A revised European–American classification of lymphoid neoplasms proposed by the international lymphoma study group. A summary version. *Am J Clin Pathol* 1995; **103**: 543–60.

7. Harris NL, Jaffe ES, Diebold J *et al.* World Health Organization classification of neoplastic disease of the haematopoietic and lymphoid tissues: report of the clinical advisory committee meeting – Airlie House, Virginia, November 1997. *J Clin Oncol* 1999; **17**: 3835–49.

8. Carter RL, McCarthy KP. Features of specific tumours, section 2. *Paediatric Oncology,* Pinkerton CR and Plowman PN, eds. 2nd edn. (Chapman & Hall Medical, London, 1997).

9. Filipovich AH, Mathur A, Kamat D *et al.* Primary immunodeficiencies: genetic risk factors for lymphoma. *Cancer Res* 1992; **52**(suppl): 5465s–7s.

10. Filipovich AH, Mathur A, Kamat D *et al.* Lymphoproliferative disorders and other tumours complicating immunodeficiencies. *Immunodeficiency* 1994; **5**: 91–112.

11. Bucsky P, Feller AC, Reiter A *et al.* Low grade malignant non-Hodgkin's lymphomas and peripheral pleomorphic T-cell lymphomas in childhood – a BFM group report. *Clin Pediatr* 1990; **202**: 258–61.

12. Ramsay A. High grade lymphomas in lymph nodes (including paediatric cases). *CPD Cell Path* 2002; **4**: 13–17.

13. Kjeldsberg CR, Wilson JF, Berard C. Non-Hodgkin's lymphoma in children. *Hum Pathol* 1983; **14**: 612–27.

14. Head D, Behm F. Acute lymphoblastic leukaemia and the lymphoblastic lymphomas of childhood. *Semin Diag Pathol* 1995; **12**: 325–34.

15. Pinto A, Hutchison RE, Grant LH *et al.* Follicular lymphomas in paediatric patients. *Mod Pathol* 1990; **3**: 308–13.

16. Shankar AG, Ashley S, Radford M *et al.* Does histology influence outcome in childhood Hodgkin's disease? Results from the United Kingdom Children's Cancer Study Group. *J Clin Oncol* 1997; **15**: 2622–30.

17. Gruss HJ, Herrmann F, Drexler HG. Hodgkin's disease: a cytokine-producing tumour – a review. *Crit Rev Oncog* 1994; **5**: 473–538.

18. Burkitt D. A sarcoma involving the jaws in African children. *Br J Surg* 1958; **46**: 218–23.

19. Levine PH, Connelly RR, McKay FW. Burkitt's lymphoma in the USA: cases reported to the American Burkitt Lymphoma Registry compared with population-based incidence and mortality data. *IARC Sci Pub* 1985; **60**: 217–24.

20. Bain BJ. The trephine biopsy in acute leukaemia. *CPD Cell Path* 2002; **4**: 39–42.

21. Levine PH, Kamaraju LS, Connelly RR. The American Burkitt's Lymphoma Registry: eight years' experience. *Cancer* 1982; **49**: 1016–22.

22. Magrath IT. Management of high-grade lymphomas. *Oncology* 1998; **12**: 40–8.

23. Campbell AGM, McIntosh N. *Forfar and Arneil's Textbook of Paediatrics.* 5th edn. (Churchill Livingstone, Edinburgh, 1998).

24. Pavlova Z, Parker JW, Taylor CR *et al.* Small noncleaved follicular center cell lymphoma: Burkitt's and non-Burkitt's variants in the U.S. *Cancer* 1987; **59**: 1892–902.

25. Perkin SL. Work-up and diagnosis of paediatric non-Hodgkin's lymphoma. *Paed Dev Path* 2000; **3**: 374–90.

26. Lones MA, Auperin A, Raphael M, McCarthy K *et al.* Mature B-cell lymphoma/leukaemia in children and adolescents: intergroup pathologist consensus with the Revised European–American Lymphoma classification. *Ann Oncol* 2000; **11**: 47–51.

27. Perkins SL, Segal GH, Kjeldsberg CR. Classification of non-Hodgkin's lymphomas in children. *Semin Diag Pathol* 1995; **12**: 303–13.

28. Miliaukas JR, Berard CW, Young RC et al. Undifferentiated non-Hodgkin's lymphoma (Burkitt's and non-Burkitt's types). The relevance of making this histologic distinction. *Cancer* 1982; **50**: 2115–21.

29. Harris NL, Jaffe ES, Stein H et al. A revised European–American classification of lymphoid neoplasms: a proposal from the International Lymphoma Study Group. *Blood* 1994; **84**: 1361–92.

30. Drillenburg P, Wielenga VJ, Kramer MH et al. CD 44 expression predicts disease outcome in localized large B cell lymphoma. *Leukaemia* 1999; **13**: 1448–55.

31. Kramer MH, Hermans J, Wijburg E et al. Clinical relevance of BCL2, BCL6, and MYC rearrangements in diffuse large B-cell lymphoma. *Blood* 1998; **92**: 3152–62.

32. Berry CL. *Paediatric pathology.* 3rd edn. (Springer-Verlag, London, 1996).

33. Mirro J Jr. Pathology and immunology of acute leukaemia. *Leukaemia* 1992; **6**(suppl 4): 13–15.

34. Raimondi SC. Current status of cytogenetic research in childhood acute lymphoblastic leukaemia. *Blood* 1993; **81**: 2237–44.

35. Warnke RA, Weiss LM, Chan JKC, Cleary ML, Dorfman RF. Tumors of the lymph nodes and spleen. *Atlas of Tumour Pathology* (Armed Forces Institute of Pathology, Washington, D.C. 1995).

36. Gordon BG, Weisenburger DD, Warkentin PI et al. Peripheral T-cell lymphoma in childhood and adolescence. A clinicopathological study of 22 patients. *Cancer* 1993; **71**: 257–63.

37. Benharroch D, Meguerian-Bedovan Z, Lamant L et al. ALK-positive lymphoma: a single disease with a broad spectrum of morphology. *Blood* 1998; **91**: 2076–84.

38. Murphy SB. Childhood non-Hodgkin's lymphoma. *New Engl J Med* 1978; **299**: 1446–8.

39. Nathwani BN, Diamond LW, Winberg CD et al. Lymphoblastic lymphoma: a clinicopathologic study of 95 patients. *Cancer* 1981; **48**: 2347–57.

40. Delsol G, al Saati T, Gatter KC et al. *Blood* 1997; **89**: 1483–90.

41. Vang R, Medeiros LJ, Warnke RA, Higgins JP, Deavers MT. Ovarian non-Hodgkin's lymphoma: a clinicopathologic study of eight primary cases. *Mod Path* 2001; **14**: 1093–9.

42. Velankar MM, Nathwani MM, Schlutz MJ et al. Indolent T-lymphoblastic proliferation: report of a case with a 16-year course without cytotoxic therapy. *Am J Surg Path* 1999; **23**: 977–81.

43. Eriksson B, Johansson AS, Roos G, Levan G, Holmberg D. Establishment and characterization of a mouse strain (TLL) that spontaneously develops T-cell lymphomas/leukemia. *Exp Hematol* 1999; **27**: 682–8.

44. Nathwani BN, Kim H, Rappaport H. Malignant lymphoma, lymphoblastic. *Cancer* 1976; **38**: 964–83.

45. The Non-Hodgkin's Lymphoma Pathologic Classification Project. National Cancer Institute sponsored study of classifications of non-Hodgkin's lymphomas: summary and description of a working formulation for clinical usage. *Cancer* 1982; **49**: 2112–35.

46. Koo CH, Rappaport H, Sheibani K, Pangalis GA, Nathwani BN, Winberg CD. Imprint cytology of non-Hodgkin's lymphomas. Based on a study of 212 immunologically characterised cases; correlation of touch imprints with tissue sections. *Hum Pathol* 1989; **20**: 1–137.

47. Orazi A, Cattoretti G, Joh K, Neiman RS. Terminal deoxynucleotidyl transferase staining of malignant lymphomas in paraffin sections. *Mod Pathol* 1994; **7**: 582–6.

48. Conde-Sterling DA, Aguilera NS, Nandedkar MA, Abbondanzo SL. Immunoperoxidase detection of CD10 in Precursor T-lymphoblastic lymphoma/leukemia: a clinicopathologic study of 24 cases. *Arch Pathol Lab Med* 2000; **124**: 704–8.

49. Hollema H, Poppema S. T-lymphoblastic and peripheral T-cell lymphomas in the northern part of The Netherlands. An immunologic study of 29 cases. *Cancer* 1989; **64**: 1620–8.

50. Czuczman MS, Dodge RK, Stewart CC et al. Value of immunophenotype in intensively treated adult acute lymphoblastic leukemia: cancer and leukemia Group B study 8364. *Blood* 1999; **93**: 3931–9.

51. Thomas X, Anglaret B, Treille-Ritouet D, Bastion Y, Fiere D, Archimbaud E. Occurrence of T-cell lymphoma in a patient with acute myelogenous leukemia. *Ann Hematol* 1996; **73**: 95–8.

52. Hirose Y, Takeshita S, Konda S, Takiguchi T. Detection of human cytomegalovirus in pleural fluid of lymphoblastic lymphoma T-cell type. *Int J Hematol* 1994; **59**: 81−9.

53. Su I, Hsieh HC, Lin KH *et al*. Aggressive peripheral T-cell lymphomas containing Epstein−Barr viral DNA: a clinicopathologic and molecular analysis. *Blood* 1991; **77**: 799−808.

54. Rabbitts TH, Boehm T, Mengle-Gaw L. Chromosomal abnormalities in lymphoid tumours: mechanism and role in tumour pathogenesis. *TIG* 1988; **4**: 300−4.

55. Okuda T, Sakamoto S, Deguchi T *et al*. Hemophagocytic syndrome associated with aggressive natural killer cell leukemia. *Mol Diagn* 1996; **1**: 139−51.

56. McCarthy KP. Molecular diagnosis of lymphomas and associated diseases. *Cancer Metastasis Rev* 1997; **16**: 109−25.

57. Jaffe ES, Harris NL, Stein H, Vardiman JW (Eds). *Pathology and Genetics of Tumours of Haematopoietic and Lymphoid Tissues*. (IARC Press, Lyon, 2001).

58. Brown L, Cheng J-T, Chen Q *et al*. Site-specific recombination of the *tal-1* gene is a common occurrence in human T-cell leukaemia. *EMBO J* 1990; **9**; 3343−51.

59. Sanchez MJ, Bockamp EO, Miller J, Gambardella L, Green AR. Selective rescue of early haematopoietic progenitors in Scl(-/-) mice by expressing Scl under the control of a stem cell enhancer. *Development* 2001; **128**: 4815−27.

60. Haung S, Brandt SJ. mSin3A regulates murine erythroleukemia cell differentiation through association with the TAL1 (or SCL) transcription factor. *Mol Cell Biol* 2000; **20**: 2248−59.

61. Robb L, Begley CG. The SCL/TAL1 gene: roles in normal and malignant haematopoiesis. *Bioessays* 1997; **19**: 607−13.

62. Davey MP, Bongiovanni KF, Kaulfersch W *et al*. Immunoglobululin and T-cell receptor gene re-arrangement and expression in human lymphoid leukemia cells at different stages of maturation. *Proc Natl Acad Sci USA* 1986; **83**: 8759−63.

63. Greaves MF, Furley AJW, Chan LC, Ford AM, Molgaard HV. Inappropriate rearrangement of immunoglobulin and T-cell receptor genes. *Immunol Today* 1987; **8**: 115−16.

64. Pelicci P-G, Knowles DM, Dall-Favera R. Lymphoid tumors displaying rearrangements of both immunoglobin and T-cell receptor genes. *J Exp Med* 1985; **162**: 1015−24.

65. Cheng GY, Minden MD, Toyonaga B, Mak TW, McCullock EA. T cell receptor and immunoglobulin gene rearrangement in acute myeloblastic leukemia. *J Exp Med* 1986; **163**: 414−24.

66. Falini B, Pileri S, Zinzani PL *et al*. ALK+ lymphoma: clinico-pathological findings and outcome. *Blood* 1999; **93**: 2697.

67. Fraga M, Brousset P, Schlaifer D *et al*. Bone marrow involvement in anaplastic large cell lymphoma. *A J Clin Pathol* 1995; **103**: 82.

68. Kadin ME. Anaplastic large cell lymphoma and its morphological variants. *Cancer Surv* 1997; **30**: 77−86.

69. Stein H, Foss H, Dürktop H *et al*. CD30⁺ anaplastic large cell lymphoma: a review of its histopathologic, genetic, and clinical features. *Blood* 2000; **96**: 3681−95.

70. Chan JKC, Buchanan R, Fletcher CDM. Sarcomatoid variant of anaplastic large cell lymphoma. *A J Surg Pathol* 1990; **14**: 383−90.

71. Frizzera G. The distinction of Hodgkin's disease from anaplastic large cell lymphoma. *Semin Diagn Pathol* 1992; **9**: 291−6.

72. Stein H. Ki-1-anaplastic large cell lymphoma: is it a discrete entity? *Leuk Lymphoma* 1993; **10**: 81−4.

73. Foss HD, Reusch R, Demael G *et al*. Frquent expression of the B-cell-specific activator protein in Reed−Sternberg cell of classical Hodgkin's disease provides further evidence for its B-cell origin. *Blood* 1999; **94**: 3108−13.

74. Benharroch D, Megueerian-Bedoyan Z, Lamant L *et al*. ALK-positive lymphoma: a single disease with a broad spectrum of morphology. *Blood* 1998; **91**: 2076−84.

75. Smith CA, Farrah T, Goodwin RG. The TNF receptor superfamily of cellular and viral proteins: activation, co-stimulation, and death. *Cell* 1994; **76**: 759−62.

76. Hittmair A, Rogatsch H, Mikuz A, Feichtinger H. CD30 expression in seminoma. *Hum Pathol* 1992; **27**: 1166−71.

77. Chiarle R, Podda A, Prolla G, Gong J, Thorbecke GJ, Inghirami G. CD30 in normal and neoplastic Cells. *Clin Immunol* 1999; **90**: 157−64.

78. Haralambieva E, Pulford K, Lamant L *et al*. Anaplastic large cell lymphomas of B-cell phenotype are anaplastic lymphoma kinase (ALK) negative and belong to the spectrum of diffuse large B-cell lymphomas. *Br J Haematol* 2000; **109**: 584–91.

79. Drexler HG, Gignac SM, von Wasielewski R, Werner M, Dirks WG. Pathobiology of *NPM-ALK* and variant fusion genes in anaplastic large cell lymphoma and other lymphomas. *Leukemia* 2000; **14**: 1533–59.

80. Paulli M, Berti E, Rosso R *et al*. CD30/Ki-1-positive lymphoproliferative disorders of the skin-clinicopathologic correlation and statistical analysis of 86 cases: a multicentric study from the European Organization for Research and Treatment of Cancer Cutaneous Lymphoma Project Group. *J Clin Oncol* 1995; **13**: 1343–54.

81. Kinney MC, Collins RD, Greer JP, Whitlock JA, Sioutos N, Kadin ME. Small-cell-predominant variant of primary Ki-1 (CD30)+ T-cell lymphoma. *A J Pathol* 1993; **17**: 859–68.

82. Stein H, Mason DY, Gerdes J *et al*. The expression of the Hodgkin disease associated antigen Ki-1 in reactive and neoplastic lymphoid tissue: evidence that Reed–Sternberg cells and histiocytic malignancies are derived from activated lymphoid cells. *Blood* 1985; **66**: 848–58.

83. Pileri S, Falini B, Delsol G *et al*. Lymphohistiocytic T-cell lymphoma (anaplastic large cell lymphoma CD30+/Ki-1+ with a high content of reactive histiocytes). *Histopathology* 1990; **16**: 383–91.

84. McCluggage WG, Walsh MY, Bhuracha H. Anaplastic large cell malignant lymphoma with extensive eosinophilic or neutrophilic infiltration. *Histopathology* 1998; **32**: 110–15.

85. Jaffe ES. Anaplastic large cell lymphoma: the shifting sands of diagnostic hematopathology. *Mod Pathol* 2001; **14**: 219–28.

86. Agnarsson BA, Kadin ME. Ki-1 positive large cell lymphoma: a morphologic and immunologic study of 19 cases. *A J Surg Pathol* 1988; **12**: 264–74.

87. Ten Berghe RL, Oudejans JJ, Pulford K, Willemze R, Mason DY, Meijer CJL. NPM-ALK expression as a diagnostic marker in cutaneous CD30-positive T-cell lymphoproliferative disorders. *J Invest Dermatol* 1998; **110**: 578.

88. Falini B, Bigerna B, Fizzotti M *et al*. ALK expression defines a distinct group of T/null lymphomas ("ALK lymphomas") with a wide morphological spectrum. *Am J Pathol* 1998; **153**: 875–86.

89. Felgar RE, Salhany KE, Macon WR, Pietra GG, Kinney MC. The expression of TIA-1+ cytolytic-type granules and other cytolytic lymphocyte-associated markers in CD30+ anaplastic large cell lymphomas (ALCL): correlation with morphology, immunophenotype, ultrastructure, and clinical features. *Hum Pathol* 1999; **30**: 228–36.

90. Krenacs L, Wellmann A, Sorbara L *et al*. Cytotoxic cell antigen expression in anaplastic large cell lymphomas of T- and null-cell type and Hodgkin's disease: evidence for distinct cellular origin. *Blood* 1997; **89**: 980–9.

91. Morris SW, Kirstein MN, Valentine MB *et al*. Fusion of a kinase gene, *ALK*, to a nucleolar protein gene, *NPM*, in non-Hodgkin's lymphoma. *Science* 1994; **263**: 1281–4.

92. Borer RA, Lehner CF, Eppenberger HM, Nigg EA. Major nucleolar proteins shuttle between nucleus and cytoplasma. *Cell* 1989; **56**: 379–90.

93. Morris SW, Naeve C, Mathew P *et al*. *ALK*, The chromosome 2 gene locus altered by the t(2;5) in non-Hodgkin's lymphoma, encodes a novel neural receptor tyrosine kinase that is highly related to leukocyte tyrosine kinase (LTK). *Oncogene* 1997; **14**: 2175–88.

94. Iwahar T, Fujimoto J, Wen DZ *et al*. Molecular characterisation of ALK, a receptor tyrosine kinase expressed specifically in the nervous system. *Oncogene* 1997; **14**: 439–49.

95. Kadin ME, Morris SW. The t(2;5) in human lymphomas. *Leuk Lymphoma* 1998; **29**: 249–56.

96. Bischof D, Pulford K, Mason DY, Morris SW. Role of the nucleophosmin (NPM) portion of the non-Hodgkin's lymphoma-associated NPM-anaplastic lymphoma kinase fusion protein in oncogenesis. *Mol Cell Biol* 1997; **17**: 2312–25.

97. Mason DY, Pulford KAF, Bischof D *et al*. Nucleolar localization of the nucleophosmin anaplastic lymphoma kinase is not required for malignant transformation. *Cancer Res* 1998; **58**: 1057–62.

98. Duyster J, Bai R, Morris SW. Translocations involving anaplastic lymphoma kinase (ALK). *Oncogene* 2001; **20**: 5623–37.

99. Stein H, Gerdes J, Schwab U *et al*. Identification of Hodgkin and Sternberg—Reed cells as a unique cell type derived from a newly-detected small-cell population. *Int J Cancer* 1982; **30**: 445.

100. Lukes R, Butler J, Hicks E. Natural history of Hodgkin's disease as related to its pathological picture. *Cancer* 1966; **19**: 317—44.

101. Lukes R, Butler J. The pathology and nomenclature of Hodgkin's disease. *Cancer Res* 1966; **26**: 1063—83.

102. Staudt LM. The molecular and cellular origins of Hodgkin's disease. *J Exp Med* 2000; **191**: 207—12.

103. Jacob J, Kelsoe G, Rajewsky K, Weiss U. Intraclonal generation of antibody mutants in germinal centers. *Nature* 1991; **354**: 389—92.

104. Kanzler H, Küppers R, Hansmann ML, Rajewsky L. Hodgkin and Reed—Sternberg cells in Hodgkin's disease represent the outgrowth of a dominant tumor clone derived from (crippled) germinal centre B cells. *J Exp Med* 1986; **184**: 389—92.

105. Bräuninger A, Hansmann ML, Strickler JG *et al*. Identification of common germinal-center B-cell precursors in two patients with both Hodgkin's disease and non-Hodgkin's lymphoma. *New Engl J Med* 1999; **340**: 1239—47.

106. Emmerich F, Meiser M, Hummel M *et al*. Overexpression of I kappa B alpha without inhibition of NF-kappa B activity and mutations in the I kappa B alpha gene in Reed—Sternberg cells. *Blood* 1999; **94**: 3129—34.

107. Marafiotic T, Hummel M, Anagnostopoulos I, Foss HD, Huhn D, Stein H. Classical Hodgkin's disease and follicular lymphoma originating from the same germinal center B cell. *J Clin Oncol* 1999; **17**: 3804—9.

108. Lukes RJ, Craver LF, Hall TC, Rappaport H, Rubin P. Report of the nomenclature committee. *Cancer Res* 1966; **26**: 1063—83.

109. MacLennan K, Bennett M, Tu A *et al*. Relationship of histopathologic features to survival and relapse in nodular sclerosing Hodgkin's disease. *Cancer* 1989; **64**: 1686—93.

110. Wijlhulzen T, Vrints L, Jairam R *et al*. Grades of nodular sclerosis (NSI-NSII) in Hodgkin's disease: are they of independent prognostic value? *Cancer* 1989; **63**: 1150—3.

111. Ferry J, Linggood R, Convery K, Efird J, Elisoeo R, Harris N. Hodgkin's disease, nodular sclerosis type: implications of histologic subclassification. *Cancer* 1993; **71**: 457—63.

112. Georgii A, Hasenclever D, Fischer R *et al*. Histopathological grading of nodular sclerosing Hodgkin's reveals significant differences in survival and relapse rather under protocol-therapy. Proceedings of the Third International Workshop on Hodgkin's Lymphoma. Kolne, Germany, 1995.

113. Colby T, Hoppe R, Warnke R. Hodgkin's disease: a clinico-pathologic study of 659 cases. *Cancer* 1981; **49**: 1848—58.

114. Ferreriro JA. Ber-H2 expression in testicular germ cell tumors. *Hum Pathol* 1994; **25**: 522—4.

115. Gruss HJ, Boiani N, Williams DE, Armitage RJ, Smith CA, Goodwin RG. Pleiotropic effects of the CD30 ligand on CD30-expressing cells and lymphoma cell lines. *Blood* 1994; **83**: 2045—56.

116. Harris NL. Hodgkin's disease: classification and differential diagnosis. *Mod Pathol* 1999; **12**: 159—76.

117. Weiss L, Chen Y, Liu X, Shibata D. Epstein—Barr virus and Hodgkin's disease: a correlative *in situ* hybridization and polymerase chain reaction study. *Am J Pathol* 1991; **139**: 1259—65.

118. Schlegelberger B, Weber-Matthiesen K, Himmler A *et al*. Cytogenetic findings and results of combined immunophenotyping and karyotyping in Hodgkin's disease. *Leukemia* 1994; **8**: 72—80.

119. Joos S, Kupper M, Ohl S *et al*. Genomic imbalances including amplification of the tyrosine kinase gene JAK2 in CD30+ Hodgkin cells. *Cancer Res* 2000; **60**: 549—52.

120. Kamel O, Chang P, Hsu F, Dolezal M, Warnke R, van der Rijn M. Clonal VDJ recombination of the immunoglobulin heavy chain gene by PCR in classical Hodgkin's disease. *Am J Clin Pathol* 1995; **104**: 419—23.

121. Tamaru J, Hummel M, Zemlin M, Kalvelage B, Stein H. Hodgkin's disease with a B-cell phenotype often shows a *VDJ* rearrangemnt and somatic mutations in the *VH* genes. *Blood* 1994; **84**: 708—15.

122. Seitz V, Hummel M, Marafioti T, Agnostopoulos I, Assaf C, Stein H. Detection of clonal T-cell receptor gamma-chain gene rearrangements in Reed—Sternberg cells of classic Hodgkin disease. *Blood* 2000; **95**: 3020—4.

123. Hansmann ML, Stein H, Fellbaum C, Hui PK, Parwaresch MR, Lennert K. Nodular paragranuloma can transform into high-grade malignant lymphoma of B type. *Human Pathol* 1989; **20**: 1169—75.

124. Miettinen M, Franssila KO, Saxén E. Hodgkin disease, lymphocytic predominance nodular. Increased risk for subsequent non-Hodgkin's lymphomas. *Cancer* 1983; **51**: 2293—300.

125. Orlandi E, Lazzarino M, Brusamolino E, Astori C, Bernasconi C. Nodular lymphocyte-predominance Hodgkin's disease (NLPHD): clinical behavior and pattern of progression in 66 patients. Proceedings of the Third International Workshop on Hodgkin's Lymphoma. Kolne, Germany, 1995.

126. Ferry JA, Zukerberg LR, Harris NL. Florid progressive transformation of germinal centers. A syndrome affecting young men, without early progression to nodular lymphocyte predominance Hodgkin's disease. *Am J Surg Pathol* 1992; **16**: 252—8.

127. Osborne BM, Butler JJ, Gresik MV. Progressive transformation of germinal centers: comparison of 23 pediatric patients to the adult population. *Mod Pathol* 1992; **5**: 135—40.

128. Falini B, Dalla Favara R, Pileri S, *et al.* bcl06 gene rearrangement and expression in Hodgkin's disease. Proceedings of the Third International Workshop on Hodgkin's Lymphoma. Kolne, Germany, 1995.

129. Poppema S. The nature of the lymphocytes surrounding Reed—Sternberg cells in nodular lymphocyte-predominance and in other types of Hodgkin's disease. *Am J Pathol* 1989; **135**: 351—7.

130. Kamel O, Gelb A, Shibuha, Warnke RA. Leu-7 (CD57) reactivity distinguishes nodular lymphocyte-predominance Hodgkin's disease from nodular sclerosing Hodgkin's disease, T-cell-rich B-cell lymphoma, and follicular lymphoma. *Am J Pathol* 1993; **142**: 541—6.

131. Delabie J, Tierens A, Wu G, Weisenburger D, Chan W. Lymphocyte-predominance Hodgkin's disease: lineage and clonality determination using a single cell assay. *Blood* 1994; **84**: 3291—8.

132. Marafioti T, Hummel I, Anagnostopoulos HD *et al.* Origin of nodular lymphocyte-predominant Hodgkin's disease from a clonal expansion of highly mutated germinal-centre B cells. *N Engl J Med* 1997; **337**: 453—8.

3

Assessment of the brain in the hospital consented autopsy

William Stewart and Susan F. D. Robinson

EXAMINATION OF THE BRAIN AT AUTOPSY – AN APPROACH

This chapter considers the pathological changes that may be found in brains examined in non-forensic autopsies, where the pathology falls within the general heading of 'natural causes'. Following recent organ-retention issues hospital consented autopsy practice has undergone marked change, resulting in a decline in the proportion of hospital deaths that come to autopsy. A recent audit in this hospital showed a fall in the autopsy rate for in-hospital deaths from 7.8% in 1997 to 3.2% in 2001, with a parallel reduction in the number of brains being retained for formal neuropathology examination within the region. In the 'Guidelines on Autopsy Practice' (2002) published by The Royal College of Pathologists it is advised that,

'All major organs (heart, lungs, brain, liver and kidneys) should be dissected in order to facilitate examination of the blood and drainage in addition to relations with adjacent structures. These organs should be separated and weighed. If permitted and clinically relevant, fixation of the intact brain, followed by a detailed examination by a neuropathologist, produces a higher detection rate of abnormalities.' [1]

Furthermore, it is suggested that occasions where the contents of the cranial cavity are not examined 'should be exceptional'. This advice is intended to support a full and thorough approach to autopsy practice at the same time as facilitating training in autopsy techniques. The established protocols whereby a brain is fixed for a number of weeks prior to a formal brain cut have had to be re-evaluated, with many more partially fixed or unfixed brains being examined such that the organ can be returned for disposal with the body. Thus, although in some instances detailed neuropathological advice may be required, a practical knowledge of the more common pathologies that may be encountered in the brain at autopsy will enable a confident approach to dissection and

Progress in Pathology Volume 7, ed. Nigel Kirkham and Neil Shepherd. Published by Cambridge University Press. © Cambridge University Press 2007.

sampling for further investigations. Information regarding specific autopsy procedures for a number of neurological conditions can be found in the British Neuropathological Society's publication 'Guidelines For Good Practice in Neuropathology' [2].

EXAMINATION OF THE FRESH BRAIN

Ideally the pathologist should take an active part in opening the skull and removing the brain. This permits an assessment of the relationship of the organ to the confines of the dura that is of particular value where brain swelling is suspected. If sterile swabs or samples of CSF are required this is best achieved prior to removal of the brain (see below). Once removed, it is advisable to weigh and dissect the brain as soon as possible, as the unfixed brain will rapidly deform.

There are several approaches to dissecting the brain with the operator advised to use the technique that they find most reproducible. Slices of unfixed brain should, ideally, be kept to a thickness of no less than 15 mm. This not only reduces the likelihood of dissection and handling artefacts which may complicate histological assessment, but also allows for adequate fixation of tissue blocks which develop an uneven, undulating surface as they fix (a consequence of differences in the densities of grey and white matter). As a general rule when selecting blocks for histology it is advisable to sample widely, preferably by taking large tissue blocks that can be trimmed to size after a period of fixation. Our local practice is that whole or half coronal slices of the cerebral hemispheres are sampled and fixed for a suitable period, following which a series of blocks are taken for histology. Using this approach, regions of interest can be sampled by careful selection of appropriate coronal slices. It is often advisable to record where individual blocks are sampled from, for future interpretation of histological features and clinicopathological correlation. With these general comments in mind the following account details the more common pathologies that may be encountered when undertaking a hospital consented autopsy.

ISCHAEMIA/INFARCTION

THE PATHOLOGY OF ISCHAEMIA

At rest, the brain consumes oxygen at a rate of approximately 50 ml/min (20% of whole body O_2 consumption) equating to a cerebral blood flow of some 750 ml/min. Within the limits of cerebral autoregulation, cerebral blood flow is maintained at a level such that oxygen delivery is not compromised. However, should intracranial pressure rise or mean arterial blood pressure fall, then the autoregulatory capacity of the cerebral circulation can be exceeded, leading to a failure in adequate oxygen delivery. This may be exacerbated by alterations in arterial blood gas levels (hypercapnia, hypoxaemia) and pre-existing cerebral damage (head injury, stroke). The consequence is the onset of the ischaemic cell process with a decreasing vulnerability from neurons through glia to microglia and blood vessels. Thus, relatively brief interruptions in blood flow will be reflected in selective neuronal necrosis, whilst cessation of flow results in infarction.

THE ISCHAEMIC NEURON

Neurons have no capacity for anaerobic respiration, hence their susceptibility to hypoxia. Once established, the ischaemic process progresses to recognisable changes that can be detected in routine histological stains within two hours or so of the precipitating event. Typically, the ischaemic neuron is described in H&E sections as having a shrunken, triangular cell body and nucleus with a bright, eosinophilic cytoplasm [3] (Fig. 3.1(a),(b)). Whilst this description is accurate, these appearances are not exclusive to ischaemia and may arise as an artefact of handling and fixation, the so-called 'dark-cell change' [4]. This must be borne in mind when diagnosing cerebral ischaemia based solely on the presence of contracted, eosinophilic neurons. In such circumstances the distribution of affected neurons should be carefully documented and correlated with the

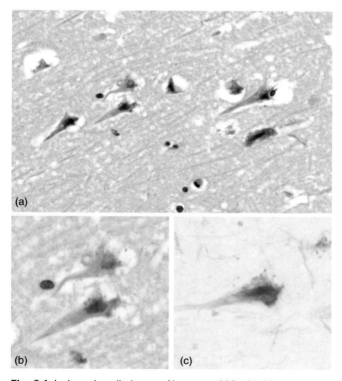

(a)

(b)   (c)

Fig. 3.1 Ischaemic cell change. Neurons within the hippocampal sector CA1 showing features of ischaemic cell change manifest in H&E sections (a, b) as contracted, eosinophilic neurons with dark nuclei. Numerous incrustations, representing swollen astrocytic foot processes, are identified around the margin of the cells in both H&E and Luxol fast blue/Cresyl violet (c).

clinical history and time course of events. Using this approach, it is possible, in most instances, to differentiate between the patterns of neuronal involvement recognised in ischaemia and post-mortem artefact. In this regard, artefact does not show evidence of a selective laminar distribution (see below), instead favouring more superficially placed neurons.

Incontrovertible evidence of irreversible ischaemia by light microscopy is presented by the detection of incrustations [5]. These are small, rounded profiles on or immediately adjacent to the somatic membrane of ischaemic neurons, which stain lightly basophilic in H&E. Although they are often better resolved in Luxol fast blue/Cresyl violet stained sections as pale purple/blue granules surrounding the soma (Fig. 3.1). They arise as a consequence of swollen astrocytic processes indenting the neuronal cell membrane. A final histological feature of the ischaemic neuron is manifest by homogenising cell change, whereby the cytoplasm becomes progressively paler and homogeneous as the nucleus becomes shrunken and fragmented. A reactive glial cell response may be present, although this can be mild if there is little neuronal necrosis.

CEREBRAL INFARCTION

Cessation or prolonged reduction of blood flow in a cerebral blood vessel culminates in cerebral infarction (stroke) manifest by necrosis of neurons, blood vessels and glia. Typically the pattern is of involvement of an entire vascular territory or, if collateral branches from adjacent vessels are present, the central region of a vascular territory. When stroke is suspected from the clinical history, close inspection of the cardiovascular system is warranted, with the majority of strokes arising as thrombo-embolic infarcts. In particular, the cardiac valves, carotid vessels, vertebral arteries and cerebral vessels should be dissected and examined for a source of embolus and/or thrombi (Fig. 3.2). Embolic infarcts are more commonly encountered in the middle cerebral artery circulation and, on naked eye inspection, often show evidence of haemorrhagic transformation (Fig. 3.3). Indeed, autopsy studies suggest the majority of haemorrhagic infarctions may be embolic in origin [6] with haemorrhagic transformation thought to follow reperfusion of the occluded vessel [7], [8].

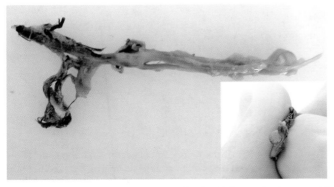

Fig. 3.2 Embolus occluding the proximal middle cerebral artery. Marantic vegetations on the mitral valve were identified at autopsy.

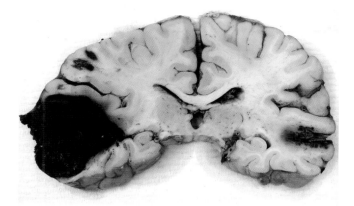

Fig. 3.3 Haemorrhagic transformation of embolic infarction. The presentation was with focal signs related to the lobar haematoma within the left temporal lobe. Further haemorrhagic lesions, including those seen here in the left parietal and right temporal lobe, were present, with the typical appearance and distribution of embolic infarcts which have undergone haemorrhagic transformation. The deceased had a prosthetic aortic valve.

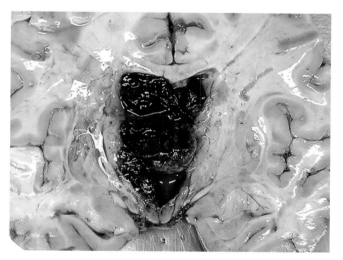

Fig. 3.4 Fresh, deeply placed haemorrhage around the deep grey nuclei and extending into the adjacent ventricles. In this case there was a history of binge drinking.

HAEMORRHAGE

Primary intracranial haemorrhage, i.e. haemorrhage in the absence of trauma, most commonly describes either intracerebral or subarachnoid haemorrhage. In turn, intracerebral haemorrhages can be subdivided into those occurring within a lobe, lobar haematomas, and those which occur more deeply (around or within the deep grey nuclei) (Fig. 3.4). This distinction is of value as, whilst hypertension remains the most common cause of non-traumatic intracerebral haemorrhage, it is much more commonly associated with deeper-placed haemorrhages (up to 80%) than lobar haematomas [9]. In keeping with this, deep haemorrhages tend to occur in a younger age group and are more common in men. An association with binge drinking [10], [11] is also documented, which is thought to be a consequence of acute hypertension [12]. As such, where a lobar haematoma is identified, other pathologies should be considered and excluded before assuming a hypertensive aetiology, such as cerebral amyloid angiopathy, vascular malformations, tumours or clotting abnormalities.

The annual incidence of non-traumatic subarachnoid haemorrhage in the UK is of the order of 10 per 100 000 population with a slight female predominance [13], [14]. The great majority of such haemorrhages are associated with rupture of a saccular aneurysm, 85–90% of which in adults are found within the anterior circulation (terminal internal carotid and vessels of anterior circle of Willis), with few located in the posterior circulation (vertebrobasilar and posterior circle of Willis). Typically, saccular aneurysms are located at arterial bifurcations, with the most common sites being at the termination of the internal carotid (40%), at the junction of anterior cerebral and anterior communicating arteries (30%), or at the bifurcation of the middle cerebral artery within the Sylvian fissure (20%) [15]. As such, associated haemorrhages are found within the basal cisterns, between the frontal lobes or within the Sylvian fissure. Occasionally, there may be haemorrhage into an adjacent lobe, producing a lobar haematoma. Thus, where a lobar haematoma arises adjacent to the Sylvian fissure or within the medial aspect of a frontal lobe, a saccular aneurysm should be considered.

CARDIO-RESPIRATORY ARREST

A consequence of the impairment of blood flow during cardiac arrest is transient global ischaemia. Examination of the brain following cardiac arrest may show little evidence of macroscopic abnormality if survival is for less than 24 hours. Despite this, careful histological examination may show evidence of widespread neuronal necrosis in vulnerable areas. If survival is for greater than 24 hours, evidence of damage within the hippocampus and neocortical ribbon (particularly within the depths of sulci) may be detected on naked eye examination.

Whilst under some circumstances neuronal necrosis may affect all layers of the neocortical ribbon, stagnant hypoxia is typically associated with selective, laminar, neuronal necrosis restricted to the mid and deeper layers of the cortex (layers III, V and VI), is more evident within the depths of sulci than the crests of gyri, and may be more marked within the occipital poles than the frontal or temporal. In the hippocampi, sectors CA1 and CA4 appear most vulnerable to ischaemic damage following cardiac arrest. Necrosis in the deep grey nuclei, cerebellum and brain stem can also occur; the last corresponding clinically to coma with absence of brainstem reflexes.

PROFOUND HYPOTENSION

In circumstances where there is profound, transient hypotension, ischaemic damage is concentrated around the arterial boundary zones. This situation may arise in a number of clinical situations, for example as a complication of anaesthesia or during haemodialysis. As with cardiac arrest if survival time is short there may be no naked eye evidence of damage. With longer survival times, macroscopic evidence of ischaemic damage is detected at the arterial boundary zones as wedge-shaped, frequently haemorrhagic, infarcts. These are often most evident in the parieto-occipital cortex, where the territories of the three cerebral arteries converge. Basal ganglia involvement may be encountered, although, in contrast to cardiac arrest, the hippocampi are generally spared. Typically, these appearances are bilateral though asymmetrical, reflecting the minor variations in calibre/distribution of the vessels comprising the circle of Willis.

'VENTILATOR BRAIN'

A number of terms have been applied to the pathology that arises as a result of a complete cessation of cerebral blood flow, reflecting either the common, although not exclusive, history of the patient having been on a ventilator prior to death (ventilator brain, respirator brain) or the underlying pathological process (permanent global ischaemia, non-perfused brain). As noted above, cerebral blood flow reflects cerebral perfusion pressure (CPP), representing the difference between mean arterial blood pressure (MABP) and intracranial pressure (ICP); adequate flow being maintained over a range of MABP through cerebral autoregulation. However, should CPP fall below approximately 50 mmHg (7 kPa), cerebral perfusion can fail. This may occur where there is a profound drop in MABP, such as in hypotension or cardiac arrest; however, in both these situations there is typically restoration of flow, which influences the pattern of ischaemic damage. Alternatively, ICP may rise, leading to failure of cerebral perfusion. Typically, this occurs where there is brain swelling, for example following trauma or with the oedema associated with cerebral infarction. In such circumstances, the brain at autopsy is soft with a dusky discolouration of the grey matter and an indistinct grey/white boundary [16]. Histologically there is autolysis with pallor of background staining and eosinophilic neurons; features which must be distinguished from those of ischaemia.

ALCOHOL

Acute alcohol intoxication in isolation results in no specific neuropathological changes. This is not to diminish the role of acute alcohol intoxication in intracranial pathology, in particular head injury, subarachnoid haemorrhage and cerebral infarction [10], [11]. In contrast, there are a number of neuropathological correlates of chronic alcohol consumption and the associated nutritional disorders.

CEREBRAL AND CEREBELLAR ATROPHY

Both imaging and post-mortem studies have documented cerebral atrophy with compensatory ventriculomegally in chronic alcoholics. Clinically, this manifests as a somewhat poorly defined cognitive impairment termed 'alcoholic dementia' [17], [18]. In contrast, the cerebellar atrophy of chronic alcohol consumption is characterised by a well-defined clinical syndrome of truncal ataxia and gait disturbance. As might be expected with these symptoms, the atrophy is primarily of the midline cerebellum, in particular the folia of the anterior superior vermis [19]. In one autopsy series the incidence of cerebellar atrophy ranged from 26.8% in chronic alcoholics to 38.6% in alcoholics with Wernike—Korsakoff syndrome [20].

WERNICKE'S ENCEPHALOPATHY

Thiamine (vitamin B_1) is a water-soluble vitamin with limited body stores that may be depleted in a number of weeks. In western countries this most often arises in chronic alcoholism, although it may be encountered in other situations where gastrointestinal absorption is disturbed. The clinical features are extraocular muscle palsies, nystagmus, ataxia, confusion and, when severe, coma. In the acute presentation there is vascular congestion with associated petechial haemorrhage involving swollen mamillary bodies and periventricular tissues (around the third and fourth ventricle and the cerebral aqueduct) [21]. Histologically, the picture is of haemorrhagic necrosis marked by oedema with extravasation of red blood cells from affected vessels which may form 'ball' microhaemorrhages. Some 24—48 hours after the acute lesion, hyperplasia of endothelial cells with capillary budding develops (subacute phase), which, over time, becomes less marked; chronic lesions are identified by gliosis and loss of myelin. In this phase a Perl's stain for haemosiderin assists in highlighting evidence of previous haemorrhage. Macroscopically the mamillary bodies of the chronic phase appear shrunken and tan/grey in colour.

CENTRAL PONTINE MYELINOLYSIS

Although central pontine myelinolysis (CPM) is included here amongst conditions associated with alcohol abuse, it may occur in many other situations such as severe liver disease, malnutrition, anorexia and human immunodeficiency virus infection [22], [23]. Whatever the associated condition, a factor common to each is altered electrolyte disturbance, most commonly hyponatraemia. More specifically, CPM appears to follow too rapid a correction of prolonged hyponatraemia. Clinically, the features are those of a rapid onset, widespread neurological impairment with flaccid paralysis. An awareness of the condition, combined with the availability of appropriate imaging has markedly improved outcome [24]. At autopsy, CPM manifests as a grey/brown, pale, granular area within the centre of the basis pontis that stops short of the pial or ventricular surfaces. Microscopy reveals a sharply demarcated region of demyelination with relative preservation of axonal profiles and the neurons of the pontine nuclei (Fig. 3.5). This latter feature is essential in differentiating the lesion from an infarct at this site. In a proportion of cases extrapontine myelinolysis may be present.

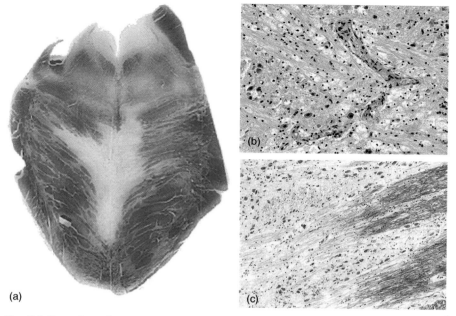

Fig. 3.5 Central pontine myelinolysis. A centrally placed region of demyelination with preservation of neurons and a moderate macrophage response is present within the pons (a, c, Luxol fast blue/Cresyl violet; b, H&E).

HEPATIC ENCEPHALOPATHY

Severe acute hepatic failure is invariably associated with a rapidly progressing encephalopathy with coma. In such cases, examination of the brain may reveal no abnormality or may show evidence of brain swelling with raised intracranial pressure and histological evidence of Alzheimer's type II astrocytes. These are most readily identified within the inner cortical layers and in the basal ganglia, and typically show enlarged, pale, often lobulated nuclei. Alzheimer's type II astrocytes are also present in chronic hepatic encaphalopathy, although they are not pathognomonic of hepatic impairment and may be found in a number of other conditions. A consequence of repeated episodes of hepatic decompensation is acquired hepatocerebral degeneration, manifest macroscopically by discolouration of the deeper cortical layers and lentiform nuclei. Histologically, the features are similar to those of hepatolenticular degeneration (Wilson's disease).

HYPOGLYCAEMIA

Profound hypoglycaemia (blood glucose levels <1.5 mM) may still occur in a number of clinical settings. As noted for ischaemic brain damage, the picture is of a selective neuronal necrosis; however, when pure and uncomplicated the pattern of involvement in hypoglycaemia differs from that in ischaemia [25]. In hypoglycaemia there is neuronal necrosis affecting the superficial cortical

Table 3.1 Common organisms associated with meningitis

Aseptic meningitis	Non-polio enteroviruses, herpes simplex virus 2, mumps, human immunodeficiency virus
Purulent meningitis	
neonates	group B Streptococci, *Escherichia coli*, *Klebsiella* spp., *Listeria monocytogenes*
adults	*Haemophilus influenzae*, *Streptococcus pneumoniae*, *Neisseria meningitidis*
Granulomatous	*Mycobacterium tuberculosis*
Immune compromised	above + fungal (*Cryptococcus neoformans*, *Candida* spp., *Aspergillus*)

layers and CA1 and the dentate fascia of the hippocampus. Furthermore, in contrast to global ischaemia, there is a distinct absence of cerebellar or brain stem involvement [26]. It should be stressed that whilst the foregoing description holds true where there is pure, isolated hypoglycaemia, in reality the situation is often complicated by coexistent global ischaemic damage consequent on hypoglycaemia associated seizures.

CNS INFECTIONS

When dealing with suspected infective conditions of the CNS, it is important to consider a number of clinical features that will influence the types of organisms involved (Table 3.1). Thus, in approaching such examinations a full clinical history should be sought, paying particular attention to information regarding the symptoms at presentation, intercurrent illnesses, immune status, prior medical history, results of all investigations and management of the acute presentation (in particular antimicrobial therapy).

AN APPROACH TO THE AUTOPSY IN SUSPECTED CNS INFECTION

Appropriate precautions regarding health and safety in the mortuary should be taken to minimise the risk of possible transmission. Many of the most common organisms encountered (including those most often implicated in meningitis or encephalitis) have a low transmission risk, and so such autopsies may be performed using standard procedures for category 1 and 2 agents within a typical hospital mortuary (ACDP report 2004) [27]. In contrast, whilst autopsies involving category 3 agents, including mycobacterium tuberculosis, human immunodeficiency virus and those associated with transmissible CJD, may be undertaken within a standard hospital mortuary, they do require additional precautions [2]. Where CJD is suspected, the case should be referred to a local neuropathologist.

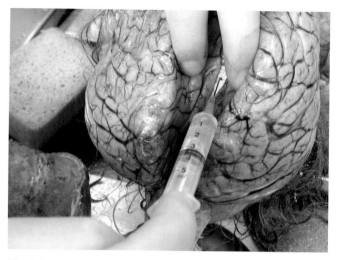

Fig. 3.6 Aspiration of CSF. On exposure of the vertex, the hemispheres can be gently parted and a sterile needle advanced through the corpus callosum into either lateral ventricle whilst applying slight negative pressure on the syringe.

SAMPLING FOR MICROBIOLOGY

There are several means of obtaining an uncontaminated CSF specimen for culture/microscopy [28]. Of these, the simplest method, with least opportunity for contamination, involves advancing a sterile needle through the corpus callosum towards either lateral ventricle whilst applying slight negative pressure to an attached syringe (Fig. 3.6). As the needle tip enters the ventricle, CSF will be aspirated. This technique is best applied immediately on reflecting the dura with the brain *in situ*. As an alternative, CSF can be aspirated under direct visualisation from the basal cisterns. In addition to CSF aspirates it is often of value to obtain swab samples from the subarachnoid space, particularly in relation to purulent exudates. Samples can be collected by passing a swab into the subarachnoid space whilst retracting the arachnoid with sterile forceps. Additional aspirates or swabs should, ideally, be obtained from any focal purulent collection. These samples are over and above those required for routine histological examination. Furthermore, where the suspicion is of a viral pathogen, tissue blocks, CSF and blood should be sampled for additional virological, ultrastructural and molecular studies.

BACTERIAL PATHOGENS

In the majority of cases CNS infections arise as a consequence of haematogenous spread, and a source of infection should be sought in the general body autopsy. In the remaining, small proportion of cases, infection may arise as a complication of a surgical procedure (including lumbar puncture) or as a consequence of local spread, such as from an infected air sinus. If death follows early in the course of the illness, the brain may be diffusely swollen with congested meningeal vessels. There is often a purulent exudate within the subarachnoid space, especially within the basal cisterns and between sulci. This exudate may have a greenish hue and be more concentrated over the parasaggital sulci in cases of pneumococcal meningitis [29]. If death follows after a longer time course, then secondary complications may be evident, such as thrombophlebitis with haemorrhagic cortical infarction and hydrocephalus (Fig. 3.7(a)). Histology shows the typical polymorphonuclear-rich inflammatory infiltrate in the sub-arachnoid space (Fig. (3.7(b)). Despite this, a search for organisms is often fruit-less because of ante mortem antimicrobial therapy. In contrast, one should be cautious of interpreting the presence of organisms within the CNS in the absence of an inflammatory cell response and/or evidence of systematised infection. An example is 'Swiss-cheese' artefact which develops post-mortem as a consequence of gas-forming, putrefactive organisms (Fig. 3.8).

In the immunosuppressed, the incidence of the more common organisms increases. Thus, following splenectomy or where humoral immunity is impaired, the risk of pneumococcal meningitis increases. In addition, organisms become increasingly identified which, in the absence of impaired humoral immunity, are rarely encountered such as *Pseudomonas aeruginosa* or *Listeria monocytogenes*. Where the impairment is in cell-mediated immunity, such as is encountered in AIDS, organ transplantation, chemotherapy or haematolymphoid malignancy, there is an increased incidence of mycobacterial meningitis. Typically this takes the form of a granulomatous meningitis; although the cellular response may be minimal in situations of severe immunological compromise.

VIRAL PATHOGENS

The most common acute necrotising encephalitis is Herpes simplex type 1 (HSV-1) infection. Typically, the history is one of fever, confusion, headache and frontotemporal localising signs. This latter feature reflects the preferential

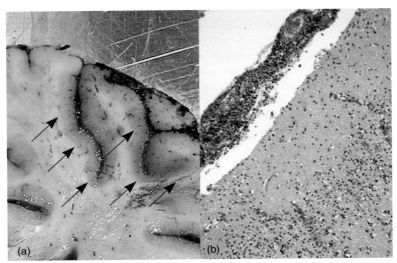

Fig. 3.7 Purulent meningitis. (a) Coronal section of a cerebral hemisphere in a case of proven streptococcal meningitis in which, at autopsy, there was evidence of meningeal thrombophlebitis and superficial cortical infarction (arrows). (b) Microscopy shows a florid meningeal inflammatory cell infiltrate (H&E).

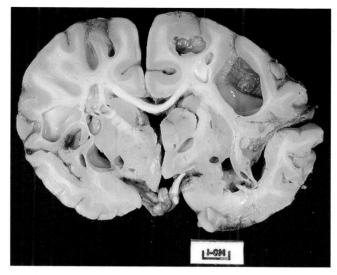

Fig. 3.8 Swiss cheese artefact. Multiple well-demarcated cysts of variable size are present throughout the specimen as a consequence of gas forming organisms. A distinctive odour is often present.

involvement of the frontal and temporal lobes that can be detected as an asymmetrical imaging abnormality on CT scanning. Examination of the brain at autopsy reveals bilateral, asymmetrical, haemorrhagic necrosis of the temporal lobes, insulae and cingulate gyrus. The corresponding histological picture is of a necrotising encephalitis, with a meningeal and parenchymal, often perivascular, macrophage-rich inflammatory cell infiltrate. This appearance should prompt a careful search within cells surrounding the necrotising focus for eosinophilic, nuclear and/or cytoplasmic viral inclusions (Fig. 3.9) [30]. Immunocytochemistry for HSV-1 can assist in the detection of viral antigen in suspected cases. If required, this can be supplemented by polymerase chain reaction for viral DNA or ultrastructural investigations for viral particles. Indeed, using PCR it is possible to detect viral DNA within paraffin-processed tissue blocks some time after the material is embedded [31].

Whilst this pattern of infection is typical in the immune competent, the picture can be modified in the immune compromised [32]. Under such circumstances there may be a less acute presentation, with involvement of sites outwith the frontal or temporal lobes. Here disease localised to the brainstem with little necrosis has been described. In addition to the increased risk of HSV-1-encephalitis, immune compromise also results in an increased susceptibility to infection with Varicella zoster virus [33] and Cytomegalovirus [34].

FUNGAL OR PROTOZOAL PATHOGENS

Rarely do fungal infections of the CNS arise in the immune competent. More often they occur in the context of impaired immunity. Indeed, the identification of such a pathogen within the CNS should lead to consideration of the immune status of the deceased as, not infrequently, fungal infection of the CNS may

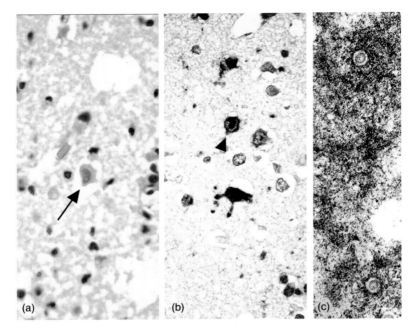

Fig. 3.9 Herpes simplex encephalitis. (a) The typical histology is of a necrotising encephalitis with scattered cells containing viral inclusions (arrow; H&E). (b) Immunocytochemistry highlights herpes simplex virus infected cells and viral inclusions (arrowhead). (c) On transmission electron microscopy, the viral particles are readily identified as targetoid profiles with a central icosahedral nucleocapsid and outer membrane.

represent the first manifestation of AIDS [35]. Of the organisms encountered in AIDS, *Cryptococcus neoformans* and *Toxoplasma gondii* are notable.

TUMOURS

Intracranial tumours are not uncommonly encountered at autopsy. No matter the origin, the range of clinical symptoms and signs is similar, with focal neurology, seizures and signs of raised intracranial pressure being typical. In addition, a small proportion of non-traumatic intracranial haemorrhages can be attributed to an underlying tumour. This is most commonly metastatic (the majority are pulmonary in origin) although haemorrhage in association with primary intracranial tumours is recognised (in particular with glioblastoma) [36], [37]. It is beyond the scope of this review to provide a detailed account of the various neoplastic lesions of the CNS, and for this the reader is directed to specialist neuropathology texts [38], [39]. Some general comment on specific lesions is, however, merited.

METASTATIC CARCINOMA

Whilst almost any tumour may metastasise to the brain, over half originate from the lung (35%) or, the breast (20%), with melanomas (10%), renal cell carcinomas (10%) and gastrointestinal carcinomas (5%) accounting for much of the remainder. In general, metastases appear as multiple lesions, are often located at the grey/white boundary, and have a predilection for the middle cerebral artery territory and watershed zones. Typically, metastases are well-demarcated lesions with surrounding oedema and a variable appearance on cut section (Fig. 3.10).

NON-METASTATIC EFFECTS OF CARCINOMA

In addition to metastatic spread to the brain, extracranial malignancy can give rise to neurological symptoms and signs as a consequence of associated systemic metabolic disturbance (such as hepatic failure, hypoglycaemia), increased susceptibility to infection through altered immunity (tumour or therapy related), and/or production of antibodies which recognise both tumour and neuronal antigens [40] (Table 3.2). This last group result in a number of paraneoplastic syndromes, giving rise to a variety of symptoms related to CNS or peripheral nerve involvement [41], [42]. These syndromes are rare, as evidenced by the incidence of disabling paraneoplastic cerebellar involvement, which is of the order 0.4% in association with pulmonary malignancies. Although mild, clinically detectable cerebellar dysfunction can be elicited in a higher proportion (up to 25%) [43]. Paraneoplastic syndromes are most commonly associated with pulmonary carcinomas, in particular small cell carcinoma; however, there are numerous series and single case reports documenting paraneoplastic syndromes in association with a wide variety of malignancies. With regard to their pathology a number of general comments are worth noting. First, the clinical syndrome may precede, follow or present concurrently with the primary malignancy. Second, even when established clinically, there may be few

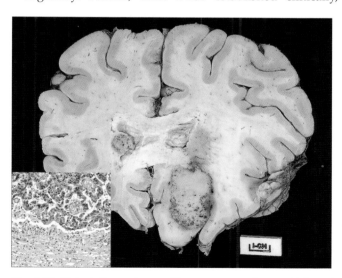

Fig. 3.10 Metastatic carcinoma. Metastases are often multiple and appear as well-demarcated lesions. The green hue is a consequence of bile pigment accumulation arising as a result of blood–brain barrier breakdown. Histology in this case shows metastatic adenocarcinoma (inset: H&E).

Table 3.2 Neurological complications of cancer

Metastatic
    mass effect
    focal deficit
    seizure
    haemorrhage

Non-metastatic
    therapy related
    infection
    metabolic/nutritional
    paraneoplastic

CNS[1]	cerebellar degeneration, limbic encephalitis, opsoclonus-myoclonus, retinopathy
PNS[2]	autonomic neuropathy, sensorimotor neuropathy
NMJ[3]	Lambert–Eaton myasthenic syndrome, myasthenia gravis

[1]*central nervous system;* [2]*peripheral nervous system;* [3]*neuromuscular junction*

histological abnormalities. Finally, the antibodies produced by any given neoplasm, and hence the associated syndromes, need not be consistent. Thus, small cell carcinoma of lung may give rise to paraneoplastic encephalomyelitis, opsoclonus-myoclonus or retinopathy, depending on which antibody is produced. Given this, it is advisable to sample widely in such cases.

NEUROEPITHELIAL TUMOURS

Neoplasms arising within the CNS are rare in adults, accounting for approximately 2% of all malignancies (up to 20% in children). Of these, the majority are neuroepithelial in origin, with glioblastoma (WHO grade IV) the most common encountered in adults. The symptomatology at presentation is largely a reflection of the site of origin of the tumour. Ultimately though, symptoms of raised intracranial pressure, such as headache, vomiting and altered conscious level supervene. Macroscopically, glioblastomas are typically solitary and show central necrosis associated with cyst formation, the margins of which are grey/brown and merge with surrounding, oedematous brain (Fig. 3.11). Histologically, the tumour is composed of highly pleomorphic, atypical astrocytes with features of malignancy evident (mitoses, endothelial hyperplasia, tumour necrosis). Immunocytochemistry for glial fibrillary acidic protein (GFAP) is, in the main, positive, and can be of use in differentiating such tumours from metastatic disease.

MENINGIOMA

The most recent WHO classification of tumours of the CNS identifies 15 subtypes based on their morphological appearance and biological behaviour [38]. They are not uncommonly encountered as an incidental finding at autopsy, and macroscopically have a broad dural base with a typically lobulated appearance on cut surface and a variable texture, from soft and fleshy to firm and gritty

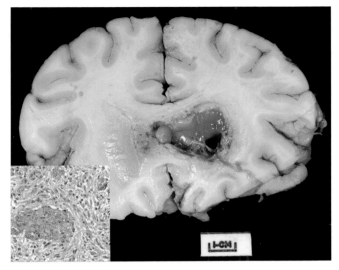

Fig. 3.11 Glioblastomas are typically solitary and show central necrosis associated with cyst formation, the margins of which are grey/brown and merge with surrounding, oedematous brain. Histologically the tumour is composed of highly pleomorphic, atypical astrocytes (inset: H&E). Mitotic figures and endothelial hyperplasia are present.

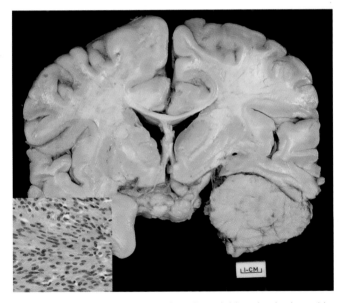

Fig. 3.12 Meningiomas often indent the neighbouring brain and have a lobulated appearance on cut surface. A variety of histological subtypes are described. In this case the tumour is composed of spindle-shaped cells with indistinct cell boundaries (inset: H&E).

(Fig. 3.12). Histologically, the 'typical' meningioma is composed of epithelioid to spindle-shaped cells with indistinct cell boundaries and scattered whorls composed of concentrically arranged clusters of cells. In the vast majority of meningiomas immunohistochemistry for EMA is positive [44].

Comment on suspected dementia is often included in clinical summaries accompanying consent forms for hospital consented autopsies of elderly patients. In many cases review of the case notes may suggest an acute confusional state rather than true cognitive impairment. Nevertheless, a thorough examination of the brain is merited to facilitate clinicopathological correlation and, where the clinical history is supportive, to fully characterise the neurodegenerative state. As has been stated, in a general, non-neuropathological autopsy there is limited opportunity to retain the whole organ for adequate fixation and dissection at a later stage. The great majority of brains are now cut fresh and sampled for histology at the time of the autopsy. A general strategy for such cases is required.

In addition to a full description of the external appearance, paying particular attention to the distribution of atrophy and state of the blood vessels, it is of value to record the weight of the detached hindbrain (cerebellum and brainstem). This can be a useful indicator of the degree of cortical atrophy, with the weight of the intact, whole brain typically 8–10 times that of the detached hindbrain. In sampling the brain for histology, a number of areas critical to the assessment of neurodegenerative conditions should be included. For practical purposes the areas of interest can be sampled by selecting half (or whole) coronal slices of the cerebral hemispheres through the frontal pole and midbrain, and sections of the brain stem from midbrain to medulla (Fig. 3.13) (see Lowe) [45]. Once fixed, these can be trimmed to appropriate sized blocks for processing and appropriate stains. Current neuropathology practice requires the use of a panel of immunohistochemical antibodies for correct diagnosis. Consideration of each of the entities included in the neurodegenerative diseases is beyond the scope of this chapter; however, comment on the pathology of the more common dementias is included.

ALZHEIMER'S DISEASE

Alzheimer's disease remains the most common of the neurodegenerative diseases (up to 70% cases). Clinically, the presentation is with memory impairment in the early stages followed by progressive symptoms of cortical dysfunction, such as speech and dressing difficulties, culminating in immobility in the late stages. Macroscopic examination reveals a reduced brain weight with a reduced whole brain/hindbrain ratio. Shrinkage of the gyri with associated widening of the sulci, particularly of the medial temporal lobe, is typical. On sectioning, compensatory ventriculomegally (hydrocephalus *ex-vacuo*) provides further evidence of atrophy; again with preferential involvement of the medial temporal lobe. Histology reveals widespread amyloid plaque deposition (Fig. 3.14(a),(b)), neuritic plaques, neurofibrillary tangles and neuronal loss with an accompanying astrocytosis. Amyloid deposited around meningeal blood vessels is also present in the majority of cases (congophillic angiopathy). As some of these features may develop with age in cognitively normal individuals, it is standard practice to make a semi-quantitative assessment of plaque

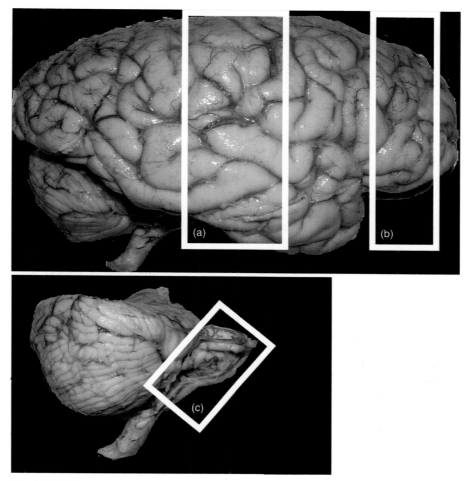

Fig. 3.13 Where dementia is suspected and it is not possible to retain the whole brain for fixation and dissection, the appropriate areas for formal assessment of the neuropathology can be sampled by selecting whole (or half) coronal slices from (a) just in front to just behind the midbrain, and (b) through the frontal pole. (c) In addition the brain stem from midbrain to upper medulla should be retained.

load and distribution, which can then be interpreted in light of the clinical information [46], [47].

DEMENTIA WITH LEWY BODIES

In hospital series between 15 and 20% of dementia is attributable to dementia with Lewy bodies, making it the second most common cause of dementia [48]. Both clinically and pathologically, the features may be similar to those of Alzheimer's disease; however, there are some key differences. Patients usually

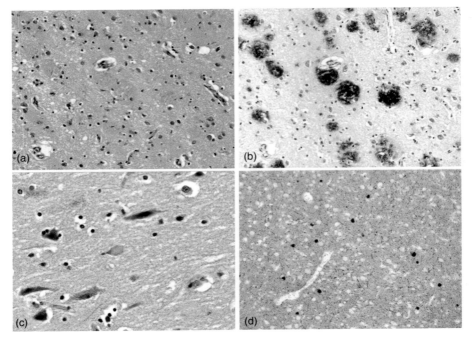

Fig. 3.14 (a)Amyloid plaques can be identified in H&E stained sections as amorphous, eosinophilic masses. (b) In an adjacent section, showing the same field, immunocytochemistry for β-amyloid highlights plaques. (c) Cortical Lewy bodies are occasionally recognisable in H&E as eosinophilic cytoplasmic inclusions. (d) Immunocytochemistry for α-synuclein reveals numerous cortical Lewy bodies in this lower power image.

present with symptoms of dementia; although in some the presentation may be with Parkinsonism or psychiatric disturbance alone [49]. A characteristic feature of dementia with Lewy bodies is a fluctuating cognitive performance and conscious level, with a particular sensitivity to neuroleptic medication [50]. Visual hallucinations are reported in up to two-thirds of patients, as are features of Parkinsonism [51]. The macroscopic appearances are similar to, if perhaps milder than, those in Alzheimer's disease. One important distinction is the presence of pallor of the substantia nigra and locus ceruleus in dementia with Lewy bodies. Histology reveals the presence of Lewy bodies in the substantia nigra (as in idiopathic Parkinson's) and in the neocortex (Fig. 3.14(c),(d)). In addition, features of Alzheimer's disease pathology, amyloid plaques and neurofibrillary tangles, may be evident.

VASCULAR DEMENTIA

A once common diagnosis, vascular dementia is now thought to be responsible for only some 8–10% of dementias in clinical practice [52]. However, a contribution from vascular disease to other forms of dementia, in particular Alzheimer's disease, is recognised [53]. Clinically, the picture is of stepwise deterioration in cognitive function and focal neurological signs. A number of pathologies may be encountered, reflecting whether the disease is mainly small or large vessel or whether there is global hypoperfusion with six possible mechanisms of dementia recognised [54]. On macroscopic examination, the brain is often of normal or slightly reduced weight with mild ventricular enlargement. Signs of ischaemic damage can be detected on coronal sections in the majority of cases, such as a pale grey and granular cerebral white matter and lacunar infarcts [55].

CONCLUSIONS

1. Wherever possible, examination of the brain should form part of a full autopsy examination.
2. In many cases it has become impractical to retain the entire organ for formal fixation and dissection. An awareness of the more common pathologies will permit a confident approach to dissection of the unfixed organ and selection of appropriate samples for further assessment.
3. An apparently normal brain on macroscopic examination may contain widespread histological abnormalities.
4. If there is any uncertainty about the approach to a specific case, a neuropathologist should be consulted.

REFERENCES

1. The Royal College of Pathologists. Guidelines on Autopsy Practice: Report of a Working Group of The Royal College of Pathologists, 2002, www.rcpath.org.
2. The British Neuropathological Society. Guidelines for Good Practice in Neuropathology, 2000, www.bns.org.uk.
3. Auer RN, Sutherland GR. Hypoxia and related conditions. In *Greenfield's Neuropathology* Graham DI, Lantos PL (Eds.) vol II. (Arnold, London, 2002), pp. 233–80.
4. Cammermeyer J. Is the solitary dark neuron a manifestation of post-mortem trauma to the brain inadequately fixed by perfusion? *Histochemistry* 1978; **56**: 97–115.
5. Hume Adams J, Graham DI. Cerebrovascular disease. In *Recent Advances in Histopathology* Anthony PP, MacSween RNM (Eds.) vol **14**. (Churchill Livingstone, London, 1989), pp. 205–22.
6. Lodder J, Krijne KB, Broekman J. Cerebral haemorrhagic infarction at autopsy: cardiac embolic cause and the relationship to the cause of death. *Stroke* 1986; **17**: 626–9.
7. Okada Y, Yamaguchi T, Minematsu K *et al.* Haemorrhagic transformation in cerebral embolism. *Stroke* 1989; **20**: 598–603.
8. Toni D, Fiorelli M, Bastianello S *et al.* Haemorrhagic transformation of brain infarct: predictability in the first 5 hours from stroke onset and influence on clinical outcome. *Neurology* 1996; **46**: 341–5.
9. Massaro AR, Sacco LR, Mohr JP *et al.* Clinical discriminators of lobar and deep haemorrhage: the Stroke Data Bank. *Neurology* 1991; **41**: 1881–5.
10. Gill JS, Shipley MJ, Tsemantzis SA. Alcohol consumption: a risk factor for hemorrhagic and non-hemorrhagic stroke. *Am J Med* 1991; **90**: 489–97.
11. Mazzaglia G, Britton AR, Altmann DR, Chenet L. Exploring the relationship between alcohol consumption and non-fatal or fatal stroke: a systematic review. *Addiction* 2001; **96**: 1743–56.
12. Delaney P, Estes M. Intracranial haemorrhage with amphetamine use. *Neurology* 1980; **30**: 1125–28.

13. Bamford J, Sandercock P, Dennis M. A prospective study of acute cerebrovascular disease in the community: the Oxfordshire Community Stroke Project — 1981—86. *J Neurol Neurosurg Psychiatry* 1990; **53**: 16—22.

14. Poberskin LH. Incidence and outcome of subarachnoid haemorrhage: a retrospective population based study. *J Neurol Neurosurg Psychiatry* 2001; **70**: 340—3.

15. Kalimo H, Kaste M, Haltia M. Vascular diseases. In *Greenfield's Neuropathology* Graham DI, Lantos PL (Eds.) vol **II**. (Arnold, London, 2002), pp. 281—355.

16. Oehmichen M. Brain death: neuropathological findings and forensic implications. *Forensic Sci Int* 1994; **69**: 205—19.

17. Victor M. Alcoholic dementia. *Can J Neurol Sci* 1994; **21**: 88—99.

18. Brun A, Anderson J. Frontal dysfunction and frontal cortical synapse loss in alcoholism — the main cause of alcoholic dementia? *Dement Geriatr Cogn* 2000; **12**: 289—294.

19. Phillips SC, Harper CG, Kril JA. A quantitative histological study of the cerebellar vermis in alcoholic patients. *Brain* 1987; **110**: 301—14.

20. Torvik A, Lindboe CF, Rodge S. Brain lesions in alcoholics. A neuropathological study with clinical correlations. *J Neurol Sci* 1982; **56**: 233—48.

21. Lindboe CF, Loberg EM. Wernicke's encephalopathy in non-alcoholics. An autopsy study. *J Neurol Sci* 1989; **90**: 125—9.

22. Lampl C, Yazdi K. Central pontine myelinolysis. *Eur Neurol* 2002; **47**: 3—10.

23. Miller RF, Harrison MJ, Hall-Craggs MA, Scaravelli F. Central pontine myelinolysis in AIDS. *Acta Neuropathol* 1998; **96**: 537—40.

24. Menger H, Jorg J. Outcome of central pontine and extrapontine myelinolysis ($n = 44$). *J Neurol* 1999; **246**: 700—5.

25. Kalimo H, Olsson Y. Effects of severe hypoglycaemia on the human brain. Neuropathological case reports. *Acta Neurol Scand* 1980; **62**: 345—56.

26. Auer RN, Hugh J, Cosgrove E, Curry B. Neuropathologic findings in three cases of profound hypoglycaemia. *Clin Neuropathol* 1989; **8**: 63—8.

27. Advisory Committee on Dangerous Pathogens. *The Approved List of Biological Agents.* (HMSO, London, 2004).

28. Love S. Autopsy approach to infections of the CNS. In Love S (Ed.) *Current Topics in Pathology. 95: Neuropathology.* (Springer, Berlin, 2001), pp. 1—50.

29. Gray F, Alonso, J-M. Bacterial infections of the central nervous system. In *Greenfield's Neuropathology* Graham DI, Lantos PL (Eds.) vol **II**. (Arnold, London, 2002), pp. 151—93.

30. Love S, Wiley CA. Viral diseases. In *Greenfield's Neuropathology* Graham DI, Lantos PL (Eds.) vol **II**. (Arnold, London, 2002), pp. 1—105.

31. Nicoll JA, Love S, Burton PA, Berry PJ. Autopsy findings in two cases of neonatal herpes simplex virus infection: detection of virus by immunohistochemistry, in situ hybridization and the polymerase chain reaction. *Histopathology* 1994; **24**: 257—64.

32. Chretien F, Belec L, Hilton DA *et al.* Herpes simplex virus type 1 encephalitis in acquired immunodeficiency syndrome. *Neuropathol Appl Neurobiol* 1996; **22**: 394—404.

33. Kleinschmidt-DeMasters BK, Amlie-Lefond C, Gilden DH. The patterns of varicella zoster virus encephalitis. *Human Pathol* 1996; **27**: 927—38.

34. Holland NR, Power C, Mathews VP, Glass JD, Forman M, McArthur JC. Cytomegalovirus encephalitis in acquired immunodeficiency syndrome (AIDS). *Neurology* 1994; **44**: 507—14.

35. Kovacs JA, Kovacs AA, Polis M *et al.* Cryptococcosis in the acquired immunodeficiency syndrome. *Ann Int Med* 1985; **103**: 533—8.

36. Yuguang L, Meng L, Shugan Z *et al.* Intracranial tumoral haemorrhage — a report of 58 cases. *J Clin Neurosci* 2002; **9**: 637—9.

37. Schrader B, Barth H, Lang EW *et al.* Spontaneous intracranial haematomas caused by neoplasms. *Acta Neurochirurgica* 2000; **142**: 979—85.

38. Kleihues P, Cavanee WK (Eds.). *Pathology and Genetics of Tumours of the Nervous System: World Health Organisation Classification of Tumours.* (IARC Press, Lyon, 2000).

39. Burger PC, Scheithauer BW, Vogel FS. *Surgical Pathology of the Nervous System and Its Coverings* 4th edn. (Churchill Livingstone, New York, 2002).

40. Darnell RB, Posner JB. Mechanisms of disease: paraneoplastic syndromes involving the nervous system. *New Engl J Med* 2003; **349**: 1543—54.

41. Giometto B, Scaravelli F. Paraneoplastic syndromes. *Brain Pathol* 1999; **9**: 247—50.

42. Scaravelli F, An SF, Groves M, Thom M. The neuropathology of paraneoplastic syndromes. *Brain Pathol* 1999; **9**: 251–60.
43. Wessel K, Diener HC, Dichgans J, Thron A. Cerebellar dysfunction in patients with bronchogenic carcinoma: clinical and posturographic findings. *J Neurol* 1988; **235**: 290–6.
44. Winek RR, Scheithauer BW, Wick MR. Meningioma, meningeal hemangiopericytoma (angioblastic meningioma), peripheral hemangiopericytoma, and acoustic schwannoma. A comparative immunohistochemical study. *Am J Surg Pathol* 1989; **13**: 251–61.
45. Lowe J. The pathological diagnosis of neurodegenerative diseases causing dementia. In Love S (Ed.) *Current Topics in Pathology. 95: Neuropathology.* (Springer, Berlin, 2001), pp. 149–77.
46. Mirra SS, Heyman A, McKeel D *et al.* The consortium to establish a registry for Alzheimer's disease (CERAD). Part II. Standardisation of the neuropathological assessment of Alzheimer's disease. *Neurology* 1991; **41**: 479–86.
47. Mirra SS, Hart MN, Terry ND. Making the diagnosis of Alzheimer's disease. *Arch Pathol Lab Med* 1993; **117**: 132–44.
48. Weiner MF. Dementia with Lewy bodies. *Arch Neurol* 1999; **56**: 1441–2.
49. Byrne EJ, Lennox G, Lowe J, Reynolds G. Diffuse Lewy body disease: the clinical features. *Adv Neurol* 1990; **53**: 283–6.
50. McKeith IG, Perry RH, Fairbairn AF, Jabeen, S, Perry EK. Operational criteria for senile dementia of Lewy body type (SDLT). *Psych Med* 1992; **22**: 911–22.
51. McKeith IG. Dementia with Lewy bodies. *Brit J Psych* 2002; **180**: 144–7.
52. Chui HC. Dementia. A review emphasizing clinicopathologic correlation and brain–behaviour relationships. *Arch Neurol* 1989; **46**: 806–14.
53. Korczyn AD. The complex nosological concept of vascular dementia. *J Neurol Sci* 2002; **203–204**: 3–6.
54. Roman GC, Tatemichi TK, Erkinjuntti T *et al.* Vascular dementia: diagnostic criteria for research studies. Report of the NINDS-AIREN International Workshop. *Neurology* 1993; **43**: 250–60.
55. Vinters HV, Ellis WG, Zarow C *et al.* Neuropathologic substrates of ischaemic dementia. *J Neuropathol Exp Neurol* 2000; **59**: 931–45.

4

The value of immunohistochemistry as a diagnostic aid in gynaecological pathology

W. Glenn McCluggage

INTRODUCTION

In recent years there has been a rapidly expanding literature investigating the value of immunohistochemistry as a diagnostic aid in gynaecological pathology [1]–[3]. The aim of this review is to provide a critical appraisal of the uses of immunohistochemistry in diagnostic gynaecological pathology that pathologists will find of practical value in their routine day-to-day practice. The value of immunohistochemical prognostic factors in various gynaecological malignancies is not covered since, although there is an extensive literature on this subject, little has found a role in routine pathological practice. Before detailing the uses of immunohistochemistry as a diagnostic aid in gynaecological pathology, several points are stressed: (a) most cases do not require immunohistochemistry, which should be reserved for those cases where there is genuine diagnostic confusion; (b) the results of immunohistochemistry should always be carefully interpreted in the context of the morphology; (c) no antibody is totally specific; and (d) in general, panels of antibodies should be used rather than relying on a single antibody. In this review I will detail what I consider to be useful applications of immunohistochemistry in gynaecological pathology site-by-site in the female genital tract.

OVARY AND PERITONEUM

ANTIBODIES OF VALUE IN DISTINGUISHING BETWEEN PRIMARY AND METASTATIC ADENOCARCINOMA

The histological distinction between a primary ovarian adenocarcinoma and a metastatic adenocarcinoma may be difficult. In some cases of metastatic

73

Progress in Pathology Volume 7, ed. Nigel Kirkham and Neil Shepherd. Published by Cambridge University Press. © Cambridge University Press 2007.

adenocarcinoma the presence of a primary neoplasm elsewhere is known, but in other instances an ovarian metastasis is the first manifestation of an adenocarcinoma. Usually, with ovarian serous adenocarcinoma there is little in the way of diagnostic difficulty, as this neoplasm generally has a characteristic histological appearance with papillary formations and psammoma bodies. However, problems may arise in distinguishing a primary ovarian mucinous, endometrioid or clear cell carcinoma from a metastasis. Similar comments pertain to peritoneal adenocarcinoma, with or without concurrent ovarian tumour.

The distinction between a primary ovarian endometrioid adenocarcinoma and a metastatic adenocarcinoma of colorectal or, rarely, small intestinal origin may be difficult. Although histological features have been described that facilitate this distinction there is much overlap [4]. Both metastatic colorectal adenocarcinoma and primary ovarian endometrioid adenocarcinoma may be bilateral. The presence of benign squamous elements or of associated endometriosis is highly suggestive of a primary ovarian endometrioid adenocarcinoma. In this distinction a panel of immunohistochemical stains, including CK7, CK20, CEA and CA125 is of value. Primary ovarian endometrioid adenocarcinomas are almost invariably CK7 (Fig. 4.1) and CA125 positive, and are usually negative with CK20 and CEA [5]–[15]. With metastatic colorectal adenocarcinoma the converse immunophenotype is usual, i.e. positivity with CK20 (Fig. 4.2) and CEA but negative staining with CK7 and CA125 [5]–[15]. Although occasional exceptions occur, this panel is of great value in distinguishing between a primary ovarian endometrioid adenocarcinoma and a metastatic colorectal adenocarcinoma.

The situation with ovarian mucinous tumours is much more problematic. It is not uncommon for metastatic mucinous tumours involving the ovary to contain very bland areas, which may closely mimic a primary benign or borderline ovarian mucinous neoplasm [16]–[18]. When dealing with a mucinous tumour of the ovary, a secondary should always be considered. Ovarian mucinous carcinomas are usually unilateral and stage I. With bilateral ovarian mucinous carcinomas or when there is extra-ovarian spread, a secondary should

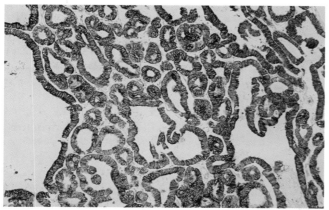

Fig. 4.1 Ovarian endometrioid adenocarcinoma exhibiting diffuse strong positivity with CK7.

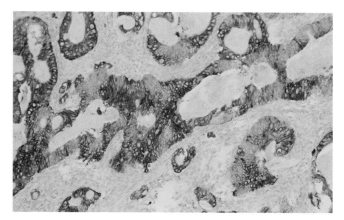

Fig. 4.2 Metastatic colorectal adenocarcinoma in ovary exhibiting diffuse strong positivity with CK20.

be strongly considered [18]. Metastatic mucinous tumours to the ovary may originate in the colorectum, appendix, pancreas, biliary tree, stomach or uterine cervix. The aforementioned panel of antibodies (CK7, CK20, CEA and CA125) may be of value but there is much overlap between primary and secondary ovarian mucinous neoplasms. In part, this overlap is because primary ovarian mucinous neoplasms, especially borderline and malignant, often exhibit intestinal differentiation, goblet cells being a common histological finding. Therefore, CK20 positivity is often found. Conversely, colorectal adenocarcinomas with abundant intracytoplasmic mucin may exhibit CK7 positivity, and this appears to be more common with poorly differentiated neoplasms [19], [20]. Generally, in primary ovarian mucinous tumours there is said to be diffuse CK7 positivity with patchy CK20 immunoreactivity [20]. The converse is true with metastatic colorectal adenocarcinomas exhibiting mucinous differentiation, i.e. diffuse CK20 and focal CK7 positivity. However, there is much immunohistochemical overlap and there should always be close correlation with the clinical and histopathological features. The true picture often manifests itself at a multidisciplinary gynaecological oncology meeting where the clinical, pathological, serological and radiological features can be integrated.

Differential cytokeratin expression is of limited value in the distinction between a primary ovarian mucinous tumour and a metastatic adenocarcinoma from sites such as pancreas, biliary tree, stomach and uterine cervix. Neoplasms arising in these sites are often CK7 positive and CK20 negative, although considerable numbers of pancreatic, biliary and gastric tumours may also exhibit CK20 positivity [10]. Cervical adenocarcinomas are usually CK7 positive and CK20 negative. Again a high index of suspicion of a metastasis is required, especially with bilateral ovarian neoplasms, even if they contain areas resembling benign and borderline tumour. As yet, there is no antibody available which definitively allows distinction between a primary ovarian adenocarcinoma and a metastatic adenocarcinoma from the pancreas or biliary tree. However, loss of Dpc4 expression may be a pointer towards a pancreatic adenocarcinoma, since this nuclear transcription factor is inactivated in many pancreatic carcinomas [20]. Conversely, primary ovarian mucinous tumours are almost invariably positive with this antibody. In addition, WT1 staining may be of value in distinguishing between an ovarian serous carcinoma, which usually exhibits nuclear positivity (see below) and a pancreaticobiliary neoplasm, which is usually negative [21].

Expression of the mucin genes MUC5AC and MUC2 may also be useful in the distinction between a primary ovarian adenocarcinoma and a metastatic colorectal adenocarcinoma [20], [22]. MUC5AC is usually expressed in ovarian mucinous tumours but is typically absent in colorectal carcinomas. However, many appendiceal and pancreatic neoplasms are also positive. In addition, there is often excessive background staining with these antibodies, and they are of limited value.

Occasionally, a clear cell carcinoma involving the ovary may be metastatic or the morphological features may raise the possibility of a secondary [23]. Primary ovarian clear cell carcinomas commonly arise in endometriosis, and endometriotic foci are often identified following extensive sampling. Furthermore, primary ovarian clear cell carcinomas often have a variegated histological appearance with a range of architectural patterns, and hobnail cells are commonly identified. Rarely, however, a metastatic renal cell carcinoma may be considered and imaging of the kidneys may be necessary. Metastatic colorectal carcinomas involving the ovary may also have a clear cell appearance [24]. In the latter case, CK7, CK20, CEA and CA125 are of value since metastatic colorectal adenocarcinoma with a clear cell appearance would be positive with CK20 and CEA but negative with CK7 and CA125 — the opposite immunophenotype of a primary ovarian clear cell carcinoma. Recently, a panel of antibodies has been devised which allows for confident distinction between an ovarian and a renal clear cell carcinoma [25]. While ovarian clear cell carcinomas are positive with CK7 and negative with CK20, renal clear cell carcinomas are usually negative with both. In addition, oestrogen receptor (ER), when positive, is a pointer towards a primary ovarian neoplasm. The renal cell carcinoma (RCC) marker and CD10, which are positive in most renal clear cell carcinomas, are almost always negative in primary ovarian neoplasms. Thus, a panel of antibodies including CK7, CK20, ER, RCC marker and CD10 is of value in distinguishing between a primary ovarian and renal clear cell carcinoma.

ORIGIN OF PSEUDOMYXOMA PERITONEI

Differential cytokeratin (CK7 and 20) staining has proven of value in helping to establish the site of origin of many cases of pseudomyxoma peritonei. This condition is characterised by the presence of abundant mucinous material throughout the abdominal and peritoneal cavity, generally containing low-grade dysplastic epithelium. In women, there may be unilateral or bilateral ovarian neoplasms, which often have the appearance of a mucinous borderline tumour. However, it is now apparent that most cases of pseudomyxoma peritonei are of large intestinal (usually appendiceal) origin [26], [27]. Although some of this evidence comes from molecular studies, differential cytokeratin staining has shown that in most cases the epithelium is positive with CK20 and negative with CK7; and when coexistant appendiceal and ovarian neoplasms are present, these generally exhibit an identical immunophenotype. With a clinical picture of pseudomyxoma peritonei, even with bilateral ovarian neoplasms, the surgeon should always remove the appendix. Even if normal on gross inspection, the appendix may contain a mucinous cystadenoma or a malignant mucinous neoplasm. In some cases identification of the appendix may be difficult, since it may be embedded within abundant mucinous material. Some cases of pseudomyxoma peritonei may also be of colorectal origin and a small number may truly be of ovarian origin. In cases with an ovarian origin, the ovarian mucinous tumour is usually strongly positive with CK20, and it has been speculated that these represent intestinal mucinous tumours arising in an ovarian teratoma [28]. Immunohistochemical expression of MUC2 and MUC5AC also supports an appendiceal origin of most cases of pseudomyxoma peritonei [29].

ANTIBODIES OF VALUE IN DISTINCTION BETWEEN SEROUS AND MESOTHELIAL PROLIFERATIONS

Benign, borderline and malignant serous proliferations may arise directly from the peritoneum, so-called primary peritoneal serous tumours of ovarian type. There may be a close morphological resemblance to reactive mesothelial proliferations or mesothelioma. In addition, primary ovarian mesothelioma or mesothelioma presenting as a primary ovarian neoplasm has been described [30]. CK7, CK20, CA125, CEA and WT1 are of no value in the distinction between serous and mesothelial lesions since, with regard to these antibodies, the immunophenotype is identical. In this distinction other antibodies may be of value [31]–[33]. Recent studies have found that the most useful of these are BerEP4 (positive in serous but negative in mesothelial lesions) and calretinin (positive in mesothelial but negative in serous lesions [32]). In one study it was stressed that, in order to be of discriminatory value, calretinin staining should be nuclear since cytoplasmic positivity is less specific [32].

ANTIBODIES OF VALUE IN DISTINCTION BETWEEN UTERINE AND OVARIAN SEROUS CARCINOMA

Uterine serous carcinoma (USC), also known as papillary serous carcinoma, is the prototype of type II endometrial cancer. USC is a highly aggressive, non-oestrogen-dependent neoplasm, usually arising in elderly women from an atrophic endometrium. It is often high stage at diagnosis, commonly with extrauterine spread and the overall prognosis is poor. Histologically USC is identical to ovarian serous carcinoma (OSC). A small USC, or its precursor lesion endometrial intraepithelial carcinoma (EIC), even when confined to the endometrium or an endometrial polyp, may disseminate widely to involve the ovaries, peritoneum and omentum without obvious myometrial infiltration. In addition, OSC commonly involves the uterus. Although in such cases the neoplasm is usually preferentially located in the outer aspect of the myometrium, tumour may also involve the endometrium, rarely even in the absence of myometrial infiltration. When a serous carcinoma involves more than one site,

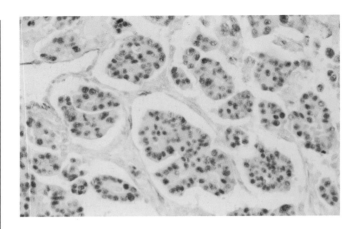

Fig. 4.3 OSC exhibiting strong nuclear positivity with WT1.

the origin of the tumour may not be apparent. Indeed, in some cases, it has been suggested that independent tumours arise within the ovary or peritoneum and within the uterus, a so-called 'field effect'. The distinction between a primary uterine and ovarian neoplasm is of significance, since adjuvant therapy, in the form of chemotherapy or radiotherapy, may differ depending on the primary site and on whether two independent tumours are present. In the distinction between USC and OSC, WT1 immunohistochemical staining may be of value [34], [35]. OSC usually exhibits diffuse nuclear positivity (Fig. 4.3) while USC is generally negative [34], [35]. One study showed 97% of OSC to be positive while all USC were negative [34]. Another study showed 94.7% of OSC to be positive [35]. However, a small number of USC were also positive, albeit usually with more focal staining (this has also been noted in abstracts presented at the United States and Canadian Academy of Pathology, Washington 2003). The results of such studies suggest that, when faced with a disseminated serous carcinoma, WT1 staining may be of value in distinguishing between an ovarian primary (usually WT1 positive) and a uterine primary (usually WT1 negative), although exceptions occur.

ANTIBODIES OF VALUE IN TYPING OF OVARIAN CARCINOMAS

There are several morphological subtypes of ovarian adenocarcinoma including serous, mucinous, endometrioid and clear cell. With well-differentiated tumours, typing is straightforward but with more poorly differentiated neoplasms this may be a problem. Although tumour behaviour is more dependent on the differentiation of the tumour than the morphological subtype, this may be of importance, since chemoresponsiveness may differ between different subtypes.

As already stated, OSC usually exhibits nuclear positivity with WT1, much more so than other morphological subtypes [36]. In cases of poorly differentiated carcinoma, widespread nuclear staining with WT1 may be a pointer towards a serous carcinoma. Clear cell carcinomas more commonly express p21 than other morphological subtypes [37].

ANTIBODIES OF VALUE IN DEMONSTRATING SEX CORD-STROMAL DIFFERENTIATION

With the exception of the fibrothecomatous group, ovarian sex cord-stromal tumours are relatively rare primary ovarian neoplasms. However, there are a wide variety of morphological subtypes, and differentiation from many other tumours may be difficult [38]. The differential diagnosis may be wide and endometrioid adenocarcinomas especially may bear a close morphological resemblance to sex cord-stromal neoplasms. In recent years several antibodies have become available that are of value in the diagnosis of ovarian sex cord-stromal tumours. The most useful of these are α-inhibin [39]–[52] and calretinin [53]–[56], but others which may be of value include CD99 [57]–[59], melan A [60], [61], mullerian inhibiting substance [62], [63], relaxin-like factor [64] and α glutathione S transferase [65]–[68]. Although the sensitivity of α-inhibin and calretinin with regards to ovarian sex cord-stromal tumours is similar (some studies have found calretinin to be slightly more sensitive [69]), α-inhibin is much more specific [69], [70]. The two antibodies may be useful in combination. Positive staining with α-inhibin is found in most morphological subtypes of ovarian sex cord-stromal neoplasm (Fig. 4.4) apart from fibromas and some poorly differentiated granulosa cell tumours, although many poorly differentiated neoplasms are positive [50]. It should be noted that β-inhibin is of no value, since positivity with this antibody is often found in ovarian adenocarcinomas and primary adenocarcinomas of other sites [71]. When using α-inhibin and other sex cord-stromal antibodies to differentiate between a sex cord-stromal tumour and a carcinoma, a panel of markers should be used. This should include epithelial membrane antigen (EMA). This is rarely positive in ovarian sex cord-stromal tumours [72] (I have noted staining in occasional sex cord-stromal neoplasms), although occasional Sertoli or Sertoli–Leydig cell neoplasms may be positive. There may be positivity with anti-cytokeratin antibodies present in sex cord-stromal neoplasms, including granulosa cell tumours, which often exhibit punctuate cytoplasmic staining [73]–[75].

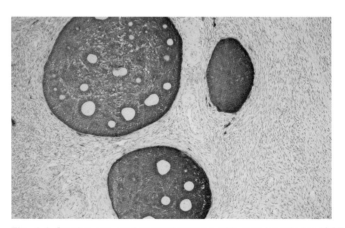

Fig. 4.4 Ovarian sex cord-stromal tumour with annular tubules (SCTAT) exhibiting strong positive staining with α-inhibin.

It should be noted that occasional ovarian carcinomas will be positive with α-inhibin, albeit usually focal and weak. In addition, activated ovarian stromal theca-like cells associated with many carcinomas and other neoplasms will be positive [76]. Therefore, close examination of the sections is necessary to ascertain which cells are positive. In some instances, especially with metastatic signet ring carcinomas, it may be difficult to ascertain which cells are positive, since there is often close intermingling of tumour cells and activated ovarian stromal cells. The presence of activated stromal cells may be the explanation for the modest increase in serum inhibin levels that can be found with some ovarian carcinomas, especially of mucinous type. It should be noted that ovarian granulosa cell tumours often result in a markedly elevated serum inhibin, and serial measurements may be useful in follow-up. An elevation in serum inhibin may indicate recurrent or metastatic tumour before this is clinically apparent.

OTHER USES OF α-INHIBIN STAINING IN GYNAECOLOGICAL PATHOLOGY

There are several other useful applications of α-inhibin staining in gynaecological pathology and this has been reviewed recently [77]. The value of α-inhibin as a marker of trophoblast will be discussed later.

Ovarian stromal hyperthecosis is a condition characterised by signs of hyperandrogenism and an elevated serum androgen. The ovaries may be grossly normal, although there is commonly associated stromal hyperplasia. α-inhibin staining may be of value in demonstrating collections of luteinised stromal cells within the ovarian cortex, which are responsible for androgen production.

Staining with α-inhibin may also be of value in fine needle aspirates of ovarian cystic lesions [78]. Usually with such specimens, the findings are non-specific, the aspirates being of low cellularity. However, occasionally these specimens are cellular and it may be difficult to distinguish granulosa from epithelial cells. The presence of granulosa cells indicates a follicular or functional cyst, which may be followed up, whereas the presence of epithelial cells is usually indicative of an epithelial lined cyst, which should probably be removed because of the risk of coexistent or subsequent malignancy. α-inhibin staining of cytological material may be useful in the confirmation of granulosa cells, and this can be used in combination with other antibodies such as EMA.

An ovarian (or more commonly paraovarian) neoplasm that may be positive with α-inhibin is the female adnexal tumour of Wolffian origin (FATWO) [45], [79]. Since this neoplasm may bear a close morphological resemblance to an ovarian sex cord-stromal tumour, there is the potential for confusion. These tumours may also stain with calretinin [79]. However, α-inhibin positivity is usually patchy and weak, in contrast to the diffuse strong immunoreactivity commonly seen in ovarian sex cord-stromal neoplasms. Immunohistochemical studies have provided evidence that FATWO is probably derived from mesonephric remnants, the pattern of staining with a wide range of antibodies being almost identical to that of benign mesonephric remnants around the ovary [45], [79], [80]. FATWO and benign mesonephric remnants generally coexpress cytokeratin and vimentin, are negative with EMA and, as already stated, are positive with α-inhibin and calretinin. CD10 may also be positive (see below).

A final tumour, which may be positive with α-inhibin and other sex cord-stromal markers, is the rare uterine tumour resembling ovarian sex cord tumour (UTROSCT) [81]–[84]. Positivity of UTROSCT with these antibodies indicates that they may exhibit true sex cord differentiation. Focal areas resembling an ovarian sex cord stromal tumour may also be seen in endometrial stromal neoplasms, and these may also be positive with sex cord stromal markers, again perhaps indicating true sex cord differentiation.

UTERUS

ANTIBODIES OF VALUE IN DISTINCTION BETWEEN TYPE I AND TYPE II ENDOMETRIAL CANCER

There are two broad categories of endometrial cancer, type I and type II. The prototype of type I endometrial cancer is endometrioid adenocarcinoma, mucinous adenocarcinoma being a less common variant. Endometrioid adeno-carcinoma usually arises in a background of atypical endometrial hyperplasia in the perimenopausal or early postmenopausal age group. The tumour is usually ER positive and well-differentiated, with presentation at an early stage. In contrast, the prototype of type II endometrial cancer is USC, a less common variant being clear cell carcinoma. USC is an aggressive neoplasm, usually arising in elderly postmenopausal women in an atrophic endometrium from a precursor known as EIC [85], [86]. It is usually ER negative and is associated with mutations in the p53 gene and consequently marked immunohistochemi-cal overexpression of p53 [87]. Usually, the morphological distinction between an endometrioid and a serous carcinoma is straightforward, although combined endometrioid and serous carcinomas occur. However, many endometrioid ade-nocarcinomas have a papillary growth pattern and a purely glandular variant of USC exists without papillary formation. In this variant there is discor-dance between the architectural pattern of well-formed glands and the nuclear features of marked pleomorphism. These are arguments for not using the term papillary serous carcinoma but rather USC. Type I cancers are usually strongly positive with ER and negative or only focally positive with p53. In contrast, type II carcinomas are usually ER negative (or weakly positive) and exhibit strong positive nuclear staining with p53 [85], [86], [88]. However, there are many exceptions. Some endometrioid carcinomas, especially grade III but occasionally grade I or II, exhibit strong positivity with p53 [89]. In addition, a proportion of USC are positive with ER, although staining is usually weak in contrast to the intense nuclear positivity seen in most low-grade endometrioid adenocarcinomas. In spite of this, ER and p53 staining may be of value, espe-cially in diagnosing the glandular variant of USC, which is usually ER negative and p53 positive (Fig. 4.5). Another scenario where ER and p53 immunostaining may be helpful is with a small fragmented biopsy where a few groups of atypical cells are present. Strong p53 and negative ER staining of these cells may assist in establishing a diagnosis of USC or EIC.

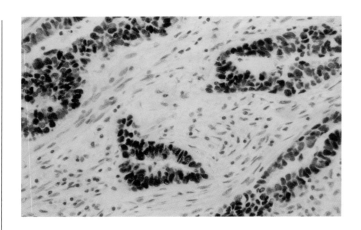

Fig. 4.5 Diffuse nuclear p53 staining in glandular variant of USC.

USC and EIC have a propensity to arise in otherwise benign endometrial polyps [88], [90], [91]. This may be a focal phenomenon, underlining the necessity for adequate sampling of large endometrial polyps in postmenopausal women. The differential diagnosis between USC and EIC arising in an endometrial polyp may include various epithelial metaplasias, such as clear cell and eosinophilic metaplasia, which may occur within polyps and which may be associated with a degree of nuclear atypia. Strong nuclear positivity with p53 and negative staining with ER would favour USC or EIC, since the metaplasias are usually ER positive. In epithelial metaplasias, p53 is usually negative or there may be focal weak heterogenous staining [92]. It has also been shown that β-catenin and E-cadherin immunostaining may assist in distinguishing between grade III endometrioid carcinoma and USC [93]. Nuclear expression of β-catenin is suggestive of an endometrioid carcinoma while E-cadherin positivity is suggestive of USC, although there may be immunohistochemical overlap

ANTIBODIES OF VALUE IN DISTINCTION BETWEEN ENDOMETRIAL AND ENDOCERVICAL ADENOCARCINOMA

In preoperative specimens when tumour is present in both endometrial and cervical biopsies, ascertaining the site of the primary may be problematic. The differential diagnosis lies between an endometrial adenocarcinoma spreading to the cervix or a cervical adenocarcinoma involving the uterus. Morphological features, such as stromal foam cells, benign squamous elements or adjacent atypical hyperplasia, favour an endometrial origin; adjacent high-grade cervical glandular intraepithelial neoplasia (HCGIN — adenocarcinoma-in-situ in WHO terminology) favours a cervical origin. In addition, the morphological features of the two tumours are subtly different. However, in some cases there is genuine diagnostic doubt. Primary surgical therapy may differ between an endometrial and an endocervical carcinoma, although in practice a modified radical hysterectomy is usually performed when it is known preoperatively that endometrial cancer has spread to the cervix. Even in the hysterectomy specimen there may be doubt as to the site of origin, and adjuvant therapies may differ between an endometrial and an endocervical adenocarcinoma. Recent studies have shown that a limited panel of antibodies, including ER, vimentin and monoclonal carcinoembryonic antigen (CEA) may assist in ascertaining the site of primary [94]–[96]. Endometrial adenocarcinoma of endometrioid type is usually diffusely positive with ER (Fig. 4.6) and vimentin (Fig. 4.7). CEA is usually negative, although there may be focal positivity and the benign squamous elements are often positive. Cervical carcinomas are usually, although not invariably, positive with CEA; vimentin is generally negative; and ER is usually negative or there is focal weak positivity. In problematic cases, in-situ hybridisation for human papilloma virus (HPV) may also be of value, since cervical adenocarcinomas are usually positive whereas endometrial adenocarcinomas are almost always negative [97]. In a recent study we have shown that p16 may also be of value in distinguishing between an endometrial and a

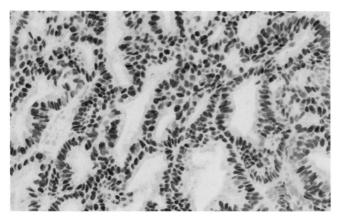

Fig. 4.6 Diffuse strong nuclear staining with ER in endometrial adenocarcinoma of endometrioid type.

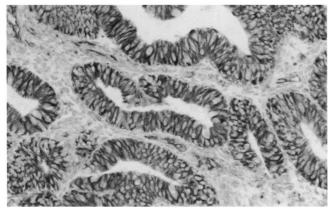

Fig. 4.7 Diffuse cytoplasmic staining with vimentin in endometrial adenocarcinoma of endometrioid type.

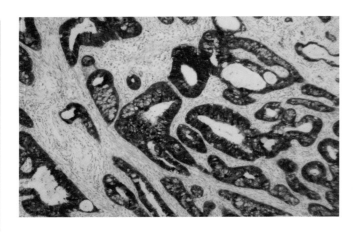

Fig. 4.8 Diffuse staining with p16 in endocervical adenocarcinoma.

cervical adenocarcinoma [98]. p16 (discussed later) is a tumour suppressor gene and diffuse strong expression of p16 is almost exclusively related to the presence of high-risk HPV subtypes. Since cervical adenocarcinomas are usually associated with high-risk HPV infection, these tumours would be expected to be positive with p16, whereas endometrial adenocarcinomas would be expected to be negative. In our study, almost all cervical adenocarcinomas exhibited intense diffuse positivity with p16 (Fig. 4.8), whereas, although endometrial adenocarcinomas were often positive, staining was usually focal [98]. Occasional endometrial adenocarcinomas exhibited diffuse positivity and the benign squamous element were often intensely positive. It is possible that those cases of endometrial carcinoma which exhibit diffuse p16 positivity are associated with high-risk HPV; and the positivity of benign squamous elements supports the hypothesis that in endometrial carcinomas, HPV, when present, is restricted to these foci [99]. It is concluded that p16 may be of value in distinguishing between a cervical and an endometrial adenocarcinoma when used as part of a panel.

Most of the aforementioned studies, investigating the immunohistochemical distinction between an endometrial and a cervical adenocarcinoma, have largely focused on endometrioid adenocarcinomas of the endometrium and usual endocervical adenocarcinomas. The question arises as to the immunophenotype of a mucinous carcinoma of the endometrium and a cervical endometrioid adenocarcinoma. I consider cervical endometrioid adenocarcinomas to be exceptionally rare, although such a diagnosis is commonly made in some institutions. This may simply reflect the tendency to categorise cervical adenocarcinomas with minimal intracytoplasmic mucin as endometrioid in type. One group addressed the question of immunophenotype in relation to site and differentiation and found that ER staining was more dependent on the site of origin, being more common in endometrial than cervical tumours. Vimentin positivity, however, was more dependent on differentiation, being more commonly positive in endometrioid than mucinous neoplasms [96]. This group also found that if a tumour was strongly ER and vimentin positive, then it was almost certainly of endometrial origin.

ANTIBODIES OF VALUE IN THE DIAGNOSIS OF UTERINE MESENCHYMAL LESIONS

With a cytologically bland cellular mesenchymal lesion composed of ovoid to spindle-shaped cells, the differential diagnosis may lie between an endometrial stromal lesion and a highly cellular leiomyomatous tumour. One of the most reliable morphological features in this distinction is the character of the blood vessels. Leiomyomatous tumours generally contain thick-walled blood vessels, whereas in endometrial stromal lesions the vessels are usually small arterioles. Myxoid and fibrous variants of endometrial stromal neoplasm, which are not unduly cellular, have also been described and may be confused with a leiomyomatous tumour [100]. A highly cellular leiomyoma may be misdiagnosed as an endometrial stromal nodule or, if the lesion has an irregular edge, as a low-grade endometrial stromal sarcoma (ESS) [101]. Traditionally, smooth muscle markers, such as desmin and α smooth muscle actin, have been used to confirm smooth muscle differentiation and exclude an endometrial stromal lesion. However, it is clear that many endometrial stromal lesions may exhibit positivity with desmin and a smooth muscle actin [102]–[104], although if there is diffuse intense desmin positivity this is in favour of a smooth muscle neoplasm. In recent years two antibodies have become available, which have been used to distinguish between smooth muscle and stromal differentiation – CD10 (a marker of endometrial stroma) and h-caldesmon (a marker of smooth muscle) [105]–[110]. These may be used in combination with desmin and α smooth muscle actin. The CD10 antibody is widely used in lymphoma panels, follicular and lymphoblastic lymphomas being positive. Staining of normal endometrial stroma and of endometrial stromal sarcomas was initially found in a study investigating CD10 immunoreactivity in a wide range of normal and neoplastic tissues [111], and additional studies have confirmed the value of CD10 as a marker of endometrial stroma. Endometrial stromal nodules and low grade ESS usually exhibit diffuse intense positivity (Fig. 4.9). However, many smooth muscle neoplasms may also be positive, albeit often focally so, and some cellular leiomyomatous tumours exhibit quite intense staining. It is stressed that immunohistochemistry should always be interpreted in the context of

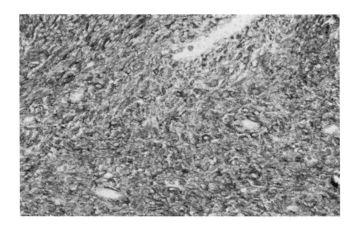

Fig. 4.9 Positive staining of low-grade ESS with CD10.

careful morphological assessment. h-caldesmon may be useful in confirming smooth muscle differentiation, although in some studies positivity has been found in a proportion of endometrial stromal neoplasms. A panel of antibodies should always be used, accepting that there may be immunophenotypic overlap.

Endometrial stroma and myometrial smooth muscle share a common progenitor cell of origin [112] and therefore it is not surprising that mixed endometrial stromal–smooth muscle neoplasms exist [113]. It is possible that positivity with CD10 in a smooth muscle neoplasm and with various muscle markers in an endometrial stromal lesion is merely a reflection of this common cell of origin.

Recent studies have also investigated the value of CD10 in demonstrating endometrial stroma at ectopic sites and in confirming a diagnosis of endometriosis [114]. While CD10 positivity of mesenchymal tissue may indicate the presence of endometriotic stroma, there are diagnostic drawbacks (discussed later).

Uterine PEComas

Recently a group of uterine mesenchymal lesions has been described characterised by epithelioid cells with abundant clear or eosinophilic cytoplasm [115]. The tumour cells are often positive with HMB45 and may be positive or negative with desmin. It is considered that these neoplasms are derived from perivascular epithelioid cells, and that they should be classified as perivascular epithelioid cell tumours (PEComas). Furthermore, it has been suggested that PEComas and epithelioid smooth muscle neoplasms are part of a histological spectrum [115]. The situation is further complicated in that undoubted epithelioid smooth muscle tumours of the uterus may exhibit HMB45 positivity [116] and normal myometrium may also be positive [117]. Further experience with uterine PEComas is necessary to ascertain whether they represent a distinct entity, or merely an unusual variant of epithelioid smooth muscle neoplasm exhibiting HMB45 positivity. Some of these tumours have occurred in patients with tuberous sclerosis. This condition is characterised by tumours such as angiomyolipoma, lymphangioleiomyomatosis, clear cell sugar tumour of the lung and various other clear cell tumours, which often exhibit dual HMB45 and desmin positivity.

CERVIX

VALUE OF PROLIFERATION MARKERS AND p16 IN THE EVALUATION OF CERVICAL SQUAMOUS LESIONS

Several studies have revealed considerable inter-and intra-observer variation in the classification of preinvasive cervical squamous lesions [118], [119]. In recent years many studies have investigated the value of proliferation markers, especially MIB1 which reacts against the Ki67 antigen, in cervical biopsies in an attempt to improve consistency [120]–[131]. Although some studies have suggested that MIB1 may be of value in the separation of koilocytosis from CIN I, in the distinction between adjacent lesions in the CIN spectrum, and in the separation of conditions, such as immature squamous metaplasia from low grade CIN, I feel this is unrealistic. The main value of proliferation markers in cervical squamous lesions is in the separation of CIN III from mimics, such as atrophic squamous epithelium, transitional metaplasia and immature squamous metaplasia. In the normal cervix nuclear MIB1 immunoreactivity is confined to the parabasal cells, whereas in CIN III there is positive nuclear staining throughout the full epithelial thickness. Atrophic squamous epithelium generally exhibits little or no proliferative activity [130], and in immature squamous metaplasia the MIB1 index is low if there is no associated CIN. MIB1 may also be of value in interpreting squamous epithelium affected by diathermy artefact at loop margins [132]. In this situation non-dysplastic squamous epithelium may mimic CIN III due to marked cautery artefact, and proliferation markers may assist.

The cyclin-dependent kinase-4 inhibitor (CDK4-I), also known as p16, is the product of the INK4A gene and specifically binds to cyclin D-cdk4/6 complexes to control the cell cycle at the G1-S interphase. Expression of p16 is regulated by retinoblastoma (Rb) expression status, which is in turn regulated by the presence of HPV E7 oncoprotein. Diffuse strong expression of p16 is found in the presence of high risk HPV [133], [134]. It has been shown that p16 is markedly overexpressed in CIN II and CIN III (due to the presence of high risk HPV) and in a proportion of CIN I lesions [133]–[136]. Preliminary studies suggest that CIN I lesions which overexpress p16 are associated with high risk HPV [136]. Clearly, if this is true, p16 may be of value as a predictor of likelihood of progression of CIN I and further studies are needed. It has also been shown that the addition of p16 immunohistochemistry improves inter- and intra-observer agreement in the interpretation of preinvasive cervical squamous lesions and may assist in identifying small CIN lesions [136].

MARKERS OF VALUE IN THE DISTINCTION OF CERVICAL GLANDULAR INTRAEPITHELIAL NEOPLASIA (CGIN) FROM BENIGN MIMICS

CGIN is the commonly used designation in the United Kingdom for the spectrum of preinvasive neoplastic cervical glandular lesions. CGIN is divided into low-grade and high-grade, which roughly correlate with glandular dysplasia and adenocarcinoma in situ (AIS) in WHO terminology. Low-grade CGIN is a poorly reproducible diagnosis, and I rarely diagnose this in the absence of high grade CGIN. The histological distinction between high grade CGIN (or even adenocarcinoma) and benign mimics, including tuboendometrial metaplasia (TEM), endometriosis and microglandular hyperplasia (MGH), may be difficult. A combination of antibodies including MIB1, p16 and bcl-2 may be of value [137]. Generally, in benign lesions only scattered nuclei are positive with MIB1, the proliferation index usually being less than 10% [138]–[141]. However, occasional benign cases will exhibit a higher proliferation index of up to 30%, and, rarely, in excess of this [140]. With high-grade

CGIN many nuclei are usually positive with MIB1, often in excess of 50%. However, occasional cases of high-grade CGIN will exhibit a low proliferation index. Although there is some overlap, MIB1 staining may be of value, in that benign lesions usually exhibit only scattered positive nuclei, whereas with high-grade CGIN many nuclei are generally positive. The proliferation index of low-grade CGIN has not been well investigated, and it is to be expected that there would be overlap in the MIB1 labelling indices between low-grade CGIN and benign mimics.

Bcl-2 may be of value in the distinction between TEM and endometriosis on the one hand, and high-grade CGIN on the other [137], [142], [143]. TEM and endometriosis generally exhibit diffuse cytoplasmic staining with bcl-2, whereas there is little or no staining of high-grade CGIN. The explanation for strong bcl-2 expression in TEM and endometriosis is not clear. However, normal proliferative endometrium and fallopian tube epithelium (which morphologically resemble endometriosis and TEM, respectively) are strongly positive with bcl-2 [144], [145]. MGH is usually negative with bcl-2.

p16 may be of value in the distinction between high-grade CGIN and benign mimics [137]. High-grade CGIN (and cervical adenocarcinoma) usually exhibits diffuse intense positivity with p16 [135], [137], [146], [147]. MGH is usually negative. Many cases of TEM and endometriosis are also immunoreactive with p16, but positivity is usually focal and patchy, in contrast to the diffuse staining seen in high-grade CGIN [137].

Vimentin may also be of value in the distinction between TEM and endometriosis and high-grade CGIN. TEM and endometriosis are positive with vimentin, in contrast to high-grade CGIN, which is usually negative [148].

Monoclonal CEA may also assist in distinguishing between neoplastic endocervical glandular lesions and benign mimics [149], [150]. Diffuse cytoplasmic staining is usual in neoplastic but not benign lesions. However, staining may be focal in cervical minimal deviation adenocarcinoma (MDA). In addition, normal endocervical glands may exhibit luminal and membranous CEA positivity, and in my experience focal cytoplasmic staining may also be seen. MGH may exhibit cytoplasmic positivity, usually restricted to areas of immature squamous metaplasia or reserve cell hyperplasia. In one study a combination of CEA, MIB1 and p53 was found to be useful in distinguishing benign from malignant endocervical glandular lesions [141].

THE VALUE OF CD10 IN CERVICAL GLANDULAR LESIONS

Recently, it has been shown that luminal CD10 positivity is usual in benign cervical mesonephric remnants, in cervical and uterine mesonephric adenocarcinomas and in other mesonephric lesions in the female genital tract, including FATWO [151], [152]. CD10 was generally negative in Mullerian-derived epithelia within the cervix and elsewhere. Another recent study has confirmed luminal CD10 positivity in most, but not all, benign cervical mesonephric remnants and mesonephric adenocarcinomas [153]. In the context of a benign cervical glandular proliferation, luminal CD10 positivity is supportive of a mesonephric lesion (Fig. 4.10). However, this study found several usual endocervical adenocarcinomas to be positive with CD10 as well as most uterine endometrioid

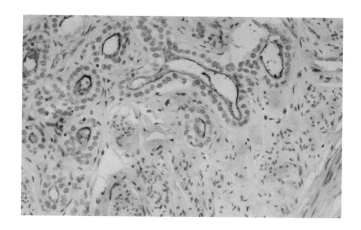

Fig. 4.10 Luminal CD10 positivity in cervical mesonephric remnants.

adenocarcinomas [153] and it was concluded that CD10 positivity in an adenocarcinoma is not evidence of a mesonephric origin.

In the aforementioned study we also found consistent positivity of cervical stroma, especially around glands, with CD10. As previously discussed, CD10 is a marker of endometrial stroma and has been used to confirm a diagnosis of endometriosis [114]. Clearly this is not reliable, since cervical stroma is also positive. Other studies have addressed whether CD10 is of value in distinguishing true myoinvasive endometrial adenocarcinoma from adenocarcinoma involving adenomyosis [154]. It would be expected that CD10 positivity around glands would be confined to areas with pre-existing adenomyosis. However, it has been shown that myoinvasive endometrial adenocarcinomas are often also surrounded by a rim of CD10 positive stromal cells and thus CD10 is of no value in this regard.

ANTIBODIES OF VALUE IN CERVICAL MDA

Cervical MDA is an extremely well-differentiated adenocarcinoma, which may be confused with a variety of benign endocervical glandular lesions. Although an endometrioid variant exists, the most common subtype is mucinous, this being referred to as adenoma malignum. Recent studies, mainly from Japanese groups, have shown that gastric mucins are present in cervical adenoma malignum and that HIK1083, a monoclonal antibody against gastric gland mucous cell mucin, is useful in making this diagnosis [155]–[157]. Normal endocervical glands are negative, although focal areas of positivity may be found in usual endocervical adenocarcinomas. The less-well-differentiated areas of adenoma malignum are usually negative. Thus, it is considered that HIK1083 can discriminate between normal endocervical glands and the well-differentiated glands of adenoma malignum. Further studies are necessary to confirm this, and to investigate whether HIK1083 can distinguish between cervical adenoma malignum and the wide range of benign endocervical glandular lesions that may mimic this. The benign endocervical glandular lesion 'lobular endocervical glandular hyperplasia' [158], which may mimic adenoma malignum, is now thought to have a pyloric gland phenotype on the basis of histochemical staining characteristics and immunohistochemistry with antibodies against pyloric gland type mucins [159]. It has even been suggested that lobular endocervical glandular hyperplasia is the benign counterpart to, or is a precursor of, adenoma malignum.

TROPHOBLASTIC DISEASE

ANTIBODIES OF VALUE IN TROPHOBLASTIC DISEASE

Well-established markers of trophoblast include β human chorionic gonadotrophin (β HCG), human placental lactogen (HPL) and placental alkaline phosphatase (PLAP). In recent years α-inhibin has been shown to be a marker of syncytiotrophoblast and of some intermediate trophoblastic cells [160]–[165]. Although rarely necessary, staining with α-inhibin may assist in confirming an intrauterine gestation by demonstrating a population of trophoblastic cells. Positive staining with α-inhibin is also usual in trophoblastic neoplasms, such as choriocarcinoma, placental site trophoblastic tumour (PSTT) and epithelioid trophoblastic tumour.

Another antibody, which has recently been shown to react with trophoblastic cells, is MelCAM (CD146) [166], [167]. This stains implantation site intermediate trophoblast, in contrast to chorion-type intermediate trophoblastic cells, which are usually negative. PSTT and exaggerated placental site are the two lesions of implantation site intermediate trophoblast. Double immunohistochemical staining with MelCAM and the proliferation marker MIB1 may be of value in distinguishing between PSTT and exaggerated placental site [167]. In exaggerated placental site the MIB1 proliferation index of trophoblastic cells is close to zero, but in PSTT it is significantly elevated. PSTT should be strongly considered if the MIB1 index in implantation site intermediate trophoblast exceeds 5%. Double staining is used since small lymphocytes may exhibit a high proliferation index. Another antibody, which may be of value in demonstrating intermediate trophoblastic cells and in the diagnosis of trophoblastic neoplasms, is HLA-G [168]. It has also been shown that CD10 is positive in all trophoblastic populations and in trophoblastic tumours [151].

The monoclonal antibody p57, a cell cycle inhibitor and tumour suppressor encoded by a strongly paternally imprinted gene, may be of value in diagnosis of a complete hydatidiform mole (CHM) [169], [170]. Since p57 is only expressed when maternal DNA is present, and since in CHM the DNA is usually entirely of paternal origin, there is no staining of the cytotrophoblast or villous mesenchyme. Positivity of decidua and extravillous implantation site intermediate trophoblast (it is not known why extravillous trophoblast stains positively) acts as an internal positive control. In contrast, normal placenta, hydropic abortion and partial hydatidiform mole exhibit positive nuclear staining of cytotrophoblast and villous mesenchyme. p57 may be useful in the diagnosis of an early CHM or when only a limited amount of tissue is present.

ANTIBODIES OF VALUE IN VULVOVAGINAL MESENCHYMAL LESIONS

A wide variety of mesenchymal lesions may arise on the vulva and vagina [171]. There is morphological overlap between these lesions, although with experience they may be distinguished. Aggressive angiomyxoma is characterised by a marked propensity for local recurrence and should be distinguished from a range of benign mesenchymal lesions, which are well-circumscribed with limited potential for recurrence. These include angiomyofibroblastoma, cellular angiofibroma, superficial angiomyxoma and fibroepithelial stromal polyp. As well as morphological overlap the immunophenotypes of many of these lesions are similar, with variable positivity with vimentin, α-smooth muscle actin, desmin, CD34, ER and PR [172]–[174]. An additional problem with aggressive angiomyxoma is recognition of its interface with adjacent normal tissues. This is important in ensuring adequacy of excision. It has been shown that the DNA architectural factor HMGA2 (formerly HMGIC), located on chromosome 12, is rearranged in aggressive angiomyxoma, resulting in aberrant HMGA2 protein expression [175]. Nuclear HMGA2 expression is usually present in aggressive angiomyxoma but not in its histological mimics [176]. In addition, normal tissues adjacent to aggressive angiomyxoma are usually negative. Clearly further work is required in this area to ascertain the full immunohistochemical distribution of HMGA2.

PAGET'S DISEASE OF THE VULVA

Vulval Paget's disease may be either primary (arising from an intra-epidermal stem cell or from cutaneous sweat glands) or secondary to a carcinoma in an internal organ, such as endometrium, cervix, urinary bladder or colorectum [177]. Positivity of Paget's cells with CAM5.2 and CEA assists in excluding mimics, such as Pagetoid Bowen's disease, melanocytic lesions and mycoses fungoides. CK7 and 20 staining may also be of value [178]–[182]. Most cases of primary vulval Paget's disease are strongly positive with CK7, while CK20 is usually negative or focally positive, although occasionally there is diffuse immunoreactivity. The only cells in the normal epidermis which are positive with CK7 are Merkel cells and Toker cells. However, a recent study has shown positive staining of pagetoid squamous cell carcinoma in situ (pagetoid Bowen's disease) with CK7, illustrating that CK7 cannot be used to distinguish this lesion from Paget's disease [183]. It should be noted that Merkel cells are also CK20 positive. With negative CK7 and strong CK20 positivity of vulval Paget's disease an underlying carcinoma of the urinary bladder or colorectum should be considered, since primary adenocarcinomas at these sites are often CK20 positive. Immunoreactivity for uroplakin III suggests Paget's disease of urothelial origin [184]. Staining with CK7 may assist in identifying small foci of invasive dermal tumour in vulval Paget's disease, and in identifying tumour cells at the surgical margins.

REFERENCES

1. McCluggage WG. Recent advances in immunohistochemistry in gynaecological pathology. *Histopathology* 2002; **40**: 309–26.
2. McCluggage WG. Recent advances in immunohistochemistry in the diagnosis of ovarian neoplasms. *J Clin Pathol* 2000; **53**: 327–34.
3. Yaziji H, Gown AM. Immunohistochemical analysis of gynaecologic tumors. *Int J Gynecol Pathol* 2001; **20**: 64–78.
4. Lash RH, Hart WR. Intestinal adenocarcinomas metastatic to the ovaries: a clinicopathologic evaluation of 22 cases. *Am J Surg Pathol* 1989; **11**: 114–21.
5. Wauters CCAP, Smedts F, Gerrits LGM *et al.* Keratins 7 and 20 as diagnostic markers of carcinomas metastatic to the ovary. *Hum Pathol* 1995; **26**: 852–55.
6. Lagendijk JA, Mullink H, van Diest PJ *et al.* Tracing the origin of adenocarcinomas with unknown primary using immunohistochemistry. Differential diagnosis between colonic and ovarian carcinomas as primary sites. *Hum Pathol* 1998; **29**: 491–7.
7. Berezowski K, Stasny JF, Kornstein MJ. Cytokeratins 7 and 20 and carcinoembryonic antigen in ovarian and colonic carcinoma. *Mod Pathol* 1996; **9**: 426–9.
8. Loy TS, Calaluce RD, Keeney GL. Cytokeratin immunostaining in differentiating primary ovarian carcinoma from metastatic colonic adenocarcinoma. *Mod Pathol* 1996; **9**: 1040–4.
9. Ueda G, Sawada M, Ogawa H *et al.* Immunohistochemical study of cytokeratin 7 for the differentiated diagnosis of adenocarcinoma in the ovary. *Gynecol Oncol* 1993; **51**: 219–23.
10. Chu PG, Weiss LM. Keratin expression in human tissues and neoplasms. *Histopathology* 2002; **40**: 403–9.
11. Park SO, Kim HS, Hong EK, Kim AWH. Expression of cytokeratins 7 and 20 in primary carcinomas of the stomach and colorectum and their value in the differential diagnosis of metastatic carcinomas to the ovary. *Hum Pathol* 2002; **33**: 1078–85.
12. Cathro HP, Stoler MH. Expression of cytokeratin 7 and 20 in ovarian neoplasia. *Am J Clin Pathol* 2002; **117**: 944–51.
13. Multhaupt HA, Arenas-Elliott CP, Warhol MJ. Comparison of glycoprotein expression between ovarian and colonic adenocarcinomas. *Arch Pathol Lab Med* 1999; **123**: 909–16.
14. Lagendijk JH, Mullink H, van Diest PJ, Meijer GA, Meijer CJ. Immunohistochemical differentiation between primary adenocarcinomas of the ovary and ovarian metastases of colon and breast origin. Comparison between a statistical and intuitive approach. *J Clin Pathol* 1999; **52**: 283–90.
15. DeCostanzo DC, Elias JM, Chumas JC. Necrosis in 84 ovarian carcinomas: a morphologic study of primary versus metastatic colonic carcinoma with a selective immunohistochemical analysis of cytokeratin subtypes and carcinoembryonic antigen. *Int J Gynecol Pathol* 1997; **16**: 245–9.
16. Young RH, Wart WR. Metastases from carcinomas of the pancreas simulating primary mucinous tumors of the ovary: a report of seven cases. *Am J Surg Pathol* 1989; **13**: 748–56.
17. Young RH, Scully RE. Ovarian metastases from carcinoma of the gallbladder and extrahepatic bile ducts simulating primary tumors of the ovary: a report of six cases. *Int J Gynecol Pathol* 1990; **9**: 60–72.
18. Lee KR, Young RH. The distinction between primary and metastatic mucinous carcinomas of the ovary: gross and histologic features in 50 cases. *Am J Surg Pathol* 2003; **27**: 281–92.
19. Kende AI, Carr NJ, Sobin LH. Expression of cytokeratins 7 and 20 in carcinomas of the gastrointestinal tract. *Histopathology* 2003; **42**: 137–40.
20. Ji H, Isacson C, Seidman JD, Kurman RJ, Ronnett BM. Cytokeratins 7 and 20, Dpc 4 and MUC5AC in the distinction of metastatic mucinous carcinomas in the ovary from primary ovarian mucinous tumors: Dpc4 assists in identifying metastatic pancreatic carcinomas. *Int J Gynecol Pathol* 2002; **21**: 391–400.
21. Goldstein NS, Bassi D, Uzieblo A. WT1 is an integral component of an antibody panel to distinguish pancreaticobiliary and some ovarian epithelial neoplasms. *Am J Clin Pathol* 2001; **116**: 246–52.

22. Albarracin CT, Jafri J, Montag AG, Hart J, Kuan S. Differential expression of MUC2 and MUC5AC mucin genes in primary ovarian and metastatic colonic carcinoma. *Hum Pathol* 2000; **31**: 672–7.
23. Young RH, Hart WR. Renal cell carcinoma metastatic to the ovary: a report of three cases emphasizing possible confusion with ovarian clear cell adenocarcinoma. *Int J Gynecol Pathol* 1992; **11**: 96–104.
24. Young RH, Hart WR. Metastatic intestinal carcinomas simulating primary ovarian clear cell carcinoma and secretory endometrioid carcinoma: A clinicopathologic and immunohistochemical study of five cases. *Am J Surg Pathol* 1998; **22**: 805–15.
25. Cameron RI, Ashe P, O'Rourke DM, Foster H, McCluggage WG. A panel of immunohistochemical stains assists in the distinction between ovarian and renal clear cell carcinoma. *Int J Gynecol Pathol* 2003; **22**: 272–6.
26. Guerrieri C, Franlund B, Fristedt S *et al*. Mucinous tumors of the vermiform appendix and ovary, and pseudomyxoma peritonei. Histogenetic implications of cytokeratin 7 expression. *Hum Pathol* 1997; **28**: 1039–45.
27. Ronnett BM, Shmookler BM, Diener-West M *et al*. Immunohistochemical evidence supporting the appendiceal origin of pseudomyxoma peritonei in women. *Int J Gynecol Pathol* 1997; **16**: 1–9.
28. Ronnett BM, Seidman JD. Mucinous tumors arising in ovarian mature teratomas: relationship to pseudomyxoma peritonei. *Mod Pathol* 2003; **16**: 209A.
29. O'Connell JT, Hacker CM, Barsky SH. MUC2 is a molecular marker for pseudomyxoma peritonei. *Mod Pathol* 2002; **15**: 958–72.
30. Clement PB, Young RH, Scully RE. Malignant mesotheliomas presenting as ovarian masses. A report of nine cases, including two primary ovarian mesotheliomas. *Am J Surg Pathol* 1996; **20**: 1067–80.
31. Ordonez NG. Role of immunohistochemistry in distinguishing epithelial peritoneal mesotheliomas from peritoneal and ovarian serous carcinomas. *Am J Surg Pathol* 1998; **22**: 1203–14.
32. Attanoos RL, Webb R, Dojcinov SD, Gibbs AR. Value of mesothelial and epithelial antibodies in distinguishing diffuse peritoneal mesothelioma in females from serous papillary carcinoma of the ovary and peritoneum. *Histopathology* 2002; **40**: 237–44.
33. Khoury N, Raju U, Crissman JD, Zarbo RJ, Greenawald KA. A comparative immunohistochemical study of peritoneal and ovarian serous tumors and mesotheliomas. *Hum Pathol* 1990; **21**: 811–19.
34. Goldstein NS, Uzieblo A. WT-1 immunoreactivity in uterine papillary serous carcinomas is different from ovarian serous carcinomas. *Am J Clin Pathol* 2002; **117**: 541–5.
35. Al-Hussaini M, Stockman A, Foster H, McCluggage WG. WT-1 assists in distinguishing ovarian from uterine serous carcinoma and in distinguishing between serous and endometrioid ovarian carcinoma. *Histopathology* 2004; **44**: 109–15.
36. Shimizu M, Toki T, Takagi Y, Konishi I, Fujii S. Immunohistochemical detection of the Wilms' tumor gene (WT1) in epithelial ovarian tumors. *Int J Gynecol Pathol* 2000; **19**: 158–63.
37. Shimizu M, Nikaido T, Toki T, Shiozawa T, Fugii S. Clear cell carcinoma has an expression pattern of cell cycle regulatory molecules that is unique among ovarian adenocarcinomas. *Cancer* 1999; **85**: 669–77.
38. Young RH, Scully RE. Ovarian sex cord-stromal tumors: problems in differential diagnosis. *Pathol Annu* 1998; **23**: 237–96.
39. McCluggage WG, Maxwell P, Sloan JM. Immunohistochemical staining of ovarian granulosa cell tumors with monoclonal antibody against inhibin. *Hum Pathol* 1997; **28**: 1034–8.
40. Zheng W, Sung CJ, Hanna I *et al*. α and β subunits of inhibin/activin as sex cord-stromal differentiation markers. *Int J Gynecol Pathol* 1997; **16**: 263–71.
41. Stewart CJR, Jeffers MD, Kennedy A. Diagnostic value of inhibin immunoreactivity in ovarian gonadal stromal tumours and their histological mimics. *Histopathology* 1997; **31**: 67–74.
42. Hildebrandt RH, Rouse RV, Longacre TA. Value of inhibin in the identification of granulosa cell tumors of the ovary. *Hum Pathol* 1997; **28**: 1387–95.

43. Costa MJ, Ames PF, Walls J, Roth LM. Inhibin immunohistochemistry applied to ovarian neoplasms: a novel, effective diagnostic tool. *Hum Pathol* 1997; **28**: 1247−54.
44. Wells M. Making sense of inhibin in ovarian tumours. *Histopathology* 1998; **32**: 81−3.
45. Kommoss F, Oliva E, Bhan AK, Young RH, Scully RE. Inhibin expression in ovarian tumors and tumor-like lesions: an immunohistochemical study. *Mod Pathol* 1998; **11**: 656−64.
46. Yamashita K, Yamoto M, Shikone T *et al.* Production of inhibin A and inhibin B in human ovarian sex cord stromal tumors. *Am J Obstet Gynecol* 1997; **177**: 1450−7.
47. Matias-Guiu X, Pons C, Prat J. Mullerian inhibiting substance, alpha-inhibin, and CD99 expression in sex cord-stromal tumors and endometrioid ovarian carcinomas resembling sex cord-stromal tumors. *Hum Pathol* 1998; **29**: 840−5.
48. Riopel MA, Perlman EJ, Seidman JD, Kurman RJ, Sherman ME. Inhibin and epithelial membrane antigen immunohistochemistry assist in the diagnosis of sex cord-stromal tumors and provide clues to the histogenesis of hypercalcaemic small cell carcinomas. *Int J Gynecol Pathol* 1998; **17**: 46−53.
49. Rishi M, Howard LN, Bratthauer GL, Tavassoli FA. Use of monoclonal antibody against human inhibin as a marker for sex cord-stromal tumors of the ovary. *Am J Surg Pathol* 1997; **21**: 583−9.
50. Flemming P, Wellmann A, Maschek H, Lang H, Georgii A. Monoclonal antibodies against inhibin represent key markers of adult granulosa cell tumors of the ovary even in their metastases. *Am J Surg Pathol* 1995; **19**: 927−33.
51. Pelkey TJ, Frierson HF Jr, Mills SE, Stoler MH. The diagnostic utility of inhibin staining in ovarian neoplasms. *Int J Gynecol Pathol* 1998; **17**: 97−105.
52. Guerrieri C, Franlund B, Malmstrom H, Boeryd B. Ovarian endometrioid carcinomas simulating sex cord-stromal tumors: a study using inhibin and cytokeratin 7. *Int J Gynecol Pathol* 1998; **17**: 266−71.
53. McCluggage WG, Maxwell P. Immunohistochemical staining for calretinin is useful in the diagnosis of ovarian sex cord-stromal tumours. *Histopathology* 2001; **38**: 403−8.
54. Doglioni C, Dei Tos AP, Laurino L. Calretinin: a novel immunocytochemical marker for mesothelioma. *Am J Surg Pathol* 1996; **20**: 1037−46.
55. Cao QJ, Jones JG, Li M. Expression of calretinin in human ovary, testis and ovarian sex cord-stromal tumors. *Int J Gynecol Pathol* 2001; **20**: 346−52.
56. Deavers MT, Malpica A, Ordonez NG, Silva EG. Ovarian steroid cell tumors: an immunohistochemical study including a comparison of calretinin with inhibin. *Int J Gynecol Pathol* 2003; **22**: 162−7.
57. Loo KT, Leung AKF, Chan JKC. Immunohistochemical staining of ovarian granulosa cell tumours with MIC2 antibody. *Histopathology* 1995; **27**: 388−90.
58. Gordon MD, Corless C, Renshaw AA *et al.* CD99, keratin and vimentin staining of sex cord-stromal tumors, normal ovary and testis. *Mod Pathol* 1998; **11**: 769−73.
59. Choi YL, Kim HS, Ahn G. Immunoexpression of inhibin alpha subunit, inhibin/activin beta subunit and CD99 in ovarian tumors. *Arch Pathol Lab Med* 2000; **124**: 563−9.
60. Stewart CJR, Nandini CL, Richmond JA. Value of A103 (melan-A) immunostaining in the differential diagnosis of ovarian sex cord tumors. *J Clin Pathol* 2000; **53**: 206−11.
61. Busam KJ, Iversen K, Coplan KA *et al.* Immunoreactivity for A103, an antibody to melan-A (Mart-1) in adrenocortical and other steroid tumors. *Am J Surg Pathol* 1998; **22**: 57−63.
62. Gustafson ML, Lee MM, Scully RE *et al.* Mullerian inhibiting substance as a marker for sex-cord tumor. *N Engl J Med* 1992; **326**: 466−71.
63. Silverman LA, Gitelman SE. Immunoreactive inhibin, mullerian inhibiting substance and activin as biochemical markers for juvenile granulosa cell tumors. *J Pediatr* 1996; **129**: 918−21.
64. Bamberger AM, Ivell R, Balvers M. Relaxin-like factor (RLF): a new specific marker for Leydig cells in the ovary. *Int J Gynecol Pathol* 1998; **18**: 163−8.
65. Sasano H, Mason JI, Sasaki E *et al.* Immunohistochemical study of 3 beta-hydroxysteroid dehydrogenase in sex cord-stromal tumors of the ovary. *Int J Gynecol Pathol* 1990; **9**: 352−62.
66. Costa MJ, Morris R, Sasano H. Sex steroid biosynthesis enzymes in ovarian sex cord-stromal tumors. *Int J Gynecol Pathol* 1994; **13**: 109−19.

67. Tiltman AJ, Ali H. Distribution of alpha glutathione S-transferase in ovarian neoplasms: an immunohistochemical study. *Histopathology* 2001; **39**: 266–72.
68. Tiltman AJ, Haffajee Z. Sclerosing stromal tumors, thecomas and fibromas of the ovary: an immunohistochemical profile. *Int J Gynecol Pathol* 1999; **18**: 254–8.
69. Mouhedi-Lankarani S, Kurman RJ. Calretinin, a more sensitive but less specific marker than alpha-inhibin for ovarian sex cord-stromal neoplasms: an immunohistochemical study of 215 cases. *Am J Surg Pathol* 2002; **26**: 1477–83.
70. Shah VI, Freites ON, Maxwell P, McCluggage WG. Inhibin is more specific than calretinin as an immunohistochemical marker for differentiating sarcomatoid granulosa cell tumour of the ovary from other spindle cell neoplasms. *J Clin Pathol* 2003; **56**: 221–4.
71. McCluggage WG, Maxwell P. Adenocarcinomas of various sites may exhibit immuno-reactivity with anti-inhibin antibodies. *Histopathology* 1999; **35**: 216–20.
72. Aquirre P, Thor AD, Scully RE. Ovarian endometrioid carcinomas resembling sex cord-stromal tumors: an immunohistochemical study. *Int J Gynecol Pathol* 1989; **8**: 364–73.
73. Otis CN, Powell JL, Barbuto D *et al*. Intermediate filamentous proteins in adult granulosa cell tumors. *Am J Surg Pathol* 1992; **16**: 962–8.
74. Czernobilsky B, Moll R, Levy R, Franke WW. Co-expression of cytokeratin and vimentin flaments in mesothelial, granulosa and rete ovarii cells of the human ovary. *Eur J Cell Biol* 1985; **37**: 175–90.
75. Costa MJ, DeRose PB, Roth LM, Brescia RJ, Zaloudek CJ, Cohen C. Immunohistochemical phenotype of ovarian granulosa cell tumors: absence of epithelial membrane antigen has diagnostic value. *Hum Pathol* 1994; **25**: 60–6.
76. Flemming P, Grothe W, Maschek H, Petry KU, Wellmann A. The site of inhibin production in ovarian neoplasms. *Histopathology* 1996; **29**: 465–8.
77. McCluggage WG. The value of inhibin staining in gynaecological pathology. *Int J Gynecol Pathol* 2001; **20**: 79–85.
78. McCluggage WG, Patterson A, White J, Anderson NH. Immunocytochemical staining of ovarian cyst aspirates with monoclonal antibody against inhibin. *Cytopathology* 1998; **9**: 336–42.
79. Devouassoux-Shisheboran M, Silver SA, Tavassoli FA. Wolffian adnexal tumor, so-called female adnexal tumor of probable Wolffian origin (FATWO): immunohistochemical evidence in support of a Wolffian origin. *Hum Pathol* 1999; **30**: 856–63.
80. Tiltman AJ, Allard U. Female adnexal tumours of probable Wolffian origin: an immuno-histochemical study comparing tumours, mesonephric remnants and paramesonephric derivatives. *Histopathology* 2001; **38**: 237–42.
81. Clement PB, Scully RE. Uterine tumors resembling ovarian sex cord tumors: a clinico-pathologic analysis of fourteen cases. *Am J Clin Pathol* 1976; **66**: 512–25.
82. Krishnamurthy S, Jungbloth AA, Busam KJ, Rosai J. Uterine tumors resembling ovarian sex-cord tumors have an immunophenotype consistent with true sex-cord differentiation. *Am J Surg Pathol* 1998; **22**: 1078–82.
83. Baker RJ, Hildebrant RH, Rouse RV, Hendrickson MR, Longacre TA. Inhibin and CD 99 (MIC2) expression in uterine stromal neoplasms with sex cord-like elements. *Hum Pathol* 1999; **30**: 671–9.
84. McCluggage WG. Uterine tumours resembling ovarian sex cord tumours: immunohisto-chemical evidence for true sex cord differentiation. *Histopathology* 1999; **34**: 373–80.
85. Ambros RA, Sherman ME, Zahn CM, Bitterman P, Kurman RJ. Endometrial intraepithelial carcinoma: distinctive lesion specifically associated with tumors displaying serous differentiation. *Hum Pathol* 1995; **26**: 1260–7.
86. Spiegel GW. Endometrial carcinoma in situ in postmenopausal women. *Am J Surg Pathol* 1995; **19**: 417–32.
87. Matias Guiu X, Catasus L, Bussaglia E *et al*. Molecular pathology of endometrial hyperplasia and carcinoma. *Hum Pathol* 2001; **32**: 569–77.
88. Wheeler DT, Bell KA, Kurman RJ, Sherman ME. Minimal uterine serous carcinoma: diagnosis and clinicopathologic correlation. *Am J Surg Pathol* 2000; **24**: 797–806.
89. Stewart RL, Royds JA, Burton JL *et al*. Direct sequencing of the p53 gene shows absence of mutations in endometrioid endometrial adenocarcinomas expressing p53 protein. *Histopathology* 1998; **33**: 440–5.

90. Silva EG, Jenkins R. Serous carcinoma in endometrial polyps. *Mod Pathol* 1990; **3**: 120—8.
91. McCluggage WG, Sumathi VP, McManus DT. Uterine serous carcinoma and endometrial intraepithelial carcinoma arising in endometrial polyps: report of five cases including two associated with tamoxifen therapy. *Hum Pathol* 2003; **34**: 939—43.
92. Quddus MR, Sung CJ, Zheny W, Lauchlan SC. p53 immunoreactivity in endometrial metaplasia with dysfunctional uterine bleeding. *Histopathology* 1999; **35**: 44—9.
93. Schlosshauer PW, Ellenson LH, Soslow RA. β-catenin and E-cadherin expression patterns in high-grade endometrial carcinoma are associated with histological subtype. *Mod Pathol* 2002; **15**: 1032—7.
94. Castrillon DH, Lee KR, Nucci MR. Distinction between endometrial and endocervical adenocarcinomas: an immunohistochemical study. *Int J Gynecol Pathol* 2002; **21**: 4—10.
95. McCluggage WG, Sumathi VP, McBride HA, Patterson A. A panel of immunohistochemical stains, including carcinoembryonic antigen, vimentin and estrogen receptor, aids the distinction between primary endometrial and endocervical adenocarcinomas. *Int J Gynecol Pathol* 2002; **21**: 11—15.
96. Kamoi S, Al Juboury MI, Akin MR, Silverberg SG. Immunohistochemical staining in the distinction between primary endometrial and endocervical adenocarcinomas: another viewpoint. *Int J Gynecol Pathol* 2002; **21**: 217—23.
97. Staebler A, Sherman ME, Zaino RJ, Ronnett BM. Hormone receptor immunohistochemistry and human papilloma virus in situ hybridization are useful for distinguishing endocervical and endometrial adenocarcinomas. *Am J Surg Pathol* 2002; **26**: 998—1006.
98. McCluggage WG, Jenkins D. p16 immunoreactivity may assist in the distinction between endometrial and endocervical adenocarcinoma. *Int J Gynecol Pathol* 2003; **22**: 231—5.
99. O'Leary JJ, Landers RJ, Crowley M *et al.* Human papillomavirus and mixed epithelial tumors of the endometrium. *Hum Pathol* 1998; **29**: 383—9.
100. Oliva E, Young RH, Clement PB, Scully RE. Myxoid and fibrous endometrial stromal tumors of the uterus. A report of 10 cases. *Int J Gynecol Pathol* 1999; **18**: 310—19.
101. Oliva E, Young RH, Clement PB, Bhan AK, Scully RE. Cellular benign mesenchymal tumors of the uterus: a comparative morphologic and immunohistochemical analysis of 33 highly cellular leiomyomas and seven endometrial stromal nodules, two frequently confused tumors. *Am J Surg Pathol* 1995; **19**: 757—68.
102. Franquemont DW, Frierson HF Jr, Mills SE. An immunohistochemical study of normal endometrial stroma and endometrial stromal neoplasms: evidence for smooth muscle differentiation. *Am J Surg Pathol* 1991; **15**: 861—70.
103. Devaney K, Tavassoli FA. Immunohistochemistry as a diagnostic aid in the interpretation of unusual mesenchymal tumors of the uterus. *Mod Pathol* 1991; **4**: 225—31.
104. Farhood AI, Abrams J. Immunohistochemistry of endometrial stromal sarcoma. *Hum Pathol* 1991; **22**: 224—30.
105. McCluggage WG, Sumathi VP, Maxwell P. CD10 is a sensitive and diagnostically useful immunohistochemical marker of normal endometrial stroma and of endometrial stromal neoplasms. *Histopathology* 2001; **39**: 273—8.
106. Chu PG, Arber PA, Weiss LM *et al.* Utility of CD10 in distinguishing between endometrial stromal sarcoma and uterine smooth muscle tumors: an immunohistochemical comparison of 34 cases. *Mod Pathol* 2001; **14**: 465—71.
107. Nucci MR, O'Connell JT, Huettner PC *et al.* h-Caldesmon expression effectively distinguishes endometrial stromal tumors from uterine smooth muscle tumors. *Am J Surg Pathol* 2001; **25**: 455—63.
108. Rash DS, Tan JY, Baergen RN *et al.* h-Caldesmon, a novel smooth muscle-specific antibody, distinguishes between cellular leiomyoma and endometrial stromal sarcoma. *Am J Surg Pathol* 2001; **25**: 253—8.
109. Agoff SN, Grieco VS, Garcia R, Gown AM. Immunohistochemical distinction of endometrial stromal sarcoma and cellular leiomyoma. *Appl Immuno Mol Morphol* 2001; **9**: 164—9.
110. Toki T, Shimizu M, Takagi Y, Ashida T, Konishi I. CD10 is a marker for normal and neoplastic endometrial stromal cells. *Int J Gynecol Pathol* 2002; **21**: 41—7.
111. Chu P, Arber DA. Paraffin-section detection of CD10 in 505 nonhematopoietic neoplasms. Frequent expression in renal cell carcinoma and endometrial stromal sarcoma. *Am J Clin Pathol* 2000; **113**: 374—82.

112. Scully RE. Smooth muscle differentiation in genital tract disorders. *Arch Pathol Lab Med* 1981; **105**: 505–7.

113. Oliva E, Clement PB, Young RH, Scully RE. Mixed endometrial stromal and smooth muscle tumors of the uterus: a clinicopathologic study of 15 cases. *Am J Surg Pathol* 1998; **22**: 997–1005.

114. Sumathi VP, McCluggage WG. CD10 is useful in demonstrating endometrial stroma at ectopic sites and in confirming a diagnosis of endometriosis. *J Clin Pathol* 2002; **25**: 391–2.

115. Vang R, Kempson RL. Perivascular epithelioid cell tumor (PEComa) of the uterus: a subset of HMB-45-positive epithelioid mesenchymal neoplasms with an uncertain relationship to pure smooth muscle tumors. *Am J Surg Pathol* 2002; **26**: 1–13.

116. Silva EG, Deavers MT, Bodurka D, Malpica A. Uterine epithelioid leiomyosarcomas with clear cells or malignant PEComas? *Mod Pathol* 2003; **16**: 211(A).

117. Zamecnik M, Michal M. HMB45+ hyalinized epithelioid tumor of the uterus is linked to epithelioid leiomyoma rather than PEC-omas. *Int J Surg Pathol* 2001; **9**: 341–3.

118. McCluggage WG, Walsh MY, Thornton CM *et al.* Inter and intraobserver variation in the histopathological reporting of cervical squamous intraepithelial lesions using a modified Bethesda grading system. *Br J Obstet Gynaecol* 1998; **105**: 206–10.

119. McCluggage WG, Bharucha H, Date A *et al.* Interobserver variation in the reporting of cervical colposcopic biopsies. Comparison of grading systems. *J Clin Pathol* 1996; **49**: 833–5.

120. McCluggage WG, Tang L, Maxwell P, Bharucha H. Monoclonal antibody MIB1 in the assessment of cervical squamous intraepithelial lesions. *Int J Gynecol Pathol* 1996; **15**: 131–6.

121. McCluggage WG, Maxwell P, Bharucha H. Immunohistochemical detection of metallothionein and MIB1 in uterine cervical squamous lesions. *Int J Gynecol Pathol* 1998; **17**: 29–35.

122. Mittal KR, Demopoulos RI, Goswami S. Proliferating cell nuclear antigen (cyclin) expression in normal and abnormal cervical squamous epithelia. *Am J Surg Pathol* 1993; **17**: 117–22.

123. Raju GC. Expression of the proliferating cell nuclear antigen in cervical neoplasia. *Int J Gynecol Pathol* 1994; **12**: 337–41.

124. Kobayashi I, Matsuo K, Ishibashi Y, Kanda S, Sati H. The proliferative activity in dysplasia and carcinoma in situ of the uterine cervix analysed by proliferating cell nuclear antigen immunostaining and silver-binding argyrophilic nucleolar organiser region staining. *Hum Pathol* 1994; **25**: 198–202.

125. Bulten J, Van der Laak JAWM, Gemmink JH, Pahlplatz MMM, de Wilde PCM, Hanselaar AGJM. MIB1, a promising marker for the classification of cervical intraepithelial neoplasia. *J Pathol* 1996; **178**: 268–73.

126. Al-Saleh W, Delvenne P, Greimers R, Fridman P, Doyen J, Boniver J. Assessment of Ki-67 antigen immunostaining in squamous intraepithelial lesions of the uterine cervix: correlation with histological grade and human papilloma virus type. *Am J Clin Pathol* 1995; **104**: 154–60.

127. Payne S, Kernohan NM, Walker F. Proliferation in the normal cervix and in preinvasive cervical lesions. *J Clin Pathol* 1996; **49**: 667–71.

128. Mittal K. Utility of proliferation – associated marker MIB1 in evaluating lesions of the uterine cervix. *Adv Anat Pathol* 1999; **6**: 177–85.

129. Kruse AJ, Baak JPA, Helliesen T, Kjellevold KH, Bol MGW, Janssen EAM. Evaluation of MIB-1 positive cell clusters as a diagnostic marker for cervical intraepithelial neoplasia. *Am J Surg Pathol* 2002; **26**: 1501–7.

130. Mittal K, Mesia A, Demopoulos RI. MIB1 expression is useful in distinguishing dysplasia from atrophy in elderly women. *Int J Gynecol Pathol* 1999; **18**: 122–4.

131. Pirog EC, Baergen RN, Soslow RA *et al.* Diagnostic accuracy of cervical low-grade squamous intraepithelial lesions is improved with MIB1 immunostaining. *Am J Surg Pathol* 2002; **26**: 70–5.

132. Mittal K. Utility of MIB1 in evaluating cauterised cervical cone biopsy margins. *Int J Gynecol Pathol* 1999; **18**: 211–14.

133. Keating JT, Cviko A, Riethdorf S *et al*. Ki-67, cyclin E and p16 (INK4) are complementary surrogate biomarkers for human papilloma virus-related cervical neoplasia. *Am J Surg Pathol* 2001; **25**: 884−91.

134. Klaes R, Friedrich T, Spitkovsky D *et al*. Over expression of p16 (INK4A) as a specific marker for dysplastic and neoplastic epithelial cells of the cervix uteri. *Int J Cancer* 2001; **92**: 276−84.

135. Murphy N, Ring M, Killalea AG *et al*. p16 INK4A as a marker for cervical dyskaryosis: CIN and CGIN in cervical biopsies and ThinPrep smears. *J Clin Pathol* 2003; **56**: 56−63.

136. Klaes R, Benner A, Friedrich T *et al*. p16INK4A immunohistochemistry improves interobserver agreement in the diagnosis of cervical intraepithelial neoplasia. *Am J Surg Pathol* 2002; **26**: 1389−99.

137. Cameron RI, Maxwell P, Jenkins D, McCluggage WG. Immunohistochemical staining with MIB1, bcl2 and p16 assists in the distinction of cervical glandular intraepithelial neoplasia from tubo-endometrial metaplasia, endometriosis and microglandular hyperplasia. *Histopathology* 2002; **41**: 313−21.

138. McCluggage WG, Maxwell P, McBride HA, Hamilton PW, Bharucha H. Monoclonal antibodies Ki-67 and MIB1 in the distinction of tuboendometrial metaplasia from endocervical adenocarcinoma and adenocarcinoma in situ in formalin fixed material. *Int J Gynecol Pathol* 1995; **14**: 209−16.

139. Van Hoeven KH, Ramondetta L, Kovatich AJ, Bibbo L, Dunton CJ. Quantitative image analysis of MIB1 reactivity in inflammatory, hyperplastic and neoplastic endocervical lesions. *Int J Gynecol Pathol* 1997; **16**: 15−21.

140. Pirog EC, Isacson C, Szabolcs MJ, Kleter B, Quint W, Richart RM. Proliferative activity of benign and neoplastic endocervical epithelium and correlation with HPV DNA detection. *Int J Gynecol Pathol* 2002; **21**: 22−6.

141. Cina SJ, Richardson MS, Austin RM, Kurman RJ. Immunohistochemical staining for Ki-67 antigen, carcinoembryonic antigen, and p53 in the differential diagnosis of glandular lesions of the cervix. *Mod Pathol* 1997; **10**: 176−80.

142. McCluggage WG, Maxwell P, Bharucha H. Immunohistochemical detection of p53 and bcl2 proteins, in neoplastic and non-neoplastic endocervical glandular lesions. *Int J Gynecol Pathol* 1997; **16**: 22−7.

143. McCluggage WG, Maxwell P. bcl-2 and p21 immunostaining of cervical tubo-endometrial metaplasia. *Histopathology* 2002; **40**: 107−8.

144. Piek JMJ, van Diest PJ, Verheijen RHM, Kenemans P. Cell cycle-related proteins p21 and bcl2: markers of differentiation in the human fallopian tube. *Histopathology* 2001; **38**: 481−2.

145. Henderson GS, Brown KA, Perkins SL, Abbott TM, Clayton F. Bcl-2 is down-regulated in atypical endometrial hyperplasia and adenocarcinoma. *Mod Pathol* 1996; **9**: 430−6.

146. Reithdorf L, Riethdorf S, Lee KR, Cviko A, Loning T, Crum CP. Human papillomavirus, expression of p16 INK4A and early endocervical glandular neoplasia. *Hum Pathol* 2002; **33**: 899−904.

147. Negri G, Egarter-Vigli E, Kasal A, Romano F, Haitel A, Mian C. p16 INK4A is a useful marker for the diagnosis of adenocarcinoma of the cervix uteri and its precursors: an immunohistochemical study with immunocytochemical correlations. *Am J Surg Pathol* 2003; **27**: 187−93.

148. Marques T, Andrade LA, Vassallo J. Endocervical tubal metaplasia and adenocarcinoma in situ: role of immunohistochemistry for carcinoembryonic antigen and vimentin in differential diagnosis. *Histopathology* 1996; **28**: 549−50.

149. Gilks CB, Young RH, Aquirre P *et al*. Adenoma malignum/minimal deviation adenocarcinoma of the uterine cervix. A clinicopathological and immunohistochemical analysis of 26 cases. *Am J Surg Pathol* 1989; **13**: 717−29.

150. Michael H, Grave L, Kraus FT. Minimal deviation endocervical adenocarcinoma: clinical and histologic features, immunohistochemical staining for carcinoembryonic antigen and differentiation from confusing benign lesions. *Int J Gynecol Pathol* 1984; **3**: 261−76.

151. Ordi J, Romagosa C, Tavassoli FA *et al*. CD10 expression in epithelial tissues and tumors of the gynaecologic tract: a useful marker in the diagnosis of mesonephric, trophoblastic and clear cell tumors. *Am J Surg Pathol* 2003; **27**: 178−86.

152. Ordi J, Nogales FF, Palacia A *et al.* Mesonephric adenocarcinoma of the uterine corpus: CD10 expression as evidence of mesonephric differentiation. *Am J Surg Pathol* 2001; **25**: 1540–5.

153. McCluggage WG, Oliva E, Herrington CS, McBride H, Young RH. CD10 and calretinin staining of endocervical glandular lesions, endocervical stroma and endometrioid adenocarcinomas of the uterine corpus: CD10 positivity is characteristic of, but not specific for, mesonephric lesions and is not specific for endometrial stroma. *Histopathology* 2003; **43**: 144–50.

154. Nascimento AF, Hirsch MS, Cviko A, Quade BJ, Nucci MR. The role of CD10 staining in distinguishing invasive endometrial adenocarcinoma from adenocarcinoma involving adenomyosis. *Mod Pathol* 2003; **16**: 22–7.

155. Ishii K, Kumagai T, Tozuka M, Ota H, Katsuyama T, Kurihara M. A new diagnostic method for adenoma malignum and related lesions: latex aglutination test with a new monoclonal antibody, HIK 1083. *Clinica Chimica Acta* 2001; **312**: 231–3.

156. Ischimura T, Koizumi T, Tateiwa H *et al.* Immunohistochemical expression of gastric mucin and p53 in minimal deviation adenocarcinoma of the uterine cervix. *Int J Gynecol Pathol* 2001; **20**: 220–6.

157. Utsugi K, Hirai Y, Takeshima N, Akiyama F, Sakurai S, Hasumi K. Utility of the monoclonal antibody HIK1083 in the diagnosis of adenoma malignum of the uterine cervix. *Gynecol Oncol* 1999; **75**: 345–8.

158. Nucci MR, Clement PB, Young RH. Lobular endocervical glandular hyperplasia, not otherwise specific: a clinicopathologic analysis of thirteen cases of a distinctive pseudo-neoplastic lesion and comparison with fourteen cases of adenoma malignum. *Am J Surg Pathol* 1999; **23**: 886–91.

159. Mikami Y, Hata S, Melamed J, Fujiwara K, Manabe T. Lobular endocervical glandular hyperplasia is a metaplastic process with a pyloric gland phenotype. *Histopathology* 2001; **39**: 364–72.

160. McCluggage WG, Ashe P, McBride H, Maxwell P, Sloan JM. Localisation of the cellular expression of inhibin in trophoblastic tissue. *Histopathology* 1998; **32**: 252–6.

161. Kommoss F, Schmidt D, Coerdt W, Olert J, Munteferig H. Immunohistochemical expression analysis of inhibin-alpha and -beta subunits in partial and complete moles, trophoblastic tumors and endometrial decidua. *Int J Gynecol Pathol* 2001; **20**: 380–5.

162. Shih IM, Seidman JD, Kurman RJ. Placental site nodule and characterisation of distinctive types of intermediate trophoblast. *Hum Pathol* 1999; **30**: 687–94.

163. Shih IM, Kurman RJ. Immunohistochemical localisation of inhibin-alpha in the placenta and gestational trophoblastic lesions. *Int J Gynecol Pathol* 1999; **18**: 144–50.

164. Pelkey TJ, Frierson HF, Mills SE, Stoler MH. Detection of the alpha-subunit of inhibin in trophoblastic neoplasia. *Hum Pathol* 1999; **30**: 26–31.

165. Shih IM, Kurman RJ. Epithelioid trophoblastic tumor – a neoplasm distinct from choriocarcinoma and placental site trophoblastic tumor simulating carcinoma. *Am J Surg Pathol* 1998; **22**: 1393–403.

166. Shih IM, Kurman RJ. The pathology of intermediate trophoblastic tumors and tumor-like lesions. *Int J Gynecol Pathol* 2001; **20**: 31–47.

167. Shih IM, Kurman RJ. Ki-67 labelling index in the differential diagnosis of exaggerated placental site, placental site trophoblastic tumor and choriocarcinoma. A double immunohistochemical staining technique using Ki-67 and mel CAM antibodies. *Hum Pathol* 1998; **29**: 27–33.

168. Singer G, Kurman RJ, McMaster MT, Shih IM. HLA-G immunoreactivity is specific for intermediate trophoblast in gestational trophoblastic disease and can serve as a useful marker in differential diagnosis. *Am J Surg Pathol* 2002; **26**: 914–20.

169. Castrillon DH, Sun DQ, Weremowicz S, Fisher RA, Crum CP, Genest DR. Discrimination of complete hydatidiform mole from its mimics by immunohistochemistry of the paternally imprinted gene product p57 (KIP2). *Am J Surg Pathol* 2001; **25**: 1225–30.

170. Fukunaga M. Immunohistochemical characterization of p57KIP2 expression in early hydatidiform moles. *Hum Pathol* 2002; **33**: 1188–92.

171. Nucci MR, Fletcher CDM. Vulvovaginal soft tissue tumours: update and review. *Histopathology* 2000; **36**: 97–108.

172. McCluggage WG, Patterson A, Maxwell P. Aggressive angiomyxoma of pelvic parts exhibits oestrogen and progesterone receptor postivity. *J Clin Pathol* 2000; **53**: 603–5.

173. Hartmann CA, Sperling M, Stein H. So-called fibroepithelial polyps of the vagina exhibiting an unusual but uniform antigen profile characterised by expression of desmin and steroid hormone receptors but no muscle-specific actin or macrophages markers. *Am J Clin Pathol* 1990; **93**: 604–8.

174. Nielsen GP, Rosenberg AE, Young RH, Lee KC, Chan JKC. Angiomyofibroblastoma of the vulva and vagina. *Mod Pathol* 1996; **9**: 284–91.

175. Nucci MR, Weremowicz S, Neskey DM *et al.* Chromosomal translocation t(8; 12) induces aberrant HMGIC expression in aggressive angiomyxoma of the vulva. *Genes Chrom Can* 2001; **32**: 172–6.

176. Nucci MR, Tallini G, Quade BJ. HMGIC expression as a diagnostic marker for vulvar aggressive angiomyxoma. *Mod Pathol* 2001; **14**: 829(A).

177. Lloyd J, Flanaghan AM. Mammary and extramammary Paget's disease. *J Clin Pathol* 2000; **53**: 742–9.

178. Goldblum JR, Wart WR. Vulvar Paget's disease: a clinicopathologic and immunohistochemical study of 19 cases. *Am J Surg Pathol* 1997; **21**: 1178–87.

179. Goldblum JR, Hart WR. Perianal Paget's disease – a histologic and immunohistochemical study of 11 cases with and without associated rectal adenocarcinoma. *Am J Surg Pathol* 1998; **2**: 170–9.

180. Crawford D, Nimmo M, Clement PB *et al.* Prognostic factors in Paget's disease of the vulva: a study of 21 cases. *Int J Gynecol Pathol* 1999; **18**: 351–9.

181. Brainard JA, Hart WR. Proliferative epidermal lesions associated with anogenital Paget's disease. *Am J Surg Pathol* 2000; **24**: 543–52.

182. Fox H, Wells M. Recent advances in pathology of the vulva. *Histopathology* 2003; **42**: 209–16.

183. Raju RR, Goldblum JR, Hart WR. Pagetoid squamous cell carcinoma in situ (Pagetoid Bowen's disease) of the external genitalia. *Int J Gynecol Pathol* 2003; **22**: 127–35.

184. Brown HM, Wilkinson EJ. Uroplakin III to distinguish primary vulvar Paget disease from Paget disease secondary to urothelial carcinoma. *Hum Pathol* 2002; **33**: 545–8.

5

The role of the pathologist in the diagnosis of cardiomyopathy: a personal view

Siân E. Hughes

INTRODUCTION

Primary cardiomyopathies are defined as diseases intrinsic to the myocardium associated with cardiac dysfunction leading to congestive heart failure, arrhythmia and sudden cardiac death. The primary cardiomyopathies are classified by their haemodynamic and morphological characteristics and include dilated cardiomyopathy (DCM), hypertrophic cardiomyopathy (HCM), restrictive cardiomyopathy (RCM), arrhythmogenic right ventricular cardiomyopathy (ARVC) and unclassified cardiomyopathy [1], [2]. A familial cause has been shown in patients with DCM, HCM and ARVC. Advances in molecular genetics have led to the identification of single gene defects and candidate disease loci responsible for these cardiomyopathies as well as previously unclassified cardiomyopathies of unknown cause, such as isolated left ventricular non-compaction (LVNC). These advances, coupled with phenotype−genotype correlation analyses, have shown that the pathology of several types of cardiomyopathy encompasses a much broader morphological spectrum than previously anticipated. This chapter will focus on recent advances in our understanding of the pathology of the inherited cardiomyopathies and the role of the pathologist in the diagnosis of cardiomyopathy at autopsy and in endomyocardial biopsy specimens.

DILATED CARDIOMYOPATHY

Idiopathic DCM is the most common cause of congestive heart failure world-wide with an estimated prevalence in a general population of 36.5 cases

101

Progress in Pathology Volume 7, ed. Nigel Kirkham and Neil Shepherd. Published by Cambridge University Press. © Cambridge University Press 2007.

per 100 000 [3]. It is characterised by progressive heart failure due to impaired contraction of the left or both ventricles accompanied by ventricular dilatation. Although the aetiology of idiopathic DCM is largely unknown [4], up to 35% of patients have familial disease [5]. This was demonstrated by detailed pedigree analyses of families of probands with DCM, coupled with the identification of single gene defects in structural proteins of the myocyte cytoskeleton, sarcolemma or nuclear membrane [5]–[7]. Acquired causes of DCM are common and include DCM secondary to ischaemic heart disease, inflammatory myocarditis, nutritional deficiency, cardiotoxins (for example, anthracycline, heavy metals), the puerpurium, excessive alcohol intake and genetic diseases of skeletal muscle (for example, Duchenne's and Becker's muscular dystrophies and myotonic dystrophy).

The mode of inheritance of familial DCM is complex and includes autosomal dominant, X-linked and autosomal recessive forms as well as mitochondrial inheritance through maternal DNA [2], [5], [6], [8], [9]. To date, there is no classification system for familial DCM but distinct clinical phenotypes have emerged [2]. The autosomal dominant forms of familial DCM are the most common and can be categorised as either a pure DCM phenotype with predominantly left ventricular dysfunction, or DCM with early cardiac conduction system disease. The rare X-linked forms of DCM include a rapidly progressive illness in adolescent males and young adults as well as Barth syndrome in male infants [10], [11].

There has been major progress in the identification of candidate chromosomal loci and specific mutations in the genes responsible for the different clinical types of familial DCM. These include mutations in the genes encoding cardiac actin, metavinculin, desmin, δ-sarcoglycan, cardiac troponin T, α-tropomyosin, lamin A/C, dystrophin and tafazzin [2], [6], [12], [13]. For example, four candidate genetic loci have been mapped for autosomal dominant DCM with cardiac conduction system disease [6], [8], [14] and five of 11 families with this clinical phenotype had mutations in the lamin A/C gene [15]. Mutations in the lamin A/C gene also cause autosomal dominant familial DCM with mild skeletal myopathy, as well as the autosomal dominant form of Emery–Dreifuss muscular dystrophy [8], [16]. The latter is associated with the development of joint contractures in childhood and may be inherited as an X-linked disease due to mutations in the protein emerin. Both emerin and lamin A/C are nuclear membrane proteins and, in contrast to the other proteins that cause DCM, do not bind to cytoskeletal proteins and maintain cytoskeletal integrity. The mechanism by which mutations in the lamin A/C gene perturb cardiac function is not known but disruption of nuclear function may cause cell death leading to cardiac disease [2], [15].

The infantile form of X-linked DCM or Barth syndrome typically presents in male infants and is characterised by neutropaenia, lactic acidosis, 3-methylglutaconic aciduria, growth retardation and mitochondrial dysfunction [10]. The cardiac manifestations encompass a diverse morphological spectrum and include left ventricular dilatation, endocardial fibroelastosis or a dilated hypertrophied left ventricle. Some patients with Barth syndrome have also been found to have LVNC. Barth syndrome is caused by mutations in the G4.5 gene. This gene encodes a protein called tafazzin, a putative acyltransferase involved in phospholipid biosynthesis. It has been proposed that defective tafazzin may produce the mitochondrial abnormalities observed in Barth syndrome by interfering with mitochondrial phospholipid metabolism [10], [17]–[20]. Late-onset X-linked DCM is a rare form of DCM occurring in males during adolescence or early adulthood with a rapidly progressive clinical course [11], [21]. Female carriers develop a mild form of DCM with onset in middle age. X-linked DCM is associated with elevated levels of creatine kinase (CK), and skeletal muscle involvement is not a feature. It is caused by mutations in the dystrophin gene [11], [21]. Mutations in the dystrophin gene are also responsible for Duchenne's and Becker's muscular dystrophies, and most patients with these skeletal myopathies will develop cardiac disease at some stage during their lives [5], [22]. The dystrophin gene is located on the X chromosome and encodes a large rod-shaped cytoskeletal protein, which stabilizes the cardiac sarcomere by attaching the actin cytoskeleton via the dystrophin-associated glycoprotein (DAG) complex to laminin-α2 and the extracellular matrix [2].

Pure familial DCM with predominantly left ventricular dysfunction is associated with mutations in multiple genes, including δ-sarcoglycan, cardiac actin, cardiac β-myosin heavy chain and troponin T [23]–[25]. Different mutations in the δ-sarcoglycan gene cause either autosomal recessive limb-girdle muscular dystrophy 2F [26] or autosomal dominant familial DCM, with a high incidence of heart failure and sudden cardiac death but without skeletal myopathy [25]. Recently, it has emerged that different mutations in the same gene can cause either an HCM or DCM phenotype. For example, mutations in troponin T, cardiac β-myosin heavy chain and α-cardiac actin genes can cause either HCM or DCM [23], [24]–[27]. These data imply that the effects of mutant sarcomeric proteins on muscle mechanics may initiate two separate series of events that remodel the heart, culminating in either DCM or HCM [23]. Thus, it appears that different mutations, which either interfere with the generation of force or affect force transmission to surrounding myocytes may cause HCM or DCM, respectively [12], [24].

Irrespective of the underlying cause of DCM the macroscopic and microscopic phenotyopes are similar. DCM is characterised by an increase in myocardial mass and thinning of the left ventricular wall, with an increase in ventricular cavity dimension accompanied by flattening and effacement of the normal trabecular architecture (Fig. 5.1(a)). The heart assumes a globular shape and there is marked ventricular chamber dilatation with diffuse endocardial thickening. The thickening of the endocardium is an adaptive response to the abnormal volume of the ventricle. Mural thrombus is often present and develops around the trabeculae of both the left and right ventricles. Atrial enlargement is invariably present and the atrial appendages usually contain thrombi. The histological changes associated with DCM are frequently non-specific. Not all the features may be present, and diagnosis should therefore be based on the presence of a combination of several macroscopic and microscopic features. Histologically, DCM is characterised by myocyte attenuation and a reduction in myocyte myofibrillary content imparting a vacuolated appearance to myocytes (Fig. 5.1(b)). The myocyte nuclei often show hypertrophy and pleomorphism. Evidence of individual myocyte death can also be observed

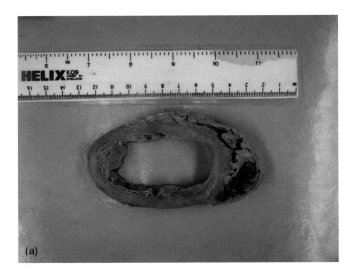

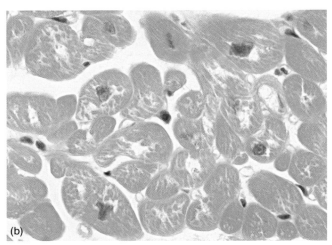

Fig. 5.1 Dilated cardiomyopathy. (a) Macroscopically DCM is characterised by dilatation of the ventricles, frequently with thrombus developing around trabeculae. (b) The histological features of DCM are non-specific. In this case there is striking loss of myofibrils imparting an empty or vacuolated appearance to myocytes.

and there is often an increase in interstitial T-lymphocytes, accompanied by accumulations of macrophages within an empty sarcolemmal sheath. A combination of fine or coarse interstitial fibrosis is usually observed depending on the duration of cardiac disease. From the pathological point of view there are no morphological features of a DCM specific for either the acquired or idiopathic forms of this disease. When index cases of idiopathic DCM are encountered at autopsy, and provided that secondary causes have been excluded, it is advisable for the pathologist to recommend cardiac screening of first-degree relatives due to the familial nature of this disease.

ISOLATED LEFT VENTRICULAR NON-COMPACTION

Isolated left ventricular non-compaction (LVNC) is an uncommon congenital myocardial disorder and was first described over a decade ago [28]. Although this disorder is acquired congenitally, the onset of symptoms is frequently delayed until adulthood [28], [29]. As a consequence, this cardiomyopathy is gaining increased recognition as an important cause of heart failure and its complications in the adult population [28]. For example, in the largest published series of isolated LVNC in adult patients, this condition was diagnosed in 17 of 37,555 echocardiograms, a prevalence of 0.05% [29].

Isolated LVNC occurs due to postnatal persistence of the embryonic pattern of myoarchitecture. It reflects the presence of abundant thread-like trabeculae with deep intertrabecular recesses (Fig. 5.2), which are characteristic of the non-compacted endocardial layer of the early fetal period before compaction is complete [30]. The apical and mid-ventricular portions of both the inferior and lateral wall of the left ventricle are usually affected and the ventricle may be dilated and/or hypertrophied.

The genetic basis for isolated LVNC is currently under investigation. In a recent study of 48 patients with isolated LVNC, a mutation in the gene G4.5 was identified in only one patient. No mutations in other genes (α-dystrobrevin, FK binding-protein 12) associated with LVNC were identified, indicating genetic heterogeneity for this disorder [31]. Undoubtedly, increased awareness of the pathological phenotype and advances in the molecular genetics of isolated LVNC will improve the diagnosis of this rare condition and facilitate its recognition as a unique cardiomyopathy.

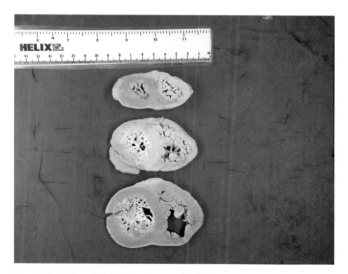

Fig. 5.2 Isolated LVNC is characterised by non-compaction of the endocardial layer of the left ventricle. The simple trabecular architecture of the normal ventricle is replaced by numerous, thread-like trabeculations with deep intertrabecular recesses extending into the hypertrophied compacted myocardial layer.

HYPERTROPHIC CARDIOMYOPATHY

Familial HCM is a common autosomal dominant genetic disorder affecting 1 in 500 of the population [32], [33] and an important cause of sudden unexpected cardiac death in the young. HCM is a disease of the cardiac contractile apparatus [34] and is caused by mutations in the genes encoding sarcomeric proteins, including cardiac β-myosin heavy chain, α-myosin heavy chain, cardiac regulatory and essential myosin light chains, myosin binding protein-C, α-cardiac actin, cardiac troponin T, cardiac troponin I, α-tropomyosin and titin [2], [6], [35], [36]. Most mutations in the sarcomeric protein genes are single-point missense mutations or small deletions or insertions [36]. The most common causes of familial HCM can be ascribed to mutations in the genes encoding cardiac β-myosin heavy chain (30%), cardiac troponin T (15%), myosin binding protein-C (20%) and α-tropomyosin (3%) [2], [35], [37].

Recently, mutations in the PRKAG2 gene, which encodes the γ2 subunit of AMP-activated-protein kinase (AMPK), have been found to cause HCM with Wolff−Parkinson−White syndrome [38]. When AMPK is activated it protects the cell from ATP depletion during hypoxic stress or increased metabolic demand. Since mutations in the known contractile protein genes are not found in up to one-third of cases of familial HCM, genes encoding proteins involved in energy homeostasis in the myocyte may account for the remaining cases. Blair *et al.* propose that energy compromise within the myocyte itself is the unifying pathogenic mechanism in all forms of HCM [38]. This view is further reinforced by biochemical and biophysical data, which show that there is no unifying abnormality of cardiac contractility due to different mutations in the sarcomeric protein genes, but all types of HCM-causing mutation share the common feature of inefficient utilization of ATP [38]. Similarly, in mitochondrial cardiomyopathy, mutations in the mitochondrial tRNA(Lys) gene (G8363A) involved in energy production, lead to HCM associated with sensorineural hearing loss and encephalomyopathy, as a consequence of altered energy production in organs with a high oxidative metabolism [39].

Genotype−phenotype correlation analyses have provided important insights into the clinical spectrum of HCM. For each gene many different mutations have been identified, and specific mutations in the same or different genes are associated with different disease severity and prognosis. For example, mutations in the troponin-T gene cause only mild or absent hypertrophy, yet are associated with a poor prognosis and a high risk of sudden cardiac death. In contrast, mutations in myosin binding protein-C gene are, in general, associated with a benign clinical course with late-onset. Similarly, genotype−phenotype correlation studies have led to the discovery of malignant mutations in the cardiac β-myosin heavy chain gene (Arg403Gln, Arg453Gln, Arg719Trp), which cause a severe form of HCM with early onset, complete penetrance and high risk of sudden cardiac death. Conversely, other mutations (Leu908Val, and Val606Met) are associated with an intermediate or a benign clinical course and a near-normal life expectancy [37], [40]−[43]. HCM also exhibits intra-familial phenotypic variation, whereby affected individuals from the same family with the same mutation exhibit unique clinical and morphological phenotypes [44]. This implies that lifestyle factors such as exercise and/or modifier genes, such as polymorphisms of the angiotensin converting enzyme (ACE) gene are likely to influence the hypertrophic response and incidence of sudden cardiac death [35], [45], [46].

Familial HCM is characterised macroscopically by unexplained left ventricular hypertrophy, which may be asymmetrical or symmetrical [47], [48]. The classical asymmetrical form of HCM was described by Donald Teare in 1958, and is characterised by hypertrophy of the basal anterior septum, which protrudes beneath the aortic valve causing sub-aortic obstruction [49]. This is accompanied by systolic anterior motion of the mitral valve, leading to endocardial fibrosis over the septum and formation of a sub-aortic mitral impact lesion. In the past, the sub-aortic mitral impact lesion has traditionally been regarded as pathognomonic of HCM [47], but this lesion may be observed in hypertrophied hearts due to hypertension, aortic stenosis and prominence of the basal septum in the hearts of elderly individuals (so-called 'sigmoid' septum) [48]. The symmetrical or diffuse form of HCM accounts for over one-third of cases, and is characterised by concentric thickening of the left ventricle with a small ventricular cavity dimension [47]. This variant is indistinguishable from cardiac hypertrophy due to hypertensive heart disease and aortic stenosis. As a consequence, a diagnosis of HCM should be deferred at autopsy until histological confirmation is obtained [48]. The right ventricle may also be involved in HCM but right ventricular hypertrophy without left ventricular involvement is not usually seen.

HCM may involve any portion of the left ventricle producing a diverse morphological spectrum. An unusual form of HCM with mid-ventricular cavity obstruction has been described, which is caused by hypertrophy of the mid-ventricular septum and papillary muscles [50]–[52]. This pattern of hypertrophy has been identified in families with both dominant [53] and recessive HCM [54] and is due to mutations in the gene encoding the essential light chain of myosin. HCM may also exclusively involve the apex of the heart [50], [55]–[57]. The apical variant was first recognised in Japan in the 1970s and occurs in up to 25% of Japanese people with HCM [58], [59]. It may also occur in Western populations but is less prevalent [58], [60], [61]. With disease duration, familial HCM may also evolve to a dilated or 'burnt-out' phase in approximately 10–15% of patients and be indistinguishable from DCM [32], [62], [63].

The principal histological hallmarks for the diagnosis of HCM are the triad of myocyte hypertrophy, disarray and interstitial fibrosis [47], [48]. Myocyte disarray occurs due to the loss of the normal parallel arrangement of myocytes. Bizarrely shaped and hypertrophied myocytes are aligned in either a 'cartwheel' (Fig. 5.3(a)) or 'herringbone' (Fig. 5.3(b)) pattern due to aberrant cell-to-cell connections around cores of collagen [47], [64]–[66]. These different histological patterns of myocyte disarray have no prognostic relevance. The myocyte nuclei are also abnormal and show nuclear hypertrophy, pleomorphism and hyperchromasia (Fig. 5.3(c)). Within the myocyte itself there is disorganisation of the myofibrillary architecture with criss-crossing of the myofibrils, which may be accentuated by a phosphotungstic acid–haematoxylin stain.

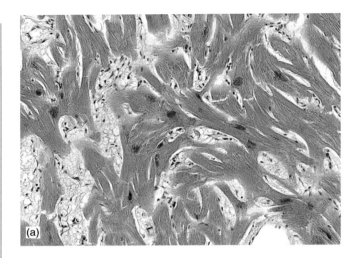

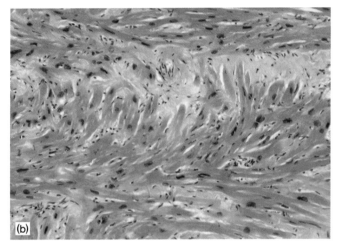

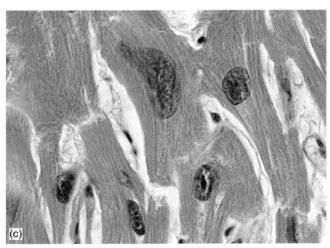

HCM is also characterised by expansion of interstitial collagen, and the fibrosis may be pericellular, patchy or coarse and can even be so extensive it may mask the disarray [67]. The small intramural coronary arteries are also abnormal in HCM and have narrow lumens due to wall thickening secondary to medial hypertrophy [68]–[70]. Small vessel disease may contribute to perfusion abnormalities and myocardial ischaemia in HCM [71] as well as replacement-type fibrosis and the DCM-like variant of HCM [70]–[72]. Pathological evidence of chronic, acute and sub-acute ischaemic damage has been documented in the hearts of a series of 19 young patients with HCM [73]. It has been proposed that the combination of myocyte disarray and/or ischaemic damage may serve as substrates for life-threatening electrical instability leading to sudden cardiac death [73].

Unfortunately, the diagnosis of HCM is not always straightforward. Myocyte disarray occurs in congenital heart disease as well as in the normal adult heart, and in isolation is not pathognomonic of HCM [74], [75]. Myocyte disarray may also be observed in the hearts of individuals with Noonan syndrome and Friedreich's ataxia [76], [77]. Noonan syndrome is caused by mutations in the gene encoding the non-receptor protein tyrosine phosphatase SHP-2 protein (PTPN11) [78]. The causative mutation in Friedreich's ataxia consists of a trinucleotide (GAA) repeat expansion in the first intron of the X25 gene encoding the mitochondrial protein frataxin, which is involved in mitochondrial iron metabolism [79]. Furthermore, in the normal adult heart, disarray may be encountered where the right ventricle interdigitates with the septum, at trabeculations, in association with areas of fibrosis, in the vicinity of blood vessels and at points of convergence of large muscle bundles. However, in these contexts, myocyte disarray is usually mild in extent [65], [80]. In most cases of HCM, provided that sufficient ventricular myocardium has been sampled, more than 20% of myocardium will exhibit disarray in at least two tissue blocks. Therefore, the detection of widespread myocyte disarray can serve as both a highly sensitive and a highly specific marker for the diagnosis of HCM [65], [66], [81].

The importance of adequate myocardial sampling at autopsy for the diagnosis of HCM cannot be overemphasised. Myocyte disarray is regional, and the disorganised myocardial architecture is not necessarily confined to those regions of the left ventricle showing maximal hypertrophy. It is advisable to sample an entire circumferential transverse slice of the heart at mid-septal level for histological examination. It is also prudent to avoid sampling the site where the right ventricle interdigitates with the interventricular septum, because myocardial disarray occurs at this region in the normal adult heart and is not indicative of HCM. Misinterpretation of junctional myocardium is a common diagnostic pitfall and may lead to an erroneous diagnosis of familial HCM.

Fig. 5.3 Hypertrophic cardiomyopathy. Myocyte disarray in HCM is characterised by hypertrophied myocytes arranged obliquely and perpendicularly with abnormal cell-to-cell connections around cores of loose connective tissue in either (a) a 'cartwheel' or (b) a 'herringbone' pattern. (c) The nuclei exhibit hypertrophy, hyperchromasia and abnormal nuclear contours. Within individual myocytes there is crisscrossing and loss of the usual parallel structure of the myofibrillar architecture.

Another area of potential diagnostic difficulty is for the pathologist to be aware that a diagnosis of HCM is not necessarily synonymous with cardiac hypertrophy. In adults, the heart may show only mild or no hypertrophy with mutations due to troponin T. Similarly, in HCM the heart tends to become structurally abnormal during the adolescent growth spurt and hypertrophy may not be evident in children. In both situations, extensive myocyte disarray is usually apparent histologically despite the absence of obvious cardiac hypertrophy. In these macroscopically 'normal' hearts, if sufficient myocardium is sampled at autopsy, it is usually possible to exclude or confirm the presence of disarray.

ARRHYTHMOGENIC RIGHT VENTRICULAR CARDIOMYOPATHY

ARVC is a disease predominantly of the right ventricular myocardium, characterised pathologically by progressive myocyte loss with fibrofatty replacement and clinically by life-threatening ventricular arrhythmias arising in either ventricle. The exact incidence and prevalence of ARVC in the general population is still unknown, but it may be the second most common cause of sudden unexpected cardiac death in previously healthy young individuals. There are several concepts surrounding the pathobiology of ARVC. These include the progressive loss of myocytes as either a consequence of programmed cell death (apoptosis) following myocyte injury or a late sequela of viral myocarditis. Apoptosis of myocytes has been detected in endomyocardial biopsy specimens and autopsy myocardium of patients with ARVC using the TUNEL technique [82], [83]. In a study by Bowles *et al.*, cardiotropic viruses (enteroviruses and adenoviruses) were identified as potential aetiologic agents in the hearts of patients with ARVC and may account for sporadic cases of this disease [84]. Clearly, it remains to be established whether viral infection is a primary event or whether the diseased myocardium is more susceptible to infection. Transdifferentiation of myocytes to mature adipocytes has also been proposed as an alternative pathogenetic mechanism in ARVC [85].

Importantly, most cases of ARVC are strongly familial and this suggests that progressive myocyte loss and atrophy may be genetically determined [86]–[88]. Genetic studies of families affected by ARVC indicate a predominantly autosomal dominant mode of inheritance with incomplete penetrance [86], [87]. Gene linkage analysis of large families affected by ARVC has revealed multiple chromosomal loci, indicating genetic heterogeneity for this disease [89], [90]. This is supported by the recent identification of mutations in both cell adhesion proteins [90]–[92] and the cardiac ryanodine receptor gene on chromosome 1q42–43 [93]. The cardiac ryanodine receptor encodes a protein (RYR2) involved in intracellular calcium homeostasis and excitation–contraction coupling in cardiac muscle. This receptor has been implicated in the onset of polymorphic ventricular arrhythmias, either in patients with a structurally normal heart or with a mild form of ARVC (ARVD2) with segmental right ventricular involvement localised to the apex [89], [93]–[97].

Several autosomal recessive variants of ARVC have been described in the literature [91], [92]. These include Naxos disease, a form of ARVC associated with palmoplantar keratoderma and woolly hair and a severe clinical course of the disease [91], [98]. This form of ARVC is due to a two-base pair deletion in the plakoglobin gene on chromosome 17, the product of which, plakoglobin, is a component of desmosomes and adherens junctions [91], [98]. Another familial syndrome of autosomal recessive ARVC due to a mutation in desmoplakin has been described in a family of Muslim-Arab origin from Israel with ARVC, pemphigus-like skin disorder and woolly hair [92]. Similarly, mutations in the desmoplakin gene (ARVD8) have recently been identified, which cause a dominant form of ARVC without skin disease [90].

Both plakoglobin and desmoplakin are integral components of adherens junctions and desmosomes. Desmosomes and adherens junctions are cell–cell adhesion complexes that work with each other to hold epithelial cells and myocytes together, and are required for maintaining the mechanical integrity of the heart and skin [91]. Desmosomes link the intermediate filament networks of neighbouring cells to the cell membrane and maintain tissue architecture. Adherens junctions, which contain classical cadherins and catenins, link the intercalated disc to cytoplasmic actin filaments and are responsible for mechanically coupling myocytes.

Irrespective of the mode of inheritance of ARVC, the identification of mutations in the cell adhesion proteins – plakoglobin and desmoplakin – favours the current working hypothesis that ARVC is a genetic disease of cell adhesion [99]. It is likely that structural abnormalities of the cell adhesion complex lead to myocyte detachment and cell death under conditions of mechanical stress. It is noteworthy that mechanical stress activates stretch-sensitive calcium permeable channels within the adherens junction [100] and also modulates calcium release from ryanodine receptor channels [101]. This provides a unifying hypothesis that impaired calcium homeostasis, due to either defective cellular junctions or receptors modulating calcium release, might trigger cell death in the different genetic forms of ARVC [90]. Repair by fibroadipose replacement occurs as a response to disruption of myocyte integrity and cell death, providing the anatomical substrate for both progressive cardiac failure and electrical instability and arrhythmias, which characterise this disease. Defective cell adhesion may also serve as a common pathogenetic mechanism underlying other familial cardiomyopathies. For example, a recessive mutation in desmoplakin causes another familial syndrome of DCM, woolly hair and a striate form of palmoplantar keratoderma. This cardiocutaneous syndrome has been identified in three families from Equador (Carvajal syndrome) [102]. In contrast to ARVC, the hearts in Carvajal syndrome lack fibrofatty infiltration or replacement of myocardium [103].

A spectrum of morphological abnormalities occurs in ARVC, ranging from an extreme phenotype characterised by diffuse dilatation of the entire right ventricle to localised aneurysms or segmental areas of wall thinning [104], which correspond to the stage of the disease. The first stage of ARVC is concealed but patients are at high risk of arrhythmic events during physical activity and sudden cardiac death. This phenotype is commonly encountered at autopsy but may be difficult to detect macroscopically in cases of sudden cardiac death [105]. The wall aneurysms or segmental areas of thinning are subtle and tend to occur in the apical, sub-tricuspid and pulmonary outflow tract regions of the right ventricle – the so-called 'triangle of dysplasia' [104], [106]–[108]. The second stage or overt electrical phase of ARVC is characterised by symptomatic ventricular arrhythmias, and is usually accompanied by obvious structural and functional abnormalities of the right ventricle. ARVC is a progressive disease, and the third phase is characterised by diffuse involvement of the right ventricle leading to right ventricular failure but with preserved left ventricular function. With disease progression there is concomitant involvement of the left ventricle. This is initially manifest as sub-epicardial posterior wall fibrosis, but with disease duration there is more extensive left ventricular involvement, culminating in an advanced stage of disease characterised by biventricular cardiomyopathy and heart failure, which may be difficult to distinguish from DCM [105], [108]–[111].

Microscopically ARVC is characterised by fibroadipose replacement, which commences from the epicardium to the endocardium in a wave-front phenomenon leading to transmural or sub-epicardial lesions (Fig. 5.4(a)). This is accompanied by myocyte atrophy and progessive myocyte loss with a segmental or diffuse distribution. Strands and islands of residual myocytes are surrounded by fibroadipose tissue (Fig. 5.4(b)). The surviving myocytes exhibit a combination of degenerative change with myocyte vacuolisation and are frequently associated with focal T-lymphocyte cell infiltrates in two thirds of cases [107], [112], [113].

Two morphological variants of ARVC have been described in the literature. These include a predominantly 'fatty' variant and a 'fibrofatty' or 'cardiomyopathic' variant [106], [107], [112]. Unfortunately, this has led to confusion amongst pathologists and a lack of a consensus concerning the pathological criteria required to fulfill the diagnosis of ARVC. The 'fatty' variant is confined to the right ventricle and is characterised by transmural infiltration of adipose tissue with a lace-like pattern of infiltration. There is sparing of the interventricular septum and left ventricle, and wall thinning is not a feature [86], [107], [112]. In contrast, the 'fibrofatty' or 'cardiomyopathic' variant is characterised by extensive replacement-type fibrosis involving the right or both ventricles [112], [113]. Several authors have challenged whether the 'fatty' variant of ARVC really exists and have proposed that the 'fatty' variant of ARVC may represent the extreme end of the normal spectrum of adipose infiltration of the right ventricle, which is observed with increasing age and body mass index [113]–[115]. Indeed, fat is a striking feature in the sub-epicardial and mediomural layer in hearts of elderly women and obese individuals. In the hearts of elderly women the right ventricular myocardium may be reduced to a thinned residual layer (Fig. 5.5(a)), accompanied by extensive fatty infiltration of the right ventricular myocardium, which is composed of residual strands of myocytes lacking fibrosis (Fig. 5.5(b),(c)). Furthermore, a retrospective study of 148 specimens of non-ischaemic causes of death (81 men and 67 women; mean age, 66 and 74 years old, respectively), demonstrated that fat with strands of myocytes was observed in 60% of cases in the subepicardial and mediomural layers of the right ventricle, irrespective of age or sex [114]. Furthermore, fibroadipose infiltration varies according to the site sampled and is far more

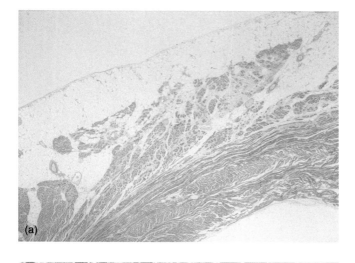

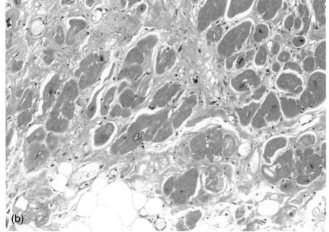

Fig. 5.4 ARVC. (a) Free wall of the right ventricle showing partial fibroadipose replacement of the myocardium ('fibrofatty' or 'cardiomyopathic' variant) in the subepicardial region. The fibroadipose replacement is advancing from the epicardium to the endocardium in a wave-front pattern. The subepicardial distribution pattern is typical of ARVC. (b) At higher magnification strands and clusters of myocytes are entrapped by fibroadipose tissue.

pronounced in the sub-tricuspid region compared with the pulmonary outflow tract. Therefore, the site of sampling of the right ventricle is critical. For example, significant fatty infiltration of the heart may be observed in the anteroapical region of the right ventricle of normal hearts, but a 15% fat replacement should be regarded as abnormal when observed in the right ventricular outflow tract [113]. It is therefore essential to adequately sample the right ventricle, and record the site from which blocks are taken, to avoid misinterpreting the significance of fatty infiltration at these sites. At autopsy the right ventricle can also be transilluminated to facilitate the detection of ARVC.

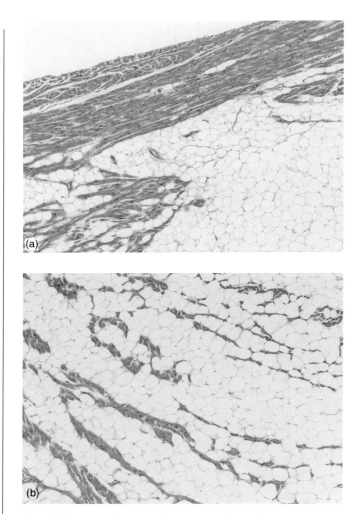

Fig. 5.5 Adipose infiltration of right ventricle. Adipose replacement is a striking feature in the sub-epicardial and mediomural layer in the hearts of elderly women and obese individuals. (a) In the heart of this elderly lady the right ventricular myocardium is reduced to a thinned residual subendocardial layer. (b) The adipose infiltration is lace-like but in contrast to 'fibrofatty' or 'cardiomyopathic' ARVC the myocytes are (c) not surrounded by fibrous tissue, which has been confirmed by a trichrome stain. Several authors have challenged whether the 'fatty' variant of ARVC really exists and have proposed that it may represent the extreme end of the normal spectrum of adipose infiltration of the right ventricle, which is observed with increasing age and body mass index.

Undoubtedly, future genetic studies will resolve the controversy surrounding the different morphological variants of ARVC, but until this issue is clarified, pathologists should exercise a degree of caution in their analysis of fatty infiltration of right ventricular myocardium when considering the diagnosis of ARVC. Indeed, Fontaliran *et al.* advocate that only the presence of fibrosis bordering or embedding surviving myocytes surrounded by fat is diagnostic of ARVC [114] and I also share this view.

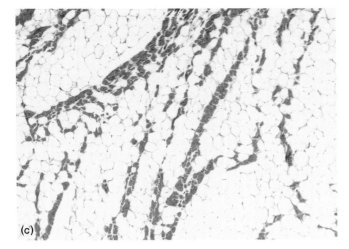

Fig. 5.5 (*cont.*)

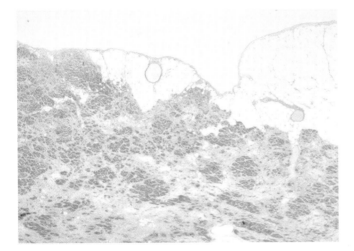

Fig. 5.6 Free wall of the left ventricle showing extensive fibroadipose replacement of myocytes in the subepicardial zone. This appearance is typical of ALVC, which can occur with or without involvement of the right ventricle.

Although ARVC is usually regarded as a disorder predominantly affecting the right ventricle, an unusual phenotype of ARVC characterised by isolated subepicardial and mediomural fibrofatty replacement confined to the left ventricular myocardium (arrhythmogenic left ventricular cardiomyopathy, ALVC) has been described in the literature [109], [110], [116]–[119]. I have observed ALVC in several cases of sudden unexpected cardiac death in previously healthy young individuals (Fig. 5.6). It is likely that ALVC is part of the ARVC spectrum rather than a distinct entity, because left ventricular sub-epicardial myocardial lesions are rare in other cardiac diseases [120] but common in ARVC. Despite extensive disease involvement of the left ventricle these patients lack congestive heart failure and their disease is concealed during life. Moreover, cases previously described as idiopathic myocardial fibrosis may well represent the ALVC spectrum. Indeed, it is my view that idiopathic myocardial fibrosis and ALVC are different terminologies describing an identical disease process. The increased recognition of the ALVC phenotype suggests that the presence of extensive left ventricular involvement is not necessarily synonymous with a final or advanced stage of ARVC, and that the phenotypic spectrum and natural history of ARVC is more complex than previously realised [105]. In accordance with Gallo et al., due to the isolated left ventricular or biventricular involvement observed with ARVC, the term 'arrhythmogenic cardiomyopathy' would more accurately reflect the different pathological variants and simplify classification of this cardiomyopathy [99], [109].

RESTRICTIVE CARDIOMYOPATHY

RCM is the least common type of primary cardiomyopathy [1] and may be classified as primary or secondary. RCM is caused by myocardial or endomyocardial diseases, which 'stiffen' the heart by infiltration or fibrosis [121]–[123]. Haemodynamically, RCM is characterised by restrictive filling and reduced diastolic volume of either or both ventricles, with relatively preserved systolic function in the early stage of disease. The ventricular wall thickness may be normal or increased, depending on the underlying aetiology of the disease.

The primary restrictive cardiomyopathies include tropical endomyocardial fibrosis (EMF), Loeffler's endocarditis and idiopathic RCM, and are less common than the secondary forms. Idiopathic RCM may occur sporadically or can occur in families where it is inherited as an autosomal dominant trait with distal skeletal myopathy and heart block. Idiopathic RCM is characterised by a lack of specific pathology in either endomyocardial biopsy or autopsy specimens. It is a non-infiltrative form of RCM, with the only detectable histological abnormality being interstitial fibrosis of the myocardium with mild-to-moderate hypertrophy [121], [122], [124], [125]. Benotti et al. were the first to describe idiopathic RCM and the diagnosis can be made by finding a characteristic 'dip and plateau' haemodynamic filling pattern [126]. Another autosomal dominant form of RCM associated with a non-hypertrophic variant of Noonan syndrome has also been described [127]. Similarly, a subset of patients with familial HCM due to troponin I mutations can also present primarily with restrictive haemodynamics [128].

EMF (Davies disease) is a restrictive obliterative cardiomyopathy and is endemic to tropical and subtropical Africa [129], [130]. EMF is an indolent disease but is a common cause of heart failure and death in young patients in endemic regions, where it is associated with mild eosinophilia [131], [132]. It is characterised by a fibrotic thickened endocardium and mural thrombi in the apices of both ventricles with partial cavity obliteration. The fibrosis involves the posterior mitral valve and encases the papillary muscles of the tricuspid valve leading to mitral and tricuspid regurgitation. Microscopically, there is a thick layer of acellular hyalinised collagen in the endocardium and granulation tissue involving the myocardium [133]. Overall, EMF carries a poor prognosis, but surgical excision of the fibrous endocardium and replacement of the mitral and tricuspid valves can ameliorate symptoms [134], [135].

Loeffler's endocarditis is an uncommon rapidly progressive disease, which tends to affect males and occurs in temperate climates. It is related to hypereosinophilic states, including idiopathic hypereosinophilic syndrome, eosinophilic leukaemia and Churg–Strauss syndrome. The initial stages of the disease are characterised by an acute inflammatory myocarditis involving the endocardium and myocardium. This is followed by the formation of thrombus over the endocardium, which is infiltrated by eosinophils. The advanced stage or fibrotic phase is identical to tropical EMF and there is extensive fibrosis of the endocardium and chronic inflammation.

Both tropical EMF and Loeffler's endocarditis share similar cardiac pathologies in advanced disease [129]. Consequently, there is general agreement that both disorders represent a continuum, whereby Loeffler's endocarditis and tropical EMF are manifestations of the same disease process but at different stages [136]–[138]. The eosinophil is central to the pathogenesis of Loeffler's endocarditis and tropical EMF, where tissue damage to the endocardium and myocardium occurs due to eosinophilic infiltration and degranulation leading to the release of toxic major basic and cationic proteins [131], [138]–[141]. Compared with its temperate zone counterpart, the more indolent course of tropical EMF may be related to the less marked eosinophilia observed with parasitic infections [136], [138].

The secondary forms of RCM are common and include the specific heart muscle diseases in which the heart is affected as part of a multisystem disorder. These can be sub-classified as either non-infiltrative or infiltrative. In RCM due to infiltrative interstitial conditions, the infiltrates localise between myocytes, whereas in infiltrative conditions due to storage disorders the deposits are found within myocytes [121]. Diseases causing secondary RCM due to interstitial infiltration include amyloidosis and cardiac sarcoidosis. Less common disorders of interstitial infiltration include Gaucher's disease, Hurler's syndrome and metastatic malignancy. Leukaemia, lymphoma, malignant melanoma, lung and breast carcinoma are the most common metastatic tumours to involve the heart [123], [142]. Infiltrative conditions of storage with myocardial involvement include haemochromatosis, glycogen storage disease and Fabry's disease. The non-infiltrative secondary causes of RCM include carcinoid heart disease and iatrogenic disease. For example, RCM may develop following radiotherapy to the mediastinum or following treatment with anthracycline [121]. In the latter conditions restrictive dynamics occur as a consequence of fibrosis.

Cardiac amyloidosis is the prototypical infiltrative secondary RCM [143] and is caused by the deposition of insoluble amyloid protein fibrils in the interstitium of the myocardium or walls of blood vessels and may be acquired or hereditary. Cardiac amyloidosis may be classified according to the type of fibril protein deposited. The most common type of amyloidosis to affect the heart is primary systemic amyloidosis (AL amyloidosis), which is due to the deposition of monoclonal kappa and lambda immunoglobulin light chains.

It is associated with plasma cell dyscrasias and multiple myeloma. Cardiac involvement is common and death due to congestive heart failure or arrhythmias occurs in more than 50% of patients with AL amyloidosis [144].

Senile cardiac amyloidosis affects more than 25% of the elderly population over the age of 80 and is a common incidental finding at autopsy [144]–[146]. It is caused by the deposition of unmutated or wild-type transthyretin (TTR) [145] in the heart. This form of cardiac amyloidosis tends to run a benign clinical course and is not associated with extracardiac manifestations [144]. However, some elderly male patients may have extensive amyloid deposits in the atria, ventricles or heart valves, producing congestive heart failure and eventual death [145]–[147].

Hereditary or familial amyloidosis is uncommon, but its recognition has important implications for patient management and genetic counselling. It is due to the deposition of mutant TTR, apoprotein AI (ApoAI) [148], [149] and apoprotein AII (ApoAII) [150]. TTR-related amyloidosis may occur sporadically but is usually inherited as an autosomal dominant trait. More than 50 mutations in the TTR gene have been described [151] and the clinical phenotype is variable depending on the type of TTR mutation. For example, peripheral and autonomic neuropathy (familial amyloid polyneuropathy, FAP) is associated with TTRMet30 mutations, [145], [152]–[154] whereas with TTRThr45, TTRMet111 and TTRLys92 mutations cardiac disease predominates [152], [155], [156].

Macroscopically, cardiac amyloidosis presents with biatrial dilatation and the ventricular wall may be of normal size or hypertrophied and simulate HCM [157]. The myocardium has a waxy appearance and a rubbery consistency (Fig. 5.7(a)). Focal nodular thickening of the valves may also occur. Microscopically there are interstitial infiltrates of eosinophilic material surrounding individual myocytes (Fig. 5.7(b)). Within the media and adventitia of the coronary vessels amyloid deposits may be observed (Fig. 5.7(c)), which may cause luminal narrowing and angina pectoris-like pain [157], [158]. Amyloid deposition occurs in the endocardium, myocardium and pericardium, and the pattern of deposition can be classified as nodular, perifibre or mixed type with or without vascular involvement. The disease extent can be graded semi-quantitatively as 1 through to 4, corresponding to less than 10%, 10–25%, 25–50% and more than 50% respectively [159]. The eosinophilic deposits display apple-green birefringence when viewed using polarised light. Further diagnostic confirmation can be obtained using immunocytochemistry and/or electron microscopy. The latter reveals the presence of linear non-branching fibrils with a diameter of 7.5 to 10 nm externally coating myocytes (Fig. 5.7(d)).

Cardiac sarcoidosis is a systemic non-caseating granulomatous disorder of unknown aetiology, which often involves the heart [160]. The granulomas are typically found in the left ventricular free wall and base of the interventricular septum, but involvement of the papillary muscles, atria and pericardium can also occur. Involvement of the cardiac conduction system is common, and arrhythmias and conduction disorders, such as heart block, may dominate the clinical picture [161]. The macroscopic and microscopic phenotype is variable, ranging from obvious massive replacement of the myocardium by coalescent granulomas to microscopic granulomas [162]. The granulomas are composed of epithelioid histiocytes with multinucleated giant cells surrounded by lymphocytes (Fig. 5.8), which over time become fibrotic [160]. The fibrotic response is responsible for irreversible organ destruction and dysfunction. The complications of cardiac sarcoidosis disease include sudden cardiac death, arrhythmias, conduction defects and heart failure. Patients with heart failure may show clinical features of either an RCM- and/or a DCM-type picture. However, sarcoid granulomas are often clinically silent and may be

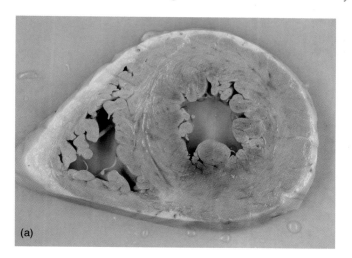

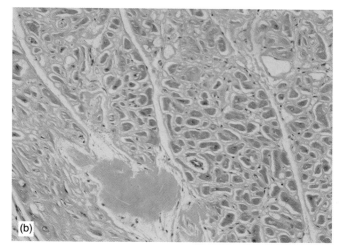

Fig. 5.7 Cardiac amyloidosis. (a) Macroscopically cardiac amyloidosis presents with biatrial dilatation and the ventricular wall may be of normal size, or hypertrophied and simulate HCM. The myocardium has a waxy appearance and a rubbery consistency. (b) In sections stained with H&E the amyloid is pale pink with a glassy appearance and surrounds individual myocytes. Large nodular eosinophilic deposits are present within the cardiac interstitium and (c) there is concomitant vascular involvement. (d) Electron microscopy can be used to confirm the diagnosis of amyloidosis. Ultrastructurally, there is fine fibrillar material coating the external surface of myocytes. The amyloid fibrils have a diameter of 7.5–10 nm. This case of extensive cardiac amylodosis was from a patient with AL amyloidosis who died from congestive heart failure.

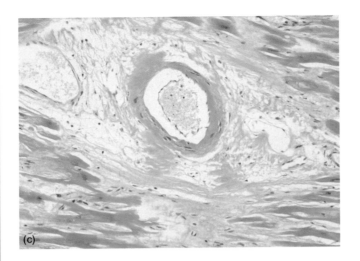

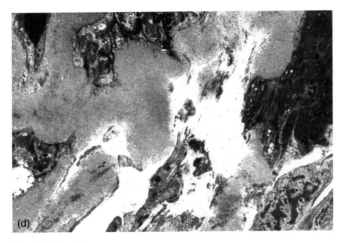

Fig. 5.7 (*cont.*)

incidentally found in the myocardium of up to 25% of patients at autopsy [162], [163].

Infiltrative cardiomyopathies causing secondary RCM include storage disorders, such as haemochromatosis, glycogen storage disease and Fabry's disease, where the deposits occur within myocytes. Haemochromatosis is an iron-storage disorder [164] and may be primary or secondary. Primary or hereditary haemochromatosis is generally inherited as an autosomal recessive disease and corresponds to multiple genetic abnormalities of iron metabolism [165]. Secondary haemochromatosis occurs due to excessive iron intake, following multiple blood transfusions or in abnormalities of haemoglobin synthesis leading to aberrant erythropoiesis. With both the primary and secondary forms there is iron deposition in multiple organs including the heart. The 'iron heart' is typically dilated with normal or increased wall thickness, and iron deposition

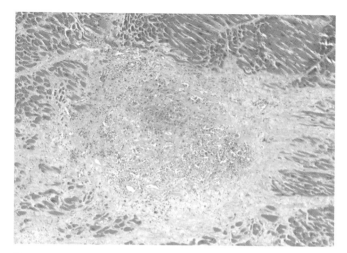

Fig. 5.8 Myocardial sarcoidosis. The granuloma is composed of epithelioid histiocytes and giant cells surrounded by a rim of lymphocytes. The granulomas typically lack necrosis. This sarcoid granuloma was an incidental finding at autopsy.

occurs within the myocyte sarcoplasm in the atria, ventricles and conduction system [166], [167].

Glycogen storage disease and Fabry's disease are autosomal recessive disorders of carbohydrate and glycolipid metabolism, respectively. Both disorders may cause RCM and are important causes of unexplained left ventricular hypertrophy. In glycogen storage disease there is deposition of glycogen in the heart and skeletal muscle. Fabry's disease is another metabolic storage disorder, whereby neutral glycosphingolipids accumulate within myocytes, and will be discussed in detail elsewhere in this chapter.

ROLE OF ENDOMYOCARDIAL BIOPSY IN THE DIAGNOSIS OF CARDIOMYOPATHY

The value of endomyocardial biopsy for the diagnosis of cardiomyopathy, especially ARVC and HCM is controversial [168]–[170]. Endomyocardial biopsy specimens usually sample the subendocardial region of the right interventricular septum, a site that is often spared in several types of cardiomyopathy. In endomyocardial biopsy specimens taken for the diagnosis of HCM, disarray is present in only one-third of these specimens, and, because of their small size and relatively non-specific pathological changes, they may be used to suggest rather than confirm a diagnosis of HCM [169], [170]. The false-negative rate of biopsies may also be high due to sampling error. Therefore, it is prudent to interpret the presence or absence of myocyte disarray in ventricular endomyocardial biopsies with caution and report the biopsy findings within the context of clinical and echocardiographic information. Although not too much emphasis should be placed on disarray in endomyocardial biopsies as a

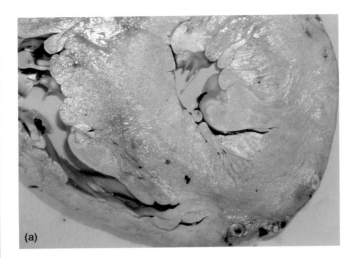

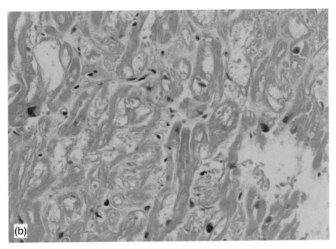

Fig. 5.9 Fabry's disease. (a) Macroscopically cardiac Fabry's disease is characterised by concentric left ventricular hypertrophy and echocardiographically simulates HCM. (b) In this endomyocardial biopsy specimen stained with H&E, the myocytes show variation in fibre size and there is prominent myocyte sarcoplasmic vacuolisation, with nuclear hypertrophy and disruption of the myofibrillary architecture. These features are not always present and evaluation of myocardium by electron microscopy is mandatory in cases of unexplained left ventricular hypertrophy to confirm or exclude the diagnosis. (c) Electron microscopy reveals the presence of concentric lamellar bodies (myelin figures) within the myocyte sarcoplasm consistent with the cardiac variant of Fabry's disease.

diagnostic criterion for HCM, they are important to confirm or exclude other diseases, which cause unexplained left ventricular hypertrophy and may mimic HCM. These include cardiac Fabry's disease, amyloidosis, mitochondrial cardiomyopathy and glycogen storage disease.

Fabry's disease is an X-linked autosomal recessive metabolic storage disorder, due to deficiency of the enzyme lysosomal α-galactosidase A [171]. This leads to the widespread accumulation of neutral glycosphingolipid in multiple organs

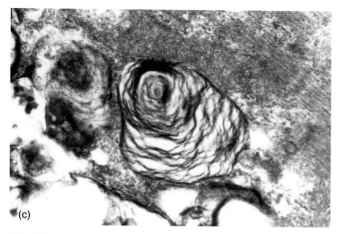

Fig. 5.9 (*cont.*)

and leads to angiokeratomas, corneal opacities and peripheral and central CNS disorders. Recently, an atypical variant of Fabry's disease has been described with late-onset. This variant predominantly affects the heart without multi-organ involvement. The prevalence of cardiac Fabry's disease was found to be between 4% and 6% of all male patients attending a tertiary referral centre for evaluation of HCM [172]. Concentric ventricular hypertrophy is the most common pattern of hypertrophy in Fabry's disease (Fig. 5.9(a)) but asymmetrical hypertrophy may also occur [171]. In endomyocardial biopsies, the histology of the myocardium in H&E stained sections shows prominent myocyte sarcoplasmic vacuolisation with nuclear hypertrophy and disruption of the myofibrillary architecture (Fig. 5.9(b)). However, this feature is not always present and evaluation of myocardium by electron microscopy is mandatory [173]–[177]. Electron microscopy demonstrates the presence of numerous concentric lamellar bodies or myelin figures within the myocyte sarcoplasm (Fig. 5.9(c)). It is possible to confirm or exclude the morphological diagnosis of Fabry's disease by measurement of α-galactosidase A activity in plasma or lecucocytes and/or genotyping [173], [175]. The latter is of relevance in heterozygous females with cardiac involvement, where the enzyme levels of these patients frequently overlap with those observed in normal individuals. The increased recognition of cardiac Fabry's disease provides further validation for the use of electron microscopy on all endomyocardial biopsy specimens from patients with suspected HCM [48].

Distinguishing HCM from cardiac amyloidosis is important because treatment and prognosis of these conditions are different [178]. In cardiac amyloidosis, endomyocardial biopsy reveals amyloid protein deposits ringing individual myocytes and the formation of a characteristic honeycomb pattern. The amyloid has an amorphous appearance. Importantly, it is possible to perform immunohistochemical studies on endomyocardial biopsy specimens to identify the amyloid fibril type [179]. It is vital to distinguish between the different types of cardiac amyloidosis because of different treatment responses and prognosis [144], [158], [180]. For example, in AL amyloidosis, cardiac function may improve after treatment and remission of the underlying plasma cell dyscrasia or myeloma may occur [122], [149], [181]. Cardiac transplantation is not generally recommended for patients with AL amyloidosis because of the progressive risk of multiorgan involvement [182], but, in contrast, orthoptic liver transplantation may be a life-saving option in patients with FAP due to mutant TTR [158]. The abnormal protein is synthesised by the liver and the new liver will produce normal circulating TTR followed by clinical improvement [183], [184].

Endomyocardial biopsy may occasionally be helpful for the detection of sarcoidosis but the diagnostic detection rate tends to be low. For example, a positive histological diagnosis was made in only 6.7% of patients in whom conduction disturbances were the major clinical feature and in 36.7% of patients with a DCM-type picture [185]. In haemochromatosis, endomyocardial biopsy and evaluation of stainable iron can provide an early diagnosis of cardiac involvement before irreversible cardiac damage has occurred (Fig. 5.10).

Endomyocardial biopsy has a limited role in the diagnosis of ARVC, since the interventricular septum is rarely involved and biopsy of the thinned right ventricle is potentially hazardous due to the high risk of perforation and cardiac tamponade [186]. Furthermore, the diagnosis of ARVC in endomyocardial biopsy specimens is notoriously difficult. The presence of adipose tissue in one fragment is almost universal when at least six myocardial fragments are taken at each biopsy session. In ARVC both the tissue area occupied by fat and the number of fragments containing fat are significantly increased compared with other conditions. However, analysis of these specimens is often compounded by age-related fatty infiltration that may be especially prominent in obese or heavily built individuals of either sex. Therefore, due to the problems encountered with the interpretation of endomyocardial biopsies and the lack of consensus between individual pathologists as to whether ARVC is present in

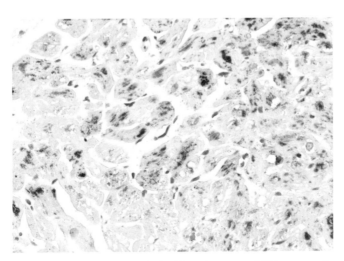

Fig. 5.10 Haemochromatosis. In this endomyocardial biopsy specimen from a patient who had received multiple transfusions, the presence of stainable iron pigment within the myocyte sarcoplasm can be confirmed by a Perl's stain.

biopsy material or not, it is probably advisable not to interpret the endomyocardial biopsy result in isolation. Other criteria such as family history and clinical investigations need to be considered before labelling a case as ARVC. Indeed, these criteria may be much more relevant than the endomyocardial biopsy, which, given its limitations, is unlikely to become the gold standard for the diagnosis of this disease.

CONCLUSION

The pathologist plays a major role in the diagnosis of cardiomyopathy. HCM and ARVC may be clinically silent. From the clinical standpoint the pathologist may be the first to encounter index cases of these cardiomyopathies at autopsy. Both HCM and ARVC have wide-ranging implications for affected families, who will require cardiac screening, genetic counselling and clinical risk stratification. It is therefore essential that the pathologist is familiar with the macroscopic and microscopic phenotypic spectrum of ARVC and HCM and can provide prompt and accurate diagnosis. Importantly, the pathology of ARVC is not fully defined and at present the diagnostic criteria to fulfill a diagnosis of ARVC are confusing. In particular, the significance of the 'fatty' versus the 'cardiomyopathic' variant of ARVC will continue to fuel diagnostic uncertainty, until future genetic studies permit confirmation of the ARVC phenotype. Recognition of these diagnostic grey areas is of considerable clinical importance, to avoid an erroneous pathological diagnosis of ARVC. The picture is further complicated by the recent recognition of the ALVC phenotype, which may present as sudden unexpected cardiac death in previously healthy young individuals. With this phenotype, disease involvement may be exclusively confined to the left ventricle. Importantly, the sub-epicardial distribution pattern of fibroadipose replacement should not be confused with fibrosis secondary to myocardial ischaemia, where lesions typically involve the sub-endocardial zone with sparing of the sub-epicardium.

The value of endomyocardial biopsy for the diagnosis of some types of cardiomyopathy, in particular ARVC and HCM, is controversial. Nevertheless, the endomyocardial biopsy is a valuable tool for the confirmation or exclusion of other diseases, which cause unexplained left ventricular hypertrophy and may clinically simulate HCM. These include cardiac Fabry's disease and amyloidosis, where effective therapeutic treatment options are available. Endomyocardial biopsy is essential to confirm the presence of amyloid, and to permit immunohistochemical studies to define the amyloid type. Similarly, the increased recognition of the cardiac variant of Fabry's disease underscores the value of performing routine electron microscopy on glutaraldehyde-fixed endomyocardial biopsy specimens from patients with suspected HCM. Indeed, the pathologist will need to be familiar with the interpretation of endomyocardial biopsy specimens at both the light microscopic and ultrastructural level.

Advances in molecular genetics have heralded the identification of candidate disease loci and a myriad of single gene defects responsible for DCM, ARVC and HCM. Attempts to define the genetic basis for isolated LVNC are still underway, but increased awareness of isolated LVNC, coupled with advances in molecular genetics, will improve diagnosis and facilitate its recognition as a distinct cardiomyopathy with unique pathological features. Although routine genetic testing of patients or relatives with cardiomyopathy is not currently available, it may become the future gold standard with major implications for understanding the pathogenesis and treatment of disease. This may ultimately lead to customised therapy for patients with different genotypes, and facilitate identification of those patients most at risk of life-threatening arrhythmic events and sudden cardiac death.

REFERENCES

1. Richardson P, McKenna WJ, Bristow M *et al.* Report of the 1995 WHO/ISFC Task Force on the definition and classification of cardiomyopathies. *Circulation* 1996; **93**: 841−2.
2. Franz W-M, Muller OJ, Katus HA. Cardiomyopathies: from genetics to the prospect of treatment. *Lancet* 2001; **358**: 1627−37.
3. Codd MB, Sugrue DD, Gersh BJ, Melton LJ. Epidemiology of idiopathic dilated and hypertrophic cardiomyopathy. A population-based study in Olmsted County, Minnesota, 1975−1984. *Circulation* 1989; **80**: 564−72.
4. Kasper EK, Agema WRP, Hutchins GM, Deckers JW, Hare JM, Baughman KL. The causes of dilated cardiomyopathy: a clinicopathologic review of 673 consecutive patients. *J Am Coll Cardiol* 1994; **23**: 586−90.
5. Grunig E, Tasman JA, Kucherer H *et al.* Frequency and phenotypes of familial dilated cardiomyopathy. *J Am Coll Cardiol* 1998; **31**: 186−94.
6. Towbin JA, Bowles NE. The failing heart. *Nature* 2002; **415**: 227−33.
7. Bowles NE, Bowles KR, Towbin JA. The "final common pathway" hypothesis and inherited cardiovascular disease. The role of cytoskeletal proteins in dilated cardiomyopathy. *Herz* 2000; **25**: 168−75.
8. Sinagra G, Di Lenarda A, Brodsky GL. Current perspective new insights into the molecular basis of familial dilated cardiomyopathy. *Ital Heart J* 2001; **2**: 280−6.
9. Arbustini E, Diegoli M, Fasani R *et al.* Mitochondrial DNA mutations and mitochondrial abnormalities in dilated cardiomyopathy. *Am J Pathol* 1998; **153**: 1501−10.
10. Barth PG, Scholte HR, Berden JA *et al.* An X-linked mitochondrial disease affecting cardiac muscle, skeletal muscle and neutrophil leucocytes. *J Neuro Sci* 1983; **62**: 327−55.
11. Muntoni F, Cau M, Ganau A *et al.* Deletion of the dystrophin muscle-promoter region associated with X-linked dilated cardiomyopathy. *N Engl J Med* 1993; **329**: 921−5.
12. Olson TM, Illenberger S, Kishimoto NY *et al.* Metavinculin mutations alter actin interaction in dilated cardiomyopathy. *Circulation* 2002; **105**: 431−7.
13. Olson T, Kishimoto N, Whitby F *et al.* Mutations that alter the surface charge of α-tropomyosin are associated with dilated cardiomyopathy. *J Mol Cell Cardiol* 2001; **33**: 723−32.
14. Brodsky GL, Muntoni F, Miocic S, Sinagra G, Sewry C, Mestroni L. Lamin A/C gene mutation associated with dilated cardiomyopathy with variable skeletal muscle involvement. *Circulation* 2000; **101**: 473−6.
15. Fatkin D, MacRae C, Sasaki T *et al.* Missense mutations in the rod domain of the lamin A/C gene as causes of dilated cardiomyopathy and conduction-system disease. *N Engl J Med* 1999; **341**: 1715−24.
16. Bonne G, Di Barletta MR, Varnous S, Becane H *et al.* Mutations in the gene encoding lamin A/C cause autosomal dominant Emery−Dreifuss muscular dystrophy. *Nat Genet* 1999; **21**: 285−8.
17. Bione S, D'Adamo P, Maestrini E *et al.* A novel X-linked gene, G4.5 is responsible for Barth syndrome. *Nat Genet* 1996; **12**: 385−9.
18. D'Adamo P, Fassone L, Gedeon A *et al.* The X-linked gene G4.5 is responsible for different infantile dilated cardiomyopathies. *Am J Hum Genet* 1997; **61**: 862−7.

19. Vreken P, Valianpour F, Nijtmans LA et al. Defective remodeling of cardiolipin and phosphatidylglycerol in Barth syndrome. *Biochem Biophys Res Commun* 2000; **279**: 378–82.
20. Bissler JJ, Tsoras HH, Goring HH et al. Infantile dilated X-linked cardiomyopathy, G4.5 mutations, altered lipids, and ultrastructural malformations of mitochondria in heart, liver, and skeletal muscle. *Lab Invest* 2002; **82**: 335–44.
21. Berko BA, Swift M. X-linked dilated cardiomyopathy. *N Engl J Med* 1987; **316**: 1186–91.
22. Cox GF, Kunkel LM. Dystrophies and heart disease. *Curr Opin Cardiol* 1997; **12**: 329–43.
23. Kamisago M, Sharma SD, DePalma SR et al. Mutations in sarcomere protein genes as a cause of dilated cardiomyopathy. *N Engl J Med* 2000; **343**: 1688–96.
24. Olson TM, Michels VV, Thibodeau SN et al. Actin mutations in dilated cardiomyopathy, a heritable form of heart failure. *Science* 1998; **280**: 750–2.
25. Tsubata S, Bowles KR, Vatta M et al. Mutations in the human δ-sarcoglycan gene in familial and sporadic dilated cardiomyopathy. *J Clin Invest* 2000; **106**: 655–62.
26. Nigro V, de Sa Moreira E, Piluso G et al. Autosomal recessive limb-girdle muscular dystrophy, LGMD2F, is caused by a mutation in the delta-sarcoglycan gene. *Nat Genet* 1996; **14**: 195–8.
27. Mogensen J, Klausen JC, Pedersen AK et al. α-cardiac actin is a novel disease gene in familial hypertrophic cardiomyopathy. *J Clin Invest* 1999; **103**: 39–43.
28. Chin TK, Perloff JK, Williams R et al. Isolated noncompaction of left ventricular myocardium. A study of eight cases. *Circulation* 1990; **82**: 507–13.
29. Ritter M, Oechslin E, Sutsch G et al. Isolated noncompaction of the myocardium in adults. *Mayo Clin Proc* 1997; **72**: 26–31.
30. Sedmera D, Pexieder T, Vuillemin M et al. Developmental patterning of the myocardium. *Anat Rec* 2000; **258**: 319–37.
31. Kenton AB, Sanchez X, Coveler KJ et al. Isolated left ventricular noncompaction is rarely caused by mutations in G4.5, α-dystrobrevin and FK Binding Protein-12. *Mol Genet and Metab* 2004; **82**: 162–6.
32. Maron BJ. Hypertrophic cardiomyopathy. A systematic review. *JAMA* 2002; **287**: 1308–20.
33. Maron BJ, Gardin JM, Flack JM, Gidding SS, Kurosaki TT, Bild DE. Prevalence of hypertrophic cardiomyopathy in a general population of young adults. Echocardiographic analysis of 4111 subjects in the CARDIA study. *Circulation* 1995; **92**: 785–9.
34. Thierfelder L, Watkins H, MacRae C et al. Alpha-tropomyosin and cardiac troponin T mutations cause familial hypertrophic cardiomyopathy: a disease of the sarcomere. *Cell* 1994; **77**: 701–12.
35. Marian AJ, Salek L, Lutucuta S. Molecular genetics and pathogenesis of hypertrophic cardiomyopathy. *Minerva Med* 2001; **92**: 435–51.
36. Bonne G, Carrier L, Richard P, Hainque B, Schwarz K. Familial hypertrophic cardiomyopathy: from mutations to functional defects. *Circ Res* 1998; **83**: 580–93.
37. Watkins H, McKenna WJ, Thierfelder L et al. Mutations in the genes for cardiac troponin T and α-tropomyosin in hypertrophic cardiomyopathy. *New Engl J Med* 1995; **332**: 1058–64.
38. Blair E, Redwood C, Ashrafian H et al. Mutations in the γ2 sub-unit of AMP-activated protein kinase cause familial hypertrophic cardiomyopathy: evidence for the central role of energy compromise in disease pathogenesis. *Hum Mol Genet* 2001; **10**: 1215–20.
39. Santorelli FM, Mak SC, El-Schahawi M et al. Maternally inherited cardiomyopathy and hearing loss associated with a novel mutation in the mitochondrial tRNA (Lys) gene (G8363A). *Am J Hum Genet* 1996; **58**: 933–9.
40. Anan R, Greve G, Thierfelder L et al. Prognostic implication of novel β cardiac myosin heavy chain gene mutations that cause familial hypertrophic cardiomyopathy. *J Clin Invest* 1994; **93**: 280–5.
41. Watkins H, Rosenzweig T, Hwang DS et al. Characteristics and prognostic implications of myosin missense mutations in familial hypertrophic cardiomyopathy. *N Engl J Med* 1992; **326**: 1106–14.
42. Vikstrom KL, Leinwand LA. Contractile protein mutations and heart disease. *Curr Opin Cell Biol* 1996; **8**: 97–105.
43. Marian AJ, Roberts R. The molecular genetic basis for hypertrophic cardiomyopathy. *J Mol Cell Cardiol* 2001; **33**: 655–70.

44. Solomon SD, Wolff S, Watkins H *et al*. Left ventricular hypertrophy and morphology in familial hypertrophic cardiomyopathy associated with mutations of the beta-myosin heavy chain gene. *J Am Coll Cardiol* 1993; **22**: 498–505.

45. Marian AJ, Yu QT, Workman R, Greve G, Roberts R. Angiotensin-converting enzyme polymorphism in hypertrophic cardiomyopathy and sudden cardiac death. *Lancet* 1993; **342**: 1085–6.

46. Brugada R, Kelsey W, Lechin M *et al*. Role of candidate modifier genes on the phenotypic expression of hypertrophy in patients with hypertrophic cardiomyopathy. *J Invest Med* 1997; **45**: 542–51.

47. Davies MJ, McKenna WJ. Hypertrophic cardiomyopathy – pathology and pathogenesis. *Histopathology* 1995; **26**: 493–500.

48. Hughes SE. The pathology of hypertrophic cardiomyopathy. *Histopathology* 2004; **44**: 412–27.

49. Teare D. Asymmetrical hypertrophy of the heart in young adults. *Br Heart J* 1958; **20**: 1–8.

50. Falicov RE, Resnekov L, Bharati S, Lev M. Mid-ventricular obstruction: a variant of obstructive cardiomyopathy. *Am J Cardiol* 1976; **37**: 432–7.

51. Fighali S, Krajcer Z, Edelman S, Leachman RD. Progression of hypertrophic cardiomyopathy into a hypokinetic left ventricle: higher incidence in patients with midventricular obstruction. *J Am Coll Cardiol* 1987; **9**: 288–94.

52. Maron BJ, Hauser RG, Roberts WC. Hypertrophic cardiomyopathy with left ventricular apical diverticulum. *Am J Cardiol* 1996; **77**: 1263–5.

53. Poetter K, Jiang H, Hassanzadeh S *et al*. Mutations in either the essential or regulatory light chains of myosin are associated with a rare myopathy in human heart and skeletal muscle. *Nature Genet* 1996; **13**: 63–9.

54. Olson TM, Karst ML, Whitby FG. Myosin light chain mutation causes autosomal recessive cardiomyopathy with mid-cavitary hypertrophy and restrictive physiology. *Circulation* 2002; **105**: 2337–40.

55. Barbosa MM, Coutinho AH, Motta MS, Fortes PR, Roza AZ, Good God EM. Apical hypertrophic cardiomyopathy: a study of 14 patients and their first degree relatives. *Int J Cardiol* 1996; **56**: 41–51.

56. Ando H, Imaizumi T, Urabe Y, Takeshita A, Nakamura M. Apical segmental dysfunction in hypertrophic cardiomyopathy: subgroup with unique clinical features. *J Am Coll Cardiol* 1990; **16**: 1579–88.

57. Wigle ED, Rakowski H, Kimball BP, Williams WG. Hypertrophic cardiomyopathy: clinical spectrum and treatment. *Circulation* 1995; **92**: 1680–92.

58. Maron BJ. Apical hypertrophic cardiomyopathy: the continuing saga. *J Am Coll Cardiol* 1990; **15**: 91–3.

59. Sakamoto T, Tei C, Murayama M, Ichiyasu H, Hada Y. Giant T wave inversion as a manifestation of asymmetrical apical hypertrophy (AAH) of the left ventricle: Echocardiographic and ultrasono-cardiotomographic study. *Jpn Heart J* 1976; **17**: 611–29.

60. Wigle ED. Cardiomyopathy. The diagnosis of hypertrophic cardiomyopathy. *Heart* 2001; **86**: 709–14.

61. Webb JG, Sasson Z, Rakowski H, Liu P, Wigle ED. Apical hypertrophic cardiomyopathy: clinical follow-up and diagnostic correlates. *J Am Coll Cardiol* 1990; **15**: 83–90.

62. Seiler C, Jenni R, Vassali G, Turina M, Hess OM. Left ventricular chamber dilatation in hypertrophic cardiomyopathy: related variables and prognosis in patients with medical and surgical therapy. *Br Heart J* 1995; **74**: 508–16.

63. Hina K, Kusachi S, Iwasaki K *et al*. Progression of left ventricular enlargement in patients with hypertrophic cardiomyopathy: incidence and prognostic value. *Clin Cardiol* 1993; **16**: 403–7.

64. Maron BJ, Wolfson JK, Roberts WC. Relation between extent of cardiac muscle cell disorganization and left ventricular wall thickness in hypertrophic cardiomyopathy. *Am J Cardiol* 1992; **70**: 785–90.

65. Maron BJ, Roberts WC. Quantitative analysis of cardiac muscle cell disorganization in the ventricular septum of patients with hypertrophic cardiomyopathy. *Circulation* 1979; **59**: 689–706.

66. Maron BJ, Anan TJ, Roberts WC. Quantitative analysis of the distribution of cardiac muscle cell disorganization in the left ventricular wall of patients with hypertrophic cardiomyopathy. *Circulation* 1981; **63**: 882−94.
67. Shirani J, Pick R, Roberts WC, Maron BJ. Morphology and significance of the left ventricular collagen network in young patients with hypertrophic cardiomyopathy and sudden cardiac death. *J Am Coll Cardiol* 2000; **35**: 36−44.
68. Maron BJ, Wolfson JK, Epstein SE, Roberts WC. Intramural ("small vessel") coronary artery disease in hypertrophic cardiomyopathy. *J Am Coll Cardiol* 1986; **8**: 545−57.
69. Maron BJ, Wolfson JK, Epstein SE, Roberts WC. Morphologic evidence for "small vessel disease" in patients with hypertrophic cardiomyopathy. *Z Kardiol* 1987; **76** Suppl 3: 91−100.
70. Takemura G, Takatsu Y, Fujiwara H. Luminal narrowing of coronary capillaries in human hypertrophic hearts: an ultrastructural morphometrical study using endomyocardial biopsy specimens. *Heart* 1998; **79**: 78−85.
71. Cannon RO, Rosing DR, Maron BJ *et al.* Myocardial ischaemia in patients with hypertrophic cardiomyopathy: contribution of inadequate vasodilator reserve and elevated left ventricular filling pressures. *Circulation* 1985; **71**: 234−43.
72. Iida K, Yutani C, Imakita M *et al.* Comparison of percentage area of myocardial fibrosis and disarray in patients with classical form and dilated phase of hypertrophic cardiomyopathy. *J Cardiol* 1998; **32**: 173−80.
73. Basso C, Thiene G, Corrado D, Buja G, Melacini P, Nava A. Hypertrophic cardiomyopathy and sudden death in the young: pathologic evidence of myocardial ischemia. *Hum Pathol* 2000; **31**: 988−98.
74. Maron BJ, Sato N, Roberts WC, Edwards JE, Chandra RS. Quantitative analysis of cardiac muscle cell disorganization in the ventricular septum. Comparison of fetuses and infants with and without congenital heart disease and patients with hypertrophic cardiomyopathy. *Circulation* 1979; **60**: 685−96.
75. Bulkley BH, Weisfeldt ML, Hutchins GM. Asymmetric septal hypertrophy and myocardial fiber disarray. Features of normal, developing and malformed hearts. *Circulation* 1977; **56**: 292−8.
76. Burch M, Mann JM, Sharland M *et al.* Myocardial disarray in Noonan syndrome. *Br Heart J* 1992; **68**: 586−8.
77. Brumback RA, Panner BJ, Kingston WJ. The heart in Friedreich's ataxia. Report of a case. *Arch Neurol* 1986; **43**: 189−92.
78. Tartaglia M, Mehler EL, Goldberg R *et al.* Mutations in PTPN11 encoding the protein tyrosine phosphatase SHP-2, cause Noonan syndrome. *Nat Genet* 2001; **29**: 465−8.
79. Rotig A, Sidi D, Munnich A *et al.* Molecular insights into Friedreich's ataxia and antioxidant-based therapies. *Trends Mol Med* 2002; **8**: 221−4.
80. Van der Bel-Kahn J. Muscle fibre disarray in common heart diseases. *Am J Cardiol* 1977; **40**: 355−64.
81. St John Sutton MG, Lie JT, Anderson KR, O'Brien PC, Frye RL. Histopathological specificity of hypertrophic obstructive cardiomyopathy. Myocardial fibre disarray and myocardial fibrosis. *Br Heart J* 1980; **44**: 433−43.
82. Valente M, Calabrese F, Thiene G *et al.* In vivo evidence of apoptosis in arrhythmogenic right ventricular cardiomyopathy. *Am J Pathol* 1998; **152**: 479−84.
83. Mallat Z, Tedgui A, Fontaliran F, Frank R, Durigon M, Fontaine G. Evidence of apoptosis in arrhythmogenic right ventricular dysplasia. *N Engl J Med* 1996; **335**: 1190−6.
84. Bowles NE, Ni J, Marcus F *et al.* The detection of cardiotropic viruses in the myocardium of patients with arrhythmogenic right ventricular dysplasia/cardiomyopathy. *J Am Coll Cardiol* 2002; **39**: 892−5.
85. D'Amati G, di Gioia CRT, Giordano C, Gallo P. Myocyte transdifferentiation. A possible pathogenetic mechanism for arrhythmogenic right ventricular cardiomyopathy. *Circulation* 2000; **124**: 287−90.
86. Corrado D, Fontaine G, Marcus FI *et al.* Arrhythmogenic right ventricular dysplasia/cardiomyopathy; need for an international registry. Study group on arrhythmogenic right ventricular dysplasia/cardiomyopathy of the working groups of myocardial and

pericardial disease and arrhythmias of the European Society of Cardiology and of the Scientific Council of Cardiomyopathies of the World Heart Federation. *Circulation* 2000; **101**: E101–16.

87. Nava A, Thiene G, Canciani B *et al.* Familial occurrence of right ventricular dysplasia: a study involving nine families. *J Am Coll Cardiol* 1988; **12**: 1222–8.

88. Nava A, Bauce B, Basso C *et al.* Clinical profile and long-term follow-up of 37 families with arrhythmogenic right ventricular cardiomyopathy. *J Am Coll Cardiol* 2000; **36**: 2226–33.

89. Tiso N, Stephan DA, Nava A *et al.* Identification of mutations in the cardiac ryanodine receptor gene in families affected with arrhythmogenic right ventricular cardiomyopathy type 2 (ARVD2). *Hum Mol Genet* 2001; **10**: 189–94.

90. Rampazzo A, Nava A, Malacrida S *et al.* Mutation in human desmoplakin binding domain binding to plakoglobin causes a dominant form of arrhythmogenic right ventricular cardiomyopathy. *Am J Hum Genet* 2002; **71**: 1200–6.

91. McKoy G, Protonotarios N, Crosby A *et al.* Identification of a deletion in plakoglobin in arrhythmogenic right ventricular cardiomyopathy with palmoplantar keratoderma and woolly hair (Naxos disease). *Lancet* 2000; **355**: 2119–24.

92. Alcalai R, Metzger S, Rosenheck S *et al.* A recessive mutation in desmoplakin causes arrhythmogenic right ventricular dysplasia, skin disorder and woolly hair. *J Am Coll Cardiol* 2003; **42**: 319–27.

93. Bauce B, Rampazzo A, Basso C *et al.* Screening for ryanodine receptor type 2 mutations in families with effort-induced polymorphic ventricular arrhythmias and sudden death. Early diagnosis of asymptomatic carriers. *J Am Coll Cardiol* 2002; **40**: 341–9.

94. Bauce B, Nava A, Rampazzo A *et al.* Familial effort polymorphic ventricular arrhythmias in arrhythmogenic right ventricular cardiomyopathy map to chromosome 1q42–43. *Am J Cardiol* 2000; **85**: 573–9.

95. Priori S, Napolitano C, Tiso N *et al.* Mutations in the cardiac ryanodine receptor gene (hRyR2) underlie catecholaminergic polymorphic ventricular tachycardia. *Circulation* 2001; **103**: 196–200.

96. Laitinen P, Brown K, Piipo K *et al.* Mutations of the cardiac ryanodine receptor (RyR2) gene in familial polymorphic ventricular tachycardia. *Circulation* 2001; **103**: 485–90.

97. Swan H, Piippo K, Viitasalo M *et al.* Arrhythmic disorder mapped to chromosome 1q42–q43 causes malignant polymorphic ventricular tachycardia in structurally normal hearts. *J Am Coll Cardiol* 1999; **34**: 2035–42.

98. Coonar AS, Protonoarius N, Tsatsopoulou A *et al.* Gene for arrhythmogenic right ventricular cardiomyopathy with diffuse nonepidermolytic palmoplantar keratoderma and woolly hair (Naxos disease) maps to 17q21. *Circulation* 1998; **97**: 2049–58.

99. Hughes SE, McKenna WJ. New insights into the pathology of inherited cardiomyopathy. *Heart* 2005; **91**: 257–64.

100. Ko KS, Arora PD, McCulloch CAG. Cadherins mediate intracellular mechanical signalling in fibroblasts by activation of stretch-sensitive calcium permeable channels. *J Biol Chem* 2001; **276**: 35967–77.

101. Petroff MGV, Kim SH, Pepe S *et al.* Endogenous nitric oxide mechanisms mediate the stretch dependence of Ca^{2+} release in cardiomyocytes. *Nat Cell Biol* 2001; **3**: 867–73.

102. Norgett EE, Hatsell SJ, Carvajal-Huerta L *et al.* Recessive mutation in desmoplakin disrupts desmoplakin-intermediate filament interactions and causes dilated cardiomyopathy, woolly hair and keratoderma. *Hum Mol Genet* 2000; **9**: 2761–6.

103. Kaplan SR, Gard JJ, Carvajal-Huerta L, Ruiz-Cabezas JC, Thiene G, Structural and molecular pathology of the heart in Carvajal syndrome. *Cardiovasc Pathol* 2004; **13**: 26–32.

104. Marcus FI, Fontaine G, Guiraudon G *et al.* Right ventricular dysplasia. A report of 24 adult cases. *Circulation* 1982; **65**: 384–98.

105. Corrado D, Basso C, Thiene G. Arrhythmogenic right ventricular cardiomyopathy: diagnosis, prognosis and treatment. *Heart* 2000; **83**: 588–95.

106. Thiene G, Nava A, Corrado D *et al.* Right ventricular cardiomyopathy and sudden death in young people. *N Engl J Med* 1988; **318**: 129–33.

107. Basso C, Thiene G, Corrado D *et al.* Arrhythmogenic right ventricular cardiomyopathy. Dysplasia, dystrophy or myocarditis? *Circulation* 1996; **94**: 983–91.

108. Corrado D, Basso C, Thiene G *et al*. Spectrum of clinicopathologic manifestations of arrhythmogenic right ventricular cardiomyopathy/dysplasia: a multicenter study. *J Am Coll Cardiol* 1997; **30**: 1512–20.

109. Gallo P, D'Amati G, Pellicia F. Pathologic evidence of extensive left ventricular involvement in arrhythmogenic right ventricular cardiomyopathy. *Hum Pathol* 1992; **23**: 948–52.

110. Pinamonti B, Sinagra GF, Salvi A *et al*. Left ventricular involvement in right ventricular dysplasia. *Am Heart J* 1992; **123**: 711–24.

111. Miani D, Pimamonti B, Bussani R, Silvestri F, Sinagra G, Camerini F. Right ventricular dysplasia: a clinical and pathological study of two families with left ventricular involvement. *Br Heart J* 1993; **69**: 151–7.

112. D'Amati G, Leone O, di Gioa CR *et al*. Arrhythmogenic right ventricular cardiomyopathy: clinicopathologic correlation based on a revised definition of pathologic patterns. *Hum Pathol* 2001; **32**: 1078–86.

113. Burke AP, Farb A, Tashko G *et al*. Arrhythmogenic right ventricular cardiomyopathy and fatty replacement of the right ventricular myocardium: are they different diseases? *Circulation* 1998; **97**: 1571–80.

114. Fontaliran F, Fontaine G, Fillette F, Aouate P, Chomette G, Grosgogeat Y. Nosologic frontiers of arrhythmogenic dysplasia. Quantitative variations of normal adipose tissue of the right heart ventricle. *Arch Mal Coeur Vaiss* 1991; **84**: 33–8.

115. Shirani J, Berezowski K, Roberts WC. Quantitative measurement of normal adipose and excessive (cor adiposum) subepicardial adipose tissue, its clinical significance and its effect on electrocardiographic QRS voltage. *Am J Cardiol* 1995; **76**: 414–18.

116. De Pasquale CG, Heddle WF. Left sided arrhythmogenic ventricular dysplasia in siblings. *Heart* 2001; **86**: 128–30.

117. Michalodimitrakis M, Papadomanolakis A, Stiakakis J, Kanaki K. Left side right ventricular cardiomyopathy. *Med Sci Law* 2002; **42**: 313–17.

118. Suzuki H, Sumiyoshi M, Kawai S *et al*. Arrhythmogenic right ventricular cardiomyopathy with an initial manifestation of severe left ventricular impairment and normal contraction of the right ventricle. *Jpn Circ J* 2000; **64**: 209–13.

119. Collett BA, Davis GJ, Rohr WB. Extensive fibrofatty infiltration of the left ventricle in two cases of sudden cardiac death. *J Forensic Sci* 1994; **39**: 1182–7.

120. Shirani J, Roberts WC. Subepicardial myocardial lesions. *Am Heart J* 1993; **125**: 1346–52.

121. Klein AL, Scalia GM. In *Textbook of Cardiovascular Medicine*, (Topol EJ ed.) Lippincott-Raven Publishers, Philadelphia, 1998.

122. Kushwaha SS, Fallon JT, Fuster V. Restrictive cardiomyopathy. *N Engl J Med* 1997; **336**: 267–76.

123. Child JS, Perloff JK. The restrictive cardiomyopathies. *Cardiol Clin* 1988; **6**: 289–316.

124. Siegel RJ, Shah PK, Fishbein MC. Idiopathic restrictive cardiomyopathy. *Circulation* 1984; **70**: 165–9.

125. Denfield SW, Rosenthal G, Gajarski RJ *et al*. Restrictive cardiomyopathies in childhood. Etiologies and natural history. *Tex Heart Inst J* 1997; **24**: 38–44.

126. Benotti JR, Grossman W, Cohn PF. Clinical profile of restrictive cardiomyopathy. *Circulation* 1980; **61**: 1206–12.

127. Cooke RA, Chambers JB, Curry PV. Noonan's cardiomyopathy: a non-hypertrophic variant. *Br Heart J* 1994; **71**: 561–5.

128. Mogensen J, Kubo T, Duque M *et al*. Idiopathic restrictive cardiomyopathy is part of the clinical expression of cardiac troponin I mutations. *J Clin Invest* 2003; **111**: 209–16.

129. Spry CJ, Take M, Tai PC. Eosinophilic disorders affecting the myocardium and endocardium: a review. *Heart Vessels Suppl* 1985; **1**: 240–2.

130. Davies JNP. Endomyocardial necrosis. A heart disease of obscure aetiology in Africans. MD thesis, Bristol University, 1948.

131. Parrillo JE. Heart disease and the eosinophil. *N Engl J Med* 1990; **323**: 1560–1.

132. Gupta PN, Valiathan MS, Balakrishnan KG *et al*. Clinical course of endomyocardial fibrosis. *Br Heart J* 1989; **62**: 450–4.

133. Chopra P, Narula J, Talwar KK *et al*. Histomorphologic characteristics of endomyocardial fibrosis: an endomyocardial biopsy study. *Hum Pathol* 1990; **21**: 613–16.

134. Mady C, Pereira Barretto AC, de Oliveira SA *et al.* Effectiveness of operative and nonoperative therapy of endomyocardial fibrosis. *Am J Cardiol* 1989; **63**: 1281−2.

135. de Oliveira SA, Pereira Barretto AC, Mady C *et al.* Surgical treatment of endomyocardial fibrosis: a new approach. *J Am Coll Cardiol* 1990; **16**: 1246−51.

136. Andy JJ. Aetiology of endomyocardial fibrosis (EMF). *West Afr J Med* 2001; **20**: 199−207.

137. Roberts WC, Buja LM, Ferrans VJ. Loeffler's fibroplastic parietal endocarditis, eosinophilic leukaema, and Davies' endomyocardial fibrosis: the same disease at different stages? *Pathol Microbiol (Basel)* 1970; **35**: 90−5.

138. Davies J, Spry CJ, Vijayaraghavan G, De Souza JA. A comparison of the clinical and cardiological features of endomyocardial disease in temperate and tropical regions. *Postgrad Med J* 1983; **59**: 179−85.

139. De Mello DE, Liapis H, Jureidini S *et al.* Cardiac localization of eosinophil-granule major basic protein in acute necrotizing myocarditis. *N Engl J Med* 1990; **323**: 1542−5.

140. Spry CJ, Tai PC. Studies on blood eosinophils. II. Patients with Loeffler's cardiomyopathy. *Clin Exp Immunol* 1976; **24**: 423−34.

141. Bigoni R, Cuneo A, Roberti MG *et al.* Cytogenetic and molecular cytogenetic characterization of 6 new cases of idiopathic hypereosinophilic syndrome. *Haematologica* 2000; **85**: 486−91.

142. Weinberg BA, Conces DJ Jr., Waller BF. Cardiac manifestations of noncardiac tumours. Part I: Direct Effects. *Clin Cardiol* 1989; **12**: 289−96.

143. Klein AL, Oh JK, Miller FA *et al.* Two-dimensional and Doppler echocardiographic assessment of infiltrative cardiomyopathy. *J Am Soc Echocardiogr* 1988; **1**: 48−59.

144. Kyle RA. Amyloidosis. *Circulation* 1995; **91**: 1269−71.

145. Westermark P, Bergstrom J, Solomon A, Murphy C, Sletten K. Transthyretin-derived senile systemic amyloidosis: clinicopathologic and structural considerations. *Amyloid* 2003; **10** Suppl I: 48−54.

146. Cornwell GG III, Murdoch W, Kyle RA, Westermark P, Pitkanen P. Frequency and distribution of senile cardiovascular amyloid. A clinicopathologic correlation. *Am J Med* 1983; **75**: 618−23.

147. Pitkanen P, Westermark P, Cornwell GG III. Senile systemic amyloidosis. *Am J Path* 1984; **117**: 391−9.

148. Hamidi Asl L, Liepnieks JJ, Hamidi Asl K *et al.* Hereditary amyloid cardiomyopathy caused by a variant apolipprotein A1. *Am J Pathol* 1999; **154**: 221−7.

149. Arbustini E, Gavazzi A, Merlini G. Fibril-forming proteins: the amyloidosis. New hopes for a disease that cardiologists must know. *Ital Heart J* 2002; **3**: 590−7.

150. Yazaki M, Liepniks JJ, Barats MS, Cohen AH, Benson MD. Hereditary systemic amyloidosis associated with a new apolipoprotein AII stop codon mutation Stop78Arg. *Kidney Int* 2003; **64**: 11−16.

151. Saraiva MJ. Transythretin mutations in health and disease. *Hum Mutat* 1995; **5**: 191−6.

152. Saito F, Nakazato M, Akiyama H *et al.* A case of late onset cardiac amyloidosis with a new transthyretin variant (Lysine 92). *Hum Pathol* 2001; **32**: 237−9.

153. Tawara S, Nakazato M, Kangawa K *et al.* Identification of amyloid prealbumin variant in familial amyloidotic polyneuropathy (Japanese type). *Biochem Biophys Res Commun* 1983; **116**: 880−8.

154. Saraiva MJM, Costa PP, Birken S, Goodman DS. Presence of an abnormal transthyretin (prealbumin) in Portugese patients with familial amyloidotic polyneuropathy. *Trans Assoc Am Phys* 1983; **96**: 261−70.

155. Saraiva MJ, Almeida M do R, Sherman W *et al.* A new transthyretin mutation associated with amyloid cardiomyopathy. *Am J Hum Genet* 1992; **50**: 1027−30.

156. Magnus JH, Stenstad K, Kolset SO *et al.* Glycosaminoglycans in extracts of cardiac amyloid fibrils from familial amyloid cardiomyopathy of Danish origin related to variant transthyretin Met 111. *Scand J Immunol* 1991; **34**: 63−9.

157. Roberts WC, Waller BF. Cardiac amyloidosis causing cardiac dysfunction: analysis of 54 necropsy patients. *Am J Cardiol* 1983; **52**: 137−46.

158. Booth DR, Tan SY, Hawkins PN *et al.* A novel variant of transthyretin, 59Thr-Lys, associated with autosomal dominant cardiac amyloidosis in an Italian family. *Circulation* 1995; **91**: 962−7.

159. Smith TJ, Kyle RA, Lie JT. Clinical significance of histopathologic patterns of cardiac amyloidosis. *Mayo Clin Proc* 1984; **59**: 547–55.

160. Newman LS, Rose CS, Maier LA. Sarcoidosis. *New Engl J Med* 1997; **336**: 1224–34.

161. Sharma OP, Maheshwari A, Thaker K. Myocardial sarcoidosis. *Chest* 1993; **103**: 253–8.

162. Silverman KJ, Hutchins GM, Bulkley BH. Cardiac sarcoid: a clinicopathologic study of 84 unselected patients with systemic sarcoidosis. *Circulation* 1978; **58**: 1204–11.

163. Perry A, Vuitch F. Causes of death in patients with sarcoidosis: a morphologic study of 38 autopsies with clinicopathologic correlations. *Arch Pathol Lab Med* 1995; **119**: 1767–72.

164. Hauser SC. Hemochromatosis and the heart. *Heart Dis Stroke* 1993; **2**: 487–91.

165. Zaahl MG, Merryweather-Clarke AT, Kotze MJ *et al*. Analysis of genes implicated in iron regulation in individuals presenting with primary iron overload. *Hum Genet* 2004; **115**: 409–17.

166. Olson LJ, Edwards WD, McCall JT *et al*. Cardiac iron deposition in idiopathic hemochromatosis: histologic and analytic assessment of 14 hearts from autopsy. *Am Coll Cardiol* 1987; **10**: 1239–43.

167. Cecchetti G, Binda A, Piperno A *et al*. Cardiac alterations in 36 consecutive patients with idiopathic hemochromatosis: polygraphic and echocardiographic evaluation. *Eur Heart J* 1991; **12**: 224–30.

168. Glazier JJ, Mortimer G, Daly KM. A clinical role for right ventricular endomyocardial biopsy. *Ir Med J* 1989; **82**: 153–5.

169. Hoshino T, Fujiwara H, Kawai C, Hamashima Y. Diagnostic value of disarray in endomyocardial biopsy specimens in hypertrophic cardiomyopathy: a critical report based on distribution of disarray in the subendocardial region of autopsied hearts. *Jpn Circ J* 1982; **46**: 1281–91.

170. Tazelaar HD, Billingham ME. The surgical pathology of hypertrophic cardiomyopathy. *Arch Pathol Lab Med* 1987; **111**: 257–60.

171. Linhart A, Palecek T, Bultas J *et al*. New insights in cardiac structural changes in patients with Fabry's disease. *Am Heart J* 2000; **139**: 1101–8.

172. Sachdev B, Takenaka T, Teraguchi H *et al*. Prevalence of Anderson–Fabry disease in male patients with late onset hypertrophic cardiomyopathy. *Circulation* 2002; **105**: 1407–11.

173. Beer G, Reinecke P, Gabbert HE, Hort W, Kuhn H. Fabry disease in patients with hypertrophic cardiomyopathy (HCM). *Z Kardiol* 2002; **91**: 992–1002.

174. Ommen SR, Nishimura RA, Edwards WD. Fabry disease: a mimic for obstructive hypertrophic cardiomyopathy? *Heart* 2003; **89**: 929–30.

175. Nakao S, Takenaka T, Maeda M *et al*. An atypical variant of Fabry's disease in men with left ventricular hypertrophy. *N Engl J Med* 1995; **333**: 288–93.

176. Nagueh SF. Fabry disease. *Heart* 2003; **89**: 819–20.

177. Frustaci A, Chimenti C, Ricci R *et al*. Improvement in cardiac function in the cardiac variant of Fabry's disease with galactose-infusion therapy. *N Engl J Med* 2001; **345**: 25–32.

178. Oh JK, Tajik AJ, Edwards WD *et al*. Dynamic left ventricular outflow tract obstruction in cardiac amyloidosis detected by continuous-wave Doppler echocardiography. *Am J Cardiol* 1987; **59**: 1008–10.

179. Hoshii Y, Takahashi M, Ishihara T, Uchino F. Immunohistochemical classification of 140 autopsy cases with systemic amyloidosis. *Pathol Int* 1994; **44**: 352–8.

180. Olson LJ, Gertz MA, Edwards WD *et al*. Senile cardiac amyloidosis with myocardial dysfunction. Diagnosis by endomyocardial biopsy and immunohistochemistry. *N Engl J Med* 1987; **317**: 738–42.

181. Nakamura M, Satoh M, Kowada S *et al*. Reversible restrictive cardiomyopathy due to light-chain deposition disease. *Mayo Clin Proc* 2002; **77**: 193–6.

182. Hosenpud JD, DeMarco T, Frazier OH *et al*. Progression of systemic disease and reduced long-term survival in patients with cardiac amyloidosis undergoing heart transplantation. Follow-up results of a multicenter survey. *Circulation* 1991; **84**(III): 338–43.

183. Holmgren G, Ericzon BG, Groth CG *et al*. Clinical improvement and amyloid regression after liver transplantation in hereditary transthyretin amyloidosis. *Lancet* 1993; **341**: 1113–16.

184. Ikeda S, Nakazato M, Ando Y *et al*. Familial transthretin-type amyloid polyneuropathy in Japan. Clinical and genetic heterogeneity. *Neurology* 2002; **58**: 1001−7.

185. Uemera A, Morimoto S, Hiramitsu S, Kato Y, Ito T, Hishida H. Histologic diagnostic rate of cardiac sarcoidosis: evaluation of endomyocardial biopsies. *Am Heart J* 1999; **138**: 299−302.

186. Angelini A, Basso C, Nava A, Thiene G. Endomyocardial biopsy in arrhythmogenic right ventricular cardiomyopathy. *Am Heart J* 1996; **132**: 203−6.

6

Metastatic adenocarcinoma of unknown origin

Karin A. Oien, Jayne L. Dennis and T. R. Jeffry Evans

INTRODUCTION

'The most important first step is to discuss the biopsy with an experienced pathologist. The pathologist may have an idea where the primary site might be, but because of lack of clinical information, has left the diagnosis open.' [1]

Most cancer patients come to clinical attention with their primary tumour. However, around 10–15% of cancer patients present with distant metastases, and in a proportion of these, the primary site cannot be identified at the time of treatment. Metastatic cancer of unknown primary site (CUP) is a common clinical problem, representing one of the ten most frequent cancer diagnoses [2]. Its prognosis is poor: the median survival time is only four months [3].

Investigation of CUP patients is aimed at diagnosing the cancer type and likely primary site, in order to identify the known tumour subsets that may respond to treatment. Most CUPs are adenocarcinomas, for which the most commonly identified primary sites are the lung and pancreas. Nevertheless, the origin remains undiagnosed in most patients, even with modern imaging, and eventually at autopsy.

Pathological assessment is an important part of the clinical work-up of such patients. Biopsy is performed to confirm malignancy, to type the tumour, and thus identify the highly chemosensitive tumours, and, increasingly, where the tumour is an adenocarcinoma, to predict the likely primary site in order to provide prognostic information and guide therapy, as well as to inform the patient. This is a large topic: this review will focus on the assessment of metastatic adenocarcinoma at biopsy, especially in the liver, although other tumour types will be discussed briefly. Immunohistochemistry plays an important role in the work-up of CUP and is discussed in depth.

For this review, Medline was searched for papers from the past five years. Cancer, carcinoma, adenocarcinoma, unknown, primary and origin were used

135

Progress in Pathology Volume 7, ed. Nigel Kirkham and Neil Shepherd. Published by Cambridge University Press. © Cambridge University Press 2007.

as keywords in various combinations. Each of the seven main primary sites was searched using marker, tumour marker and general immunohistochemical keywords. Each individual tumour marker identified was then separately searched for its tissue and tumour expression. Additional papers were identified from the reference lists of the literature retrieved.

This review is aimed primarily at trainees in histopathology, although it may also be of interest to consultant staff.

NATURE OF THE PROBLEM

The clinical management of patients with CUP has been the subject of a number of excellent recent reviews, which have formed the basis of this section [2]–[9].

DEFINITION

Cancer of unknown primary site (CUP) has been known by a range of other terms: unknown or occult primary tumour; carcinoma or adenocarcinoma of unknown primary; metastases of unknown origin; etc [2]. CUP is currently the most widely accepted comprehensive term. The definition of CUP within a study context has varied over time and with the inclusion criteria used [2]: improvements in imaging and in pathology mean that more primary tumours can be identified now than in the past [10]. In essence, CUP encompasses patients presenting with metastatic disease for which the site of origin cannot be identified at the time of diagnosis and/or therapy, despite a detailed medical history, clinical examination and diagnostic work-up. Most but not all studies require histological confirmation of metastases [2], [9]. These criteria may in fact be less stringent than previously: in the early 1970s, autopsy demonstration of the absence of any identifiable primary tumour was regarded as essential for the diagnosis of CUP, a requirement which would obviously be difficult to fulfil in the current climate. It is worth remembering that these tumours are heterogeneous in terms of histology, prognosis and treatment [11]: this aspect is highlighted throughout.

EPIDEMIOLOGY

In a general medical oncology service historically (up to the 1970s), CUP constituted as much as 10–15% of patients referred with solid tumours [12]. Although the site of origin can now be more frequently identified, CUP remains a significant problem, currently constituting 3–4% of all malignant neoplasms [2], [10], [13]. CUP is thus one of the ten most frequent cancer diagnoses [2], and in a population-based study, CUP was the sixth most common cancer presentation in both men and women [13]. Looking at absolute numbers, in the Netherlands, with a population of 16 million, almost 2500 new CUP patients are diagnosed annually, giving an age-standardised incidence rate of 6.7 per 100 000 for males and 5.3 per 100 000 for females [2].

Table 6.1 Types of tumour presenting as metastases of unknown origin

Tumour type	Frequency (%)
Adenocarcinoma	47, 50, 60, 61, 77
Poorly differentiated adenocarcinoma or undifferentiated carcinoma	12, 29, 30, 30, 44
Squamous	5, 5, 6, 7, 15
Undifferentiated	2, 5, 5, 5
Neuroendocrine	4, 7

Assembled from references [2], [6], [11], [13]–[15]

Patients with CUP have a median age of 60 years [2]. There is a slight gender bias towards men: figures of 53% male and 47% female are typical [13]. CUP is very rare in children, making up less than 1% of solid tumours [2].

PROGNOSIS

The prognosis for patients with CUP is poor: their median survival is four months [3], [13]. A study from The Netherlands, which was population-based rather than using tertiary referral patients, who tend to do better, found that only 15% of 1024 patients studied between 1984 and 1992 were still alive after one year. Interestingly, by 1999, seven years after the study ended, 25 (2.4%) patients were still alive, but further details of their cases were not given [13].

TUMOUR TYPES

The tumours of CUP are heterogeneous [11], with different histopathological types and anatomical locations: these two parameters govern the investigative and therapeutic strategies [8]. Looking first at the histopathological type, most studies of CUP exclude lymphoma, metastatic melanoma and metastatic sarcoma [9], [11]. Instead, the focus is on epithelial malignancies: adenocarcinoma, squamous carcinoma, poorly differentiated (adeno-)carcinoma and neuroendocrine carcinoma. The relative frequencies of these are presented in Table 6.1, [2], [6], [11], [13]–[15] which clearly shows that the most common CUP tumour is adenocarcinoma. The table includes listings for so-called 'undifferentiated carcinomas' and 'undifferentiated tumours': these diagnoses may largely be historical, since most could now be more specifically characterised by immunohistochemistry. The 'neuroendocrine' category is small because some studies included these with undifferentiated tumours. In most studies, squamous or 'epidermoid' carcinoma also includes basal cell and transitional tumours [10]. In childhood, most of the rare cases of CUP are embryonal ('small blue cell') tumours [2].

Karin A. Oien, Jayne L. Dennis and T. R. Jeffry Evans

SITES OF METASTASIS

Moving now to the anatomical location, metastatic disease presents most commonly in solid organs, lymph nodes and serous fluids. The main solid organs are liver, lung, bone and brain; the main lymph node groups are cervical, supraclavicular, axillary, inguinal and mediastinal/retroperitoneal; and the serous cavities are pleural and peritoneal. In the population-based study of CUP from The Netherlands, 26% of patients presented with disease disseminated to three or more sites; the rankings thereafter were 24% liver, 12% lung/pleura, 11% lymph nodes, 9% peritoneum, 8% bone, 2% brain and 8% elsewhere [13]. Further details about the individual metastatic sites are provided in the review by Pavlidis and colleagues [2].

SITES OF ORIGIN

The question as to which primary sites most commonly give rise to CUP is intrinsically difficult to answer. Even with extensive diagnostic work-up, the number of patients for whom a site of origin is identified during life is low, ranging from below 20% to 25% [2], [3].

Later, at autopsy, the primary site is found in between 30% and 80% of patients [2], [3], [5], [12]. The two most common sites of origin are lung and pancreas: the figures for each range between 16% and 37% [3], [5], [12], [14], [15]. The next most common primary sites include: colon and rectum (9–18%); stomach (6–8%); ovary (4–6%); liver (5–11%); kidney (6%); breast (2–5%); and prostate (4%) [5], [12], [15]. Other tumour types listed in an older study included melanoma at 6% and lymphoma at 4% [15], but these should now be excluded at an early stage on pathology.

SITES AND MODES OF METASTATIC PRESENTATION COMBINED

Table 6.2 presents the most common combinations of tumour type, metastatic site and primary site in CUP. These simple patterns assist in the prediction of the site of origin and are important for prognostic and therapeutic purposes. Let us look more closely at liver metastasis, which is one of the most common subgroups of CUP, as shown in Fig. 6.1: isolated hepatic spread accounts for approximately 25% of patients, and liver involvement is present in most of the 50% of patients with multiple organ involvement [2]. Liver metastasis is associated with a poor prognosis, which is similar whether other organs are involved or not [15]. The tumour is usually a moderately or poorly differentiated adenocarcinoma. The presence of neuroendocrine features is associated with a better therapeutic response and thus longer survival [2].

UNIQUE CHARACTERISTICS OF CUP

At this stage it is worth emphasising that whilst (adeno)carcinomas of unknown primary are heterogeneous in type and site, these tumours do share certain fundamental, and unusual, characteristics. First, the primary tumour is absent

Table 6.2 Tumour types, metastatic sites and primary sites in CUP

Site of metastatic tumour	Likely type and primary site
Liver	Adenocarcinoma
Lung	Adenocarcinoma Exclude germ cell tumour
Bone	Adenocarcinoma especially breast or prostate Renal cell and thyroid carcinoma
Brain	Adenocarcinoma from lung, breast or gastrointestinal tract Squamous cell carcinoma
Lymph node (cervical)	Squamous cell carcinoma from head and neck, oesophagus or bronchus Thyroid carcinoma
Lymph node (supraclavicular) (Virchow's node, Troisier's sign)	Squamous cell carcinoma, as above Adenocarcinoma especially breast or upper gastrointestinal tract
Lymph node (axillary)	Adenocarcinoma from breast
Lymph node (inguinal)	Squamous or other carcinoma from genitourinary tract (Melanoma)
Lymph node (mediastinal/ retroperitoneal, midline)	Poorly differentiated carcinoma/ germ cell tumour (male)
Peritoneal fluid (also periumbilical adenopathy or mass — Sister Mary Joseph's node)	Papillary serous adenocarcinoma: ovary (or primary peritoneal) Non-serous adenocarcinoma from gastrointestinal tract or elsewhere
Pleural effusion	Adenocarcinoma from lung, breast or ovary (Mesothelioma)

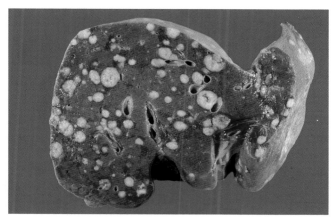

Fig. 6.1 Gross picture of adenocarcinoma metastatic to the liver.

139

in terms of clinical signs and symptoms and on investigation, and thus the cancer has disseminated early [2]. If identified later on, the primary tumour is usually small [3]. Second, and related to the first, this disease is aggressive: the clinical history at presentation is short, usually less than three months, and progression thereafter is rapid [3]. Lastly, the pattern of cancer spread in patients presenting with metastases is surprisingly different from those with an identified primary [12]. Bone metastases will be used as an example. These are very common in patients with known lung cancer, 30–50% of whom have osseous involvement at autopsy; by contrast, in patients whose lung cancer is found first at post-mortem, bony metastases are seen in only 4% at diagnosis and 11% after death. Similarly, prostatic cancer lacking a demonstrable primary has a three-fold lower incidence of bone metastases compared with patients with a known primary [2]. Conversely, 28% of patients with autopsy-diagnosed pancreatic cancer had bone involvement at initial presentation, compared with only 5–10% at autopsy in those with a known primary [12]. No explanation for these differences has yet been found.

PROGNOSTIC FEATURES AND THERAPY

By definition, patients with CUP have metastatic malignancy. In the past, the prognosis has been regarded as uniformly poor but this is no longer the case. Clinical subgroups which have better outcomes and respond to therapy have been identified, and their early recognition is the main aim of diagnostic work-up, including pathological assessment. This treatable cohort has expanded, even over the past two years, with improvements in chemotherapy for specific adeno-carcinomas, especially from the gastrointestinal tract. However, as previously discussed, the median survival for patients with CUP is four months. Within The Netherlands population-based study of 1024 patients, the 'treatable' subgroups accounted for approximately 30%, with the remaining patients receiving supportive care only [13].

What then constitutes these favourable subgroups? Individual positive and negative factors have been recognised: histopathological type; anatomical site (lymph node presentation is favourable, except for supraclavicular); the number of metastatic sites involved (one or two is favourable); and the patient's overall performance status [2], [5]. These individual factors can then be used to define subsets of CUP sensitive to either loco-regional treatment or systemic chemo-therapy, often with curative intent [2]. These subsets are detailed in Table 6.3 [2]. Loco-regional treatment with surgery and/or radiation is used for metastatic squamous carcinoma in lymph nodes and metastatic adenocarcinoma in axillary lymph nodes, and may be considered for isolated metastases in solid organs. Platinum-based chemotherapy is effective for poorly differentiated carcinomas involving the mediastinal-retroperitoneal nodes in males (extragonadal germ cell tumour), peritoneal papillary serous adenocarcinoma in females and poorly differentiated neuroendocrine carcinoma [2].

Most CUP patients, however, fall into unfavourable subsets: liver metastasis in general, except perhaps for an isolated deposit likely to be from colorectum; multiple metastases in any single solid organ (liver, lung, bone and brain); malignant ascites with adenocarcinoma which is not serous papillary; and

Table 6.3 Favourable subsets of CUP and their treatment

Favourable subset of CUP	Treatment as for equivalent stage of
Squamous carcinoma in cervical lymph node	Head and neck cancer Locoregional therapy: surgery and/or irradiation 35–50% 5-year survival
Squamous carcinoma in inguinal lymph node	Genito-urinary tumour Locoregional therapy: surgery and/or irradiation
Adenocarcinoma in axillary lymph node (female)	Breast cancer Locoregional then systemic therapy 75% 5-year survival
Extragonadal germ cell tumour in lymph node or lung (male)	Poor prognosis germ cell tumour Platinum-based chemotherapy 10–15% 5-year survival
Serous papillary adenocarcinoma in peritoneum (female)	Ovarian cancer Taxane/platinum-based chemotherapy 11–24% 5-year survival
Neuroendocrine carcinoma	Platinum or paclitaxel/carboplatin based chemotherapy 10–15% 5-year survival
Adenocarcinoma in bone with high PSA (male)	Prostate cancer with hormonal therapy
Single small metastasis in solid organ (liver, lung, brain)	Consider local treatment with resection and/or radiation, and/or systemic chemotherapy

pleural effusion [2]. These patients are relatively resistant to systemic therapy and have short survival times. Patients who are either very elderly or who have a poor performance status are best managed with symptomatic care. However, some may benefit from chemotherapy, which has long been the treatment of choice for patients with CUP. Almost all cytotoxic drugs have been tried either as single agents or in combination [2], usually empirically, and currently the use of a taxane, e.g. paclitaxel, in combination with a platinum agent, may provide the best treatment option for patients in unfavourable CUP groups [2].

Most of the unfavourable tumours are adenocarcinomas. Specific and effective treatments are already established for tumours originating in the breast, ovary and prostate. The emergence of new, more targeted therapies for the previously insensitive adenocarcinomas makes prediction of primary site more important. Consider the gastrointestinal adenocarcinomas: colonic, pancreatic and gastro-oesophageal. Until the past decade, 5-fluorouracil (5-FU)-based therapy was standard for all of these tumours [7]. Now, however, a more tailored approach is taken: e.g. 5-FU/leucovorin with irinotecan or oxaliplatin for colon, gemcitabine for pancreas, and epirubicin, cisplatin and 5-FU (ECF) for gastro-oesophageal cancers [7], [15].

While identification of the primary site provides important prognostic information and may facilitate specific antitumour treatment [14], these are not the only reasons for the search. Even if no proven treatment is available, patients and their families are often confused and frustrated to find out that the origin of their tumour is unknown, and they often want to learn the nature and source of their cancer, perhaps in an effort to come to terms with their disease: this wish should be respected [16].

The diagnostic and therapeutic nihilism of the past in searching for the unknown primary is thus disappearing. Concomitantly, identification of the likely primary site and the role of the histopathologist therein are becoming more important [7].

CLINICAL WORK-UP AND NON-INVASIVE INVESTIGATIONS

Most patients with CUP in the UK present first to their primary care physician and are then referred for investigation to a hospital specialist. Such a referral is usually on an elective basis, but this may become acute if the patient's disease progresses. Obviously, different symptoms and signs will lead to referral to different clinicians: e.g. gastrointestinal surgeon, respiratory physician, ear nose and throat surgeon, or gynaecologist. Typically, patients have symptoms and signs related to the site of metastatic cancer: many also have constitutional symptoms [6]. Liver spread, in particular, is often associated with non-specific symptoms including anorexia, weight loss, malaise and abdominal discomfort.

The initial evaluation often leads to a strong suspicion of metastatic cancer [6]. Subsequent investigations are aimed at confirming this diagnosis and identifying a primary site where possible. A detailed clinical history and physical examination are important, including examination of the rectum, pelvis, testes, thyroid and skin. Useful non-invasive tests include: full blood count, serum biochemistry, urinalysis and faecal occult blood testing. The results will guide further investigations which may include the following: cytology, radiology, serum tumour markers, endoscopy and biopsy.

CYTOLOGY

The first investigation of palpable lymphadenopathy is likely to be fine needle aspiration cytology. Likewise, effusion cytology will be performed early in patients with ascites or pleural effusions. For these presentations, the likely tumour types and primary sites have been discussed above.

RADIOLOGY

For non-specific abdominal symptoms, especially with abnormal liver function tests, liver ultrasound may be the test of choice. With respiratory symptoms, a chest X-ray will usually be performed. Frequently, the diagnosis of suspected malignancy will be made through these preliminary investigations.

Thereafter, CT scanning of chest, abdomen and pelvis is a useful tool for disease staging and may identify the site of origin. In patients with CUP, abdominal and pelvic CT scans identify a primary site in 30–35% [2], mostly in the pancreas [3]. CT scanning may also guide the selection of the best site for biopsy. Liver biopsy is one of the most common specimens received in this scenario, and it is important to be aware that on both ultrasound and CT scan, the typical multiple nodules of metastatic malignancy may in some cases be difficult to differentiate from the nodular liver of cirrhosis.

In women with metastatic adenocarcinoma involving axillary lymph nodes, the likely primary site is clearly the breast. Mammography has been proposed although its sensitivity is only around 20% [2]. Where a mammogram does not help, magnetic resonance imaging (MRI) may contribute [2].

SERUM TUMOUR MARKERS

Once the diagnosis of metastatic malignancy is made, serum tumour markers will usually be measured. Four markers may be useful in guiding the clinician towards a primary site, and in the follow-up of response to therapy in treatable subsets of CUP: prostate-specific antigen (PSA) in men with mainly bony metastases; CA125 in women with malignant ascites; and beta human chorionic gonadotrophin (bHCG) and alpha feto protein (AFP) in young men with mediastinal/retroperitoneal adenopathy or lung metastases [3]. Thyroid cancer is likely to be diagnosed by other means but it is worth remembering that the diagnosis is likely in CUP patients with bone metastases and high levels of serum thyroglobulin [2]. Perhaps surprisingly to us as pathologists, studies have shown that the sensitivity and specificity of most other available epithelial serum tumour markers (CEA, CA15-3 (breast) and CA19-9) are too low to be reliably diagnostic of a CUP primary site [3], although clinically they are still often used for this purpose and for monitoring treatment response.

ENDOSCOPY

Endoscopy is used for the evaluation of CUP patients with specific clinical presentations; for example, ENT endoscopy with isolated cervical lymph nodes, bronchoscopy with respiratory symptoms, gastrointestinal endoscopy with abdominal symptoms or positive FOB tests, and proctoscopy and/or colposcopy in patients with inguinal lymphadenopathy [2].

PROGRESSION TO BIOPSY

Studies have shown that this routine work-up is sufficient to identify the primary site in most patients in whom it will be possible by clinical means; more exhaustive invasive investigations, such as endoscopies not guided by symptomatology, only discomfort the patient and do not increase the yield of primary sites identified, alter treatment or lead to improved survival [15]. A limited diagnostic approach aiming to recognise patients with good prognostic features is now considered the best policy [2], [9].

If no primary site is identified clinically, the usual course of action is then to proceed to biopsy the metastasis, to (a) confirm malignancy and (b) subtype the tumour. In patients with poor performance status, it is common practice not to perform a biopsy but to diagnose CUP on clinical grounds alone: such clinical diagnosis constitutes around 20% [13]. Compared to those with histologically confirmed disease, these patients were older, received less cancer therapy and had a shorter median survival of 7 weeks [13]: the diagnosis of malignancy is clearly supported by the shorter survival time.

HISTOPATHOLOGY

'By far the most important step in the diagnostic procedure is biopsy of the most accessible lesion for pathological examination.' [3]

STANDARD HISTOPATHOLOGY

So, how should we as pathologists approach cancers of unknown primary site? Our focus is on clearly metastatic tumours, for which adenocarcinomas are the most common. However, other tumours may enter the differential diagnosis through unusual presentations or inadequate clinical information, so it is important to consider, and usually to exclude, other tumour types.

For this, a simple, logical and comprehensive approach is best. From basic pathology, the main forms of cancer are: carcinoma, melanoma, sarcoma, leukaemia and lymphoma, neuro-glial tumours and germ cell tumours. Taking these in turn, neuro-glial tumours almost never metastasise, and leukaemia and lymphoma are regarded as potentially systematised ab initio, although they must still be considered in the differential diagnosis. Germ cell tumours are rare but important, because, like haematological tumours, they may be highly chemosensitive: and epithelial differentiation in teratomas simulates carcinoma. Metastatic melanomas and sarcomas may occur without an obvious primary, but usually do so in lymph nodes and lung respectively.

Outwith these situations, almost all CUPs are carcinomas, which may be divided into: squamous (and transitional cell) tumours; adenocarcinomas; and carcinomas of solid organs, including liver, kidney and endocrine glands. These three groups can generally be separated on histological grounds, and with the help of mucin stains, but immunohistochemistry, particularly for specific cytokeratins, may be of value for confirmation and with poorly differentiated tumours.

Let us then return to the focus of this review. Most adenocarcinomas presenting as metastases are from seven main primary sites: breast, colon, lung, ovary, pancreas, prostate and stomach [12]. A shared glandular morphology is the basis on which the diagnosis is made. Thereafter, as Hammar stated, 'Experienced pathologists are aware of morphological patterns of many metastatic adenocarcinomas and, based on this experience, the primary site of some . . . can be stated with a significant degree of certainty on histological evaluation of neoplasms in H&E stained sections.' [16] Informative histology includes: 'dirty necrosis' in glands lined by columnar epithelium, which makes a colonic origin likely, as shown in Fig. 6.2; the presence of calcispherites, suggesting ovary; and 'signet ring' cells, which usually indicate stomach or breast (or colon).

The contribution of morphology to the prediction of site of origin was studied by Sheahan and colleagues [17]. Two pathologists evaluated one hundred metastatic adenocarcinomas of known primary site. The cases were viewed first without and then with knowledge of gender and metastatic site. Morphology alone enabled prediction of the correct primary site as choice 1 in 26% of cases for both pathologists, and as choices 1–3 in 50% and 43%. When gender and metastatic site were added, the correct prediction was choice 1 in 50% and 55% and choices 1–3 in 74% and 67% [17]. Accuracy was highest for prostatic, ovarian and breast and lowest for upper gastrointestinal and pancreatico-biliary tumours. The underlying clinical baseline was provided by a 1970s study, which showed that when a clinician developed a working diagnosis of a specific primary site in CUP, this was correct in less than 50% when compared with the autopsy findings [12].

Where distinctive morphological features of primary site are lacking, additional pathological procedures are undertaken. The most useful of these is immunohistochemistry: other techniques are discussed briefly below.

ELECTRON MICROSCOPY AND CYTOGENETICS

Electron microscopy is of use in distinguishing broad categories of tumours, e.g. carcinoma versus sarcoma, and the identification of neuroendocrine tumours.

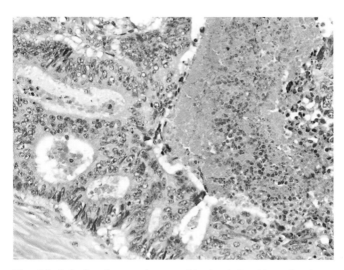

Fig. 6.2 Colonic adenocarcinoma with glands lined by tall columnar epithelium and dirty necrosis (top right) (H&E).

For prediction of the primary site of adenocarcinomas, certain features have been reported to be helpful: microvillous morphology and intracellular lamellar bodies suggest lung; intracellular neolumens containing projecting microvilli suggest breast; and outpouchings of the cell cytoplasm bearing rather short microvilli and a glycocalyx suggest serous papillary carcinoma of ovary or peritoneum [16]. In general, however, electron microscopy has little to contribute to this diagnostic challenge.

The same is true for cytogenetics, both conventional and molecular [2]. However, cytogenetics is a valuable diagnostic tool in lymphoma, sarcoma, small blue cell tumours and extragonadal germ cell tumours (which may show the i(12p) abnormality), and therefore appropriate sampling should be considered when biopsying a tumour of unknown origin [2].

IMMUNOHISTOCHEMISTRY

IMMUNOHISTOCHEMISTRY FOR PREDICTION OF PRIMARY SITE

Immunohistochemistry was first introduced into routine pathology practice in the late 1970s, and in tumour diagnosis was first used to separate broad categories, e.g. lymphoma versus carcinoma versus sarcoma [18]. Now, immunohistochemistry is the established method for clinically relevant tumour subtyping in lymphoma [19]. We are gradually progressing towards the same end with adenocarcinomas, and the field has been reviewed using Medline, as outlined above. Markers proposed to be of value in the distinction between primary sites have been identified and selected on the basis of sensitivity and specificity, and papers profiling their expression at each site sought. The literature comprises: comprehensive studies of established markers in adenocarcinomas from the 1990s [20]–[25]; reviews on cytokeratins 7 and 20 [26], [27]; and papers on individual markers [28]–[39]. The data are summarised in Table 6.4 which includes the markers CK7, CK20, CDX2, CEA, CA19-9, TTF1, GCDFP-15, ER, CA125, mesothelin and PSA.

INTERPRETATION OF MARKERS OF PRIMARY SITE

We will shortly look at each marker in detail. For each antibody, further information can be obtained, not only from the primary literature, but also from: textbooks [18]; the website Immunoquery.com, which is an excellent resource in many diagnostic dilemmas; and the commercial antibody suppliers (especially Novocastra, Dako and Serotec) through their websites, catalogues, datasheets and literature on techniques and applications. Interestingly, most antibodies used in pathology departments still carry the rider, 'For research use only: not for diagnostic use'!

For our purposes, the ideal marker would be highly sensitive (and thus identify most tumours from the target site) and specific (and thus would not stain tumours from sites other than the target). However, even markers with rather low values may be useful in specific situations, for example if the differential diagnosis has already been narrowed down to two or three sites only.

Table 6.4 Expression of markers of primary site in adenocarcinomas

Tumour site	(% Positivity of marker)										
	CK20	CDX2	CEA	CA19–9	CK7	TTF1	GCDFP-15	ER	CA125	Mesothelin	PSA
Colon	65, 73, 84, 88, 92, 92, 93, 100	90, 99	58, 86, 96, 98, 98, 99, 100, 100, 100	71, 76, 79, 85	5, 6, 7, 9, 16, 23, 38	0, 0, 0	0, 0, 0, 0, 0, 0, 0	0, 0, 0, 0, 13	4, 4, 9, 10, 13, 18	4, 22	0, 0
Stomach	30, 41, 50, 51, 54, 68	20, 70	67, 72, 75, 80	56, 71	38, 51, 60, 71	0, 0	0, 0, 3	0, 2	7, 11	10, 29	0
Pancreas	0, 35, 39, 44, 62	0, 32	50, 81, 88, 92, 98	85, 85	87, 92, 95	0, 0, 0	0, 0, 0	0, 0	48, 48	75, 86	0
Lung	0, 8, 9, 10, 10	0, 0	54, 63, 88, 90, 91	13, 30, 32, 69	96, 100, 100	66, 75, 75	0, 0, 0, 4, 6	0, 0, 3, 11	20, 20, 20, 35	22, 24	9
Breast	0, 0, 0, 0, 4, 7, 19	0, 0	32, 37, 40, 57, 71	6, 11, 24, 45	70, 89, 93, 93, 96	0, 0	33, 52, 62, 67, 72, 74, 77	32, 33, 58, 60, 63, 73	13, 13, 13, 23, 24	3, 6	0
Ovary (non-mucinous)	0, 0, 4, 19	0, 0	0, 0, 21, 37, 40	41, 57	83, 89, 91, 100, 100	0, 0	0, 0, 0, 0, 4, 4	4, 12, 34, 50	61, 63, 74, 80, 91, 96	95, 100	0, 0
Ovary (mucinous)	50, 61, 68	20, 64	67, 80	78	—	—	0	50	17, 35	—	—
Prostate	0, 0, 21	1, 4	0, 14	6	0, 5, 12, 29	0, 0	10, 15	10	2, 2, 5	0, 0	86, 96
Renal	0, 0, 3, 14	0, 0	0, 5	8, 27	11, 14, 29	0, 0	0, 3, 3, 14	0, 2, 29	0, 0	0, 0	0

Assembled from refs. [20], [22]–[39]

The nature of these proposed markers of primary site varies: some are nuclear proteins such as transcription factors, directly regulating cell differentiation; others are structural intermediate filaments; and yet others are specific cellular products, expressed on the surface or secreted. In assessing whether an antibody is positive or negative, it is therefore imperative to know where the staining is expected to be − nuclear, cytoplasmic and/or membranous − so that only true staining is accepted. Considering the location of staining, it is equally necessary to ensure that only tumour tissue is evaluated; for example, alveolar cells adjacent to or entrapped within a tumour will be TTF1-positive and potentially confounding in an adenocarcinoma metastatic to lung. Lastly, while immunohistochemical staining is generally uniform in any given normal cell type, tumours are more heterogeneous [26]: the resulting variability may be more problematic with small biopsy samples. This is only amplified by the existence of significant tumour subtypes, for example, in breast, ovarian and gastric cancer, which may or may not be studied separately.

The intensity of the immunohistochemical staining is also important. Some diagnostic markers, such as PSA and TTF1, tend to be either strongly positive or absent. However, other markers, including cytokeratins and ER, may be more graduated, with weak and moderate, as well as strong, staining [40]. Interpretation of these markers is more complex, which should be borne in mind when reviewing the literature: the threshold used for reactivity varies between studies, and obviously, as it is raised, the number of 'positive' cases decreases [40]. This is even without introducing the issue of 'random' intra- and inter-observer variation in interpretation [26]. Regarding thresholds, most studies tend to ignore weak, focal staining [23], [24], [41].

As a slight aside, immunohistochemistry may be successful even in necrotic tumours. Obviously, such material has to be evaluated with great care to avoid misinterpreting non-specific staining as positive, and careful inspection of and comparison with the positive and negative controls is important. With these caveats, we have found immunohistochemistry to be surprisingly useful on occasion, even when H&E yields only amorphous eosinophilic necrotic tissue.

METHODOLOGICAL CONSIDERATIONS

Immunohistochemistry is often regarded as a straightforward technique, but in fact its performance is as complex as its interpretation, and variation may arise at many stages [20], [26]. For each marker, there are usually multiple antibodies: these may be polyclonal or monoclonal and may have been raised against the whole marker (glyco-) protein or using a range of different smaller epitopes. Each antibody has an optimal dilution and method of antigen retrieval, if needed, whether heat or enzymatic. Specimen processing, particularly fixation conditions and time, also affects tissue antigenicity [20]. All of these issues must be considered when introducing and evaluating new markers.

SPECIFIC MARKERS AND THEIR ANTIBODIES

Our focus is on adenocarcinomas and, to a lesser extent, other epithelial tumours: squamous (and transitional) carcinomas and those of solid organs. While other cancers, including germ cell tumours, melanomas, sarcomas, lymphomas and leukaemias, may present to pathologists as metastases of unknown origin, as discussed above, it is assumed that these have been excluded already [8]: a full discussion of immunohistochemical markers for these tumours is outwith the scope of this review and readers are referred to standard textbooks [18], [42].

CYTOKERATINS

Basic biology of cytokeratins

Cytokeratins (CKs) are the principal positive marker for carcinomas. Chu and Weiss recently published an excellent review [43]. These proteins play a structural role within cells, being the intermediate filaments (IF) specific to epithelia. They are divided into Type I and Type II IFs. Twenty different keratin subunits exist and their molecular weights (MW) lie between 40 and 70 kDa. Keratins are divided by MW into low and high forms, and they are also split into acidic and basic forms [43]. Type I cytokeratins are low MW and acidic, and are numbered CK10−20; Type II cytokeratins are high MW and basic, and are numbered CK1−9. In cells, keratin filaments contain at least one Type I subunit and one Type II subunit, as a pair. Each cell type expresses only certain cytokeratins, which vary during development and differentiation.

A number of antibody mixtures are commonly used. AE1/3 is a mixture of the AE1 and AE3 clones, of which AE1 recognises the type I keratins CK10, CK15−16 and CK19, while AE3 recognises the type II keratins CK1−6 and CK8; AE1/3 is thus a pan-specific cocktail for cytokeratins which should stain all carcinomas [43]. CAM 5.2 reacts with CK8 and CK18, which are present in most secretory and parenchymatous epithelia; it thus stains adenocarcinomas as well as liver and renal carcinomas [43].

CK7 is widely expressed in simple glandular epithelium, generally from ducts, including pancreas, biliary tract and renal collecting duct, and in transitional epithelium. CK20 is expressed in gastrointestinal and transitional epithelium and some neuro-epithelial cells [9]: specifically, it is found in gastric foveolar epithelium, endocrine cells in pyloric glands, intestinal villous and crypt epithelium, cutaneous and oral Merkel cells, taste buds and urothelial umbrella cells [43]. CK5 is present in basal cells of squamous and glandular epithelia, myoepithelium and mesothelium, and hyperproliferative squamous epithelia contains CK6. A CK5/6 antibody mix is popular: it stains squamous and transitional epithelia, plus mesothelium, but not glandular epithelium [43].

Cytokeratins in carcinomas

Squamous carcinomas are usually identifiable as such on histology, but poorly differentiated tumours may be distinguished by immunohistochemistry.

Unlike the main adenocarcinomas (except prostate), and unlike transitional cell carcinomas, squamous carcinomas are usually negative for both CK7 and CK20 [8], [43]. Squamous carcinomas are also generally negative for CAM5.2, unlike adenocarcinomas [43]. In contrast, almost all squamous carcinomas are positive with CK5/6: the same is true of two-thirds of transitional cell carcinomas, and most biphasic mesotheliomas, whereas adenocarcinomas lack CK5/6 [43].

Carcinomas of solid organs include hepatocellular, renal, thyroid and other endocrine. Their presentation as true metastases of unknown origin is now much less common than in previous decades, because of improvements in imaging. Both hepatocellular and standard renal (clear) cell carcinomas are negative with CK7 and CK20. AE1/3 is positive in both [43]. CAM5.2 is generally positive only in the liver tumours, because renal cell carcinomas lack CK8 and CK18 [43]. Although conventional renal carcinomas are CK7-negative, papillary, collecting duct and chromophobe renal carcinomas are CK7+ [43].

A hepatocellular tumour can be confirmed as such using polyclonal CEA (or CD10) to outline canaliculi. More recently, the antibody Hep Par 1 (hepatocyte paraffin 1, hepat) has emerged as a positive marker of hepatocytes. Fan *et al.* studied 676 tumours: 95% of hepatocellular carcinomas were positive, but so were half of the gastric carcinomas. Only small numbers of adenocarcinomas from other sites, including colon and ovary, expressed the antigen [44]. The demonstration of alpha-fetoprotein production by immunohistochemistry or by raised serum levels is found in around 25% and 75% respectively of hepatocellular carcinomas.

Thyroid carcinomas are generally CK7+/CK20−. Thyroglobulin is a specific marker which is found only in thyroid follicular epithelium and related neoplasms, and is useful in confirming the origin of metastatic papillary carcinoma in cervical lymph nodes or of bone metastases [20]. Thyroid transcription factor 1 (TTF1) is obviously found in most thyroid carcinomas, including all those of follicular origin [9], [28], [32]: TTF1 regulates thyroglobulin transcription. Thyroid medullary carcinomas are distinguished by their expression of calcitonin [8].

Metastatic neuroendocrine tumours, including poorly differentiated large-cell carcinomas with neuroendocrine features, are not uncommon [11]. Their recognition is important because of their good response to chemotherapy. Metastatic neuroendocrine tumours are relatively common in the liver, where they may resemble a hepatocellular lesion and can be distinguished using the neuroendocrine markers chromogranin, synaptophysin, CD56 and PGP9.5 [8]. Note that CK7 may be positive in 20−40% of neuroendocrine neoplasms [43].

Cytokeratins 7 and 20 in adenocarcinomas

In combination, CK7 and CK20 expression in adenocarcinomas is characteristic of certain primary sites, as summarised in Table 6.5. CK7 is restricted to a subset of adenocarcinomas of glandular epithelial origin [43]. The vast majority of adenocarcinomas of lung, (non-mucinous) ovary, endometrium, breast, pancreas and biliary tract and salivary gland are CK7 positive [43]. Almost all colorectal tumours are CK7 negative [43].

Table 6.5 Combined expression of cytokeratins 7 and 20 in carcinomas

	CK7 positive	CK7 negative
CK20 positive	*GI and GU adenocarcinomas* Pancreas and biliary tract (two-thirds) Stomach (one-third) Ovary (mucinous) Transitional cell carcinoma (two-thirds)	*GI adenocarcinomas* Colon and rectum Stomach (one-third) Merkel
CK20 negative	*Range of adenocarcinomas* Breast Lung (adenocarcinoma) Ovary (serous and endometrioid) Pancreas and biliary tract (one-third) Stomach (19%) Endometrium Salivary Thyroid Transitional cell carcinoma (one-third) Malignant mesothelioma (two-thirds)	*Prostatic and other adenocarcinomas* Prostate Stomach (14%) Hepatocellular carcinoma Renal (clear) cell carcinoma Adrenal carcinoma Squamous carcinoma Small cell carcinoma (but one-quarter CK7 positive) Malignant mesothelioma (one-third)

Assembled from refs. [8], [16], [43]

CK20 is positive in almost all colon carcinomas and in half of gastric and pancreatic adenocarcinomas [43]. CK20 is often found in ovarian mucinous tumours, but tumours primary to the ovary are usually also CK7 positive [43], [45]. Amongst other tumours, CK20 is found in 68% of transitional cell carcinomas (alongside CK7) and 86% of Merkel cell tumours [43]. CK20 is essentially absent from skin, breast, respiratory epithelium, salivary gland and liver [43].

The CK20+/CK7− phenotype strongly favours a colonic primary while CK20−/CK7+ narrows the differential to lung, breast, biliary, pancreatic, ovarian and endometrial carcinomas [9]. CK20+/CK7+ indicates a gastrointestinal or mucinous ovarian adenocarcinoma, or transitional cell carcinoma. Of the seven common adenocarcinomas, only prostate is usually CK7−/CK20−. The CK7/CK20 expression pattern in gastric carcinomas varies considerably, perhaps reflecting the range of expression in normal gastric mucosa, where the superficial and foveolar epithelial cells are CK20 positive and mucous neck cells are CK7 positive [38].

CK20 (along with CDX2) is valuable in evaluating the likely primary site of signet ring cell adenocarcinomas [46], [47]. These can obviously originate from breast (lobular carcinoma) and stomach (diffuse carcinoma) as well as, rarely, colon. Tot found that all gastrointestinal signet ring cell carcinomas (all of 22) were CK20 positive compared with almost none from the breast (2/79) [46]. The positive breast marker was ER.

PSA

Pathologists will be familiar with prostate specific antigen (PSA) [48]. PSA is a serine protease present at high levels in semen. It is an extremely specific and sensitive marker of normal prostatic epithelial cells and prostatic adenocarcinoma [20]. PSA is also found in peri-urethral and peri-anal glands and may occasionally be expressed in salivary and breast tumours [9].

TTF1

Thyroid transcription factor 1 (TTF1) is expressed in the nucleus of lung and thyroid epithelial cells, including C-cells [9], [28], [32], [49]. Cytoplasmic staining has been reported and should be disregarded. In the lung, TTF1 is found in respiratory epithelium, especially Type II pneumocytes and Clara cells [28]. TTF1 is a transcription factor involved in developmental regulation, and so it contains a homeobox domain.

The tissue-specific expression of TTF1 is generally maintained in the corresponding carcinomas [49]. TTF1 is expressed by 68–75% of non-mucinous lung adenocarcinomas and 40–50% of non-neuroendocrine lung large cell carcinomas [9], [28], [32]. Mucinous adenocarcinomas, principally bronchiolo-alveolar, unlike other pulmonary adenocarcinomas, are usually negative for TTF1: they may also stain with CK20 [32], [39], [49]. Only a minority of lung squamous carcinomas stain with TTF1: figures vary from 0 to 25% [32]. Tumours from other sites, except obviously thyroid, do not express TTF1 [28], [32]. Previously, surfactant proteins A and B had been proposed as markers of lung origin [9]. In this function, they have been superseded by TTF1, which is not surprising since TTF1 controls their transcription. TTF1 is both more sensitive and more specific in adenocarcinomas of lung origin than either of the surfactant proteins, and TTF1 is always absent from mesotheliomas [50]. When the tumour under investigation is in the lung itself, TTF1 positivity should be evaluated carefully to ensure that it is in tumour cells and not in entrapped normal respiratory epithelium [32].

Most small-cell carcinomas (around 90%) and large-cell neuroendocrine carcinomas are positive for TTF1, whether they originate in lung or elsewhere [28].

ER

Like TTF1, oestrogen receptor (ER) positivity is assessed on nuclear staining [51]. Intuitively, one would expect that ER expression would be restricted to carcinomas of the breast, ovary and elsewhere in the gynaecological tract [20]. This has certainly been our personal experience, and this agrees with the recent literature as seen in Table 6.4. However, previous reports have suggested that a number of other tumour types, including prostatic, gastric, lung, thyroid and transitional cell carcinomas, may express ER by immunohistochemistry [20], [33]. The methodology in the early reports varied: a range of primary antibodies against ER was used in both frozen and fixed tissues [20], [33]. This, together with variability in the threshold used for positivity (for example, whether weak staining is included), may account for these discrepancies. ER is composed of alpha and beta subunits: the former is the target of most currently used antibodies.

Note that ER is useful in evaluating the likely primary site of signet ring cell adenocarcinomas [46], [47]. These can obviously originate from breast (lobular carcinoma) and stomach (diffuse carcinoma) as well as, more rarely, colon. Some 81% of signet ring breast cancers are ER-positive, compared with none of the gastrointestinal tumours [46], [47]. CK20 and CDX2 are useful positive markers for a gastrointestinal origin.

GCDFP-15

Gross cystic disease fluid proteins (GCDFPs) were first identified in fluid from macroscopic breast cysts [35]. They are also detectable in the plasma of patients with breast cancer [35]. GCDFPs form a family that are named by their molecular weights: GCDFP-15, GCDFP-24, GCDFP-44 and GCDFP-70. Of these, GCDFP-15 is the most commonly found in breast cancer [35]. GCDFP-15 is expressed by cells with apocrine characteristics and is present in 62–75% of breast carcinomas, with only minor differences among the histological subtypes [9], [20]. GCDFP-15 is also found in normal and cancerous salivary glands, sweat glands, bronchial glands, prostate and seminal vesicle [35]. GCDFP-15 immunoreactivity takes the form of cytoplasmic staining [35]. The presence of GCDFP-15 in a tumour does not correlate with ER positivity: Wick and colleagues found that GCDFP-15 was present in 11 of 21 cases of breast cancer that lacked ER, thus it provides information supplementary to ER alone regarding a likely breast origin [35].

CA125

CA125 was characterised as a membrane glycoprotein in ovarian carcinoma cells nearly 20 years ago [20]. Thereafter it was recognised also to be expressed by mesothelial cells and mesotheliomas [20]. Other than the latter, CA125 is expressed in gynaecological malignancies: in 62%, 61% and 94% of adenocarcinomas of endocervix, ovary and endometrium, respectively [36]. Around one-half of pancreatico-biliary carcinomas and one-quarter of lung adenocarcinomas are also CA125-positive, but it is uncommon in adenocarcinomas from other sites, as shown in Table 6.4 [36].

MESOTHELIN

Like CA125, mesothelin is a glycoprotein [31], [34]. It is the 40 kd carboxy terminal component of a 69 kDa precursor protein, whose amino portion is the secreted cytokine known as megakaryocyte-potentiating factor. Mesothelin's function is unknown but a role in cell adhesion has been postulated [34]. Mesothelin is normally expressed in normal mesothelium and in some epithelial cells of the kidney, tonsil, trachea and fallopian tube [34]. The immunoreactivity is predominantly membranous but may also be cytoplasmic [34]. In tumours, mesothelin is expressed in most ovarian serous and pancreatic ductal adenocarcinomas [31], [34], as with CA125. Mesothelin is expressed at lower levels in lung, gastro-oesophageal and colonic adenocarcinomas [34].

CEA

Although carcinoembryonic antigen (CEA) is recognised principally as a serological marker for the follow-up of patients with colon cancer [52], it is expressed by many other adenocarcinomas, as shown in Table 6.4. CEA has a membranous and cytoplasmic distribution. It is a member of the immunoglobulin gene superfamily and is therefore a large glycoprotein, with common domains shared between family members, as well as smaller regions, which may be tissue-restricted and recognised only by a subset of antibodies [20]. The wide range of results seen in studies of CEA and its expression in tumours, as shown in Table 6.4, reflects this antigenic complexity. In general, clearly identified, monoclonal anti-CEA preparations are preferred and good results have been obtained with the well characterised clone II-7 [33]. It is especially useful in the differentiation of adenocarcinoma from mesothelioma: CEA is absent from the latter [53].

CA19-9

CA19-9 is an epitope located specifically on Sialyl Lewis^a glycolipids [20], [54]. The antibody targeting CA19-9 was raised against a colonic adenocarcinoma cell line and produces membrane staining. CA19-9 is similar to CA50 and is expressed in most carcinomas of the gastrointestinal tract, pancreas, biliary tree, ovaries and endometrium. Other adenocarcinomas are said to be rarely positive [20], although results vary as shown by Table 6.4. Hepatocellular and renal carcinomas are usually negative for CA19-9 [20]. CA19-9 has been used as a serum marker for the diagnosis and follow-up of gastrointestinal and especially pancreatic cancer, but it is also expressed in benign pancreatic disease including chronic pancreatitis [54].

CDX2

CDX2, like TTF1, is a homeobox protein transcription factor: it is named for its homology with the Drosophila gene *caudal*. CDX2 is normally expressed in intestinal epithelial cells from the proximal duodenum to distal rectum, where it plays an important role in epithelial differentiation and maintenance [29], [55]. Positive staining is therefore nuclear: cytoplasmic staining may occur but should be disregarded [55].

Over 90% of colonic adenocarcinomas show CDX2 staining which is strong and diffuse, that is, present in most cells, as shown in Fig. 6.3 [29], [30]. The same is true of duodenal adenocarcinomas [29]. CDX2 expression is lower in gastro-oesophageal and pancreatico-biliary carcinomas: Werling *et al.* described more heterogeneous CDX2 expression, with most tumours showing CDX2 in a minority of cells, with a substantial minority of completely negative cases and a

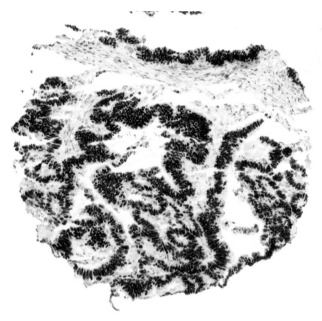

Fig. 6.3 Colonic adenocarcinoma in a tissue microarray core, stained for CDX2 which is located in the epithelial nuclei.

smaller minority uniformly positive [29]; whereas Moskaluk *et al.* found widespread CDX2 staining in only 20–30% of gastro-oesophageal adenocarcinomas, with pancreatico-biliary tumours being essentially negative [30]. The only other cancers to show high-level expression of CDX2 are ovarian mucinous adenocarcinomas (64%) and, interestingly, primary bladder adenocarcinomas (100%) [29].

Thus CDX2 is a highly sensitive and highly, but incompletely, specific marker for gastrointestinal adenocarcinomas, and strong, uniform and diffuse staining is seen primarily in tumours of colonic origin. There appears to be little, if any, association between the expression levels of nuclear transcription factors and the state of differentiation of the tumour, thus 74 out of 75 colonic adenocarcinomas were CDX2-positive, regardless of their grade [29], unlike CK20 [38], [49].

CDX2 might also be helpful in predicting the primary site of neuroendocrine tumours. In general, their CDX2 expression resembles that of non-neuroendocrine carcinomas from the same anatomical location [30]. Thus, out of 30 neuroendocrine tumours studied, 8 of 9 midgut carcinoids and 4 of 9 hindgut carcinoids displayed extensive CDX2 staining, whereas carcinoids of stomach, biliary tract and lung showed no or only focal CDX2 expression [30]. Out of 14 pancreatic islet cell tumours, 13 also showed little or no CDX2 staining [30].

OTHER NEW MARKERS

Other markers with potential utility in the assessment of adenocarcinomas of unknown origin emerge regularly. For example, where the differential diagnosis lies between pancreatico-biliary and ovarian carcinomas, CK17 and WT1 (Wilm's tumour 1) proteins may help. Goldstein and Bassi have shown that, in this situation, cytokeratin 17 is specific for pancreatico-biliary tumours (staining 42%, versus none of the ovarian) and WT1 is specific for serous ovarian tumours (staining 54%, versus none of the pancreatico-biliary) [40].

EXTENSION OF MARKERS FROM PRIMARY TUMOURS TO METASTASES

Most genes proposed as markers of primary site are in fact involved in the differentiation and function of the corresponding normal tissue. It is their retained expression during carcinogenesis which is of diagnostic use. Many markers have been evaluated predominantly in primary tumours, yet their principal clinical utility may be in metastatic disease. It is often assumed but not always verified that primary and metastatic tumours share similar expression profiles [49], but happily the few immunohistochemical studies which have been performed show general concordance [22], [23], [56].

USE OF PANELS OF MULTIPLE MARKERS

In routine diagnostic practice, immunohistochemical markers are generally used not in isolation but as part of a larger panel. However, while the individual markers described above have been investigated in depth, the utility of comprehensive antibody panels (other than cytokeratins) in predicting the primary site of adenocarcinomas has been addressed by surprisingly few primary studies and review articles: most are included in Table 6.4 [9], [16], [20]−[24], [49], [57].

One of the first papers on the subject was by Ellis and Hitchcock in 1988. They evaluated CEA, EMA, CA125 and CA19−9. Although they did not identify any 'distinctive results ... for a particular site of origin', they stated that, 'Some patterns of consistent positivity or negativity for the panel of antisera used were seen, however, which if applied to metastatic deposits have the potential to assist prediction of the site of origin' [57].

In 1997, Perry et al. investigated 68 consecutive biopsies from brain metastases where the primary site was known [23]. Spread to the brain commonly occurs with lung, breast and gastrointestinal adenocarcinomas, and with renal cancers. The helpful markers were: GCDFP-15, ER and CK7 for breast; CK20 for gastrointestinal; and CK7 for lung [23]. GCDFP-15 and ER were relatively specific but insensitive markers, whereas CK7 and CK20 scored highly on both parameters [23]. CAM 5.2, wide-spectrum keratins and progesterone receptor (PR) were unhelpful [23].

Brown et al. studied 128 metastatic adenocarcinomas from five sites of origin (breast, colon, lung, ovary and upper gastrointestinal tract) in 1998. They tested eight markers and selected four: CEA, CA19−9, CA125 and BCA225 (breast cancer antigen 225). Using these, the primary site was correctly predicted in 66% [24], as follows: BCA225+, CEA− and CA125− for breast; CEA+, BCA− and CA125− for colon; BCA225+, CEA+ and CA19−9− for lung; CA125+ and CEA− for ovary and CEA+, CA19−9+ and CA125+ for upper gastrointestinal tract [24]. The four markers tested but discarded were: GCDFP-15, B72.3, DF3 (CA15-3) and ER [24]. Again, GCDFP-15 and ER were found to be specific but with low sensitivity [24]. This was the only recent study to evaluate BCA225. While it was very sensitive for breast, staining over 95%, it was also present in ovary (67%), lung (78%) and upper gastrointestinal tract (28–47%) [24]. Because of this lack of specificity, BCA225 was omitted from Table 6.4.

Lagendijk *et al.* studied primary and metastatic adenocarcinomas from three sites (colon, breast and ovary) in order better to distinguish ovarian primary from secondary tumours. The use of six markers (CK7, CK20, CA125, CEA, ER and GCDFP-15) yielded correct classification in 80–90% [21], [22]. CEA identified tumours metastatic to the ovary. GCDFP-15 led to the identification of 70–80% of breast carcinomas with no false positives. CA125 was commonly expressed in ovarian primaries and rarely found in colonic carcinomas.

DeYoung and colleagues studied over 2800 epithelial malignancies (a wide range including germ cell tumours, mesotheliomas and solid carcinomas) in 2000. Many immunohistochemical markers were evaluated. A panel of 14 were selected and incorporated into a diagnostic algorithm, resembling a flow-chart, and including the site-specific markers PSA, GCDFP-15, CEA-M, CA125, CA19–9, CK20 and ER [20]. In cases of clinical metastatic cancer of unknown origin, where the primary site later became evident, their prediction using the algorithm agreed in 66% [20].

Our focus has been on adenocarcinomas presenting as metastases in the classical sites, such as liver. Obviously, other locations, such as ovary, as discussed above, and bladder, may harbour metastatic malignancy [21], [22], [25]. Their evaluation lies outwith the scope of this review. It is worth, however, highlighting ovarian mucinous tumours. They are well-recognised to show gastric, intestinal and pancreatic differentiation and so it is no surprise that their expression profile overlaps with those of gastrointestinal tumours, as shown in Table 6.4 and elsewhere [58]. This makes the distinction of primary from secondary difficult and, indeed, it is likely that many mucinous tumours regarded as originating in the ovary in fact represent metastasis from a (hitherto occult) gastrointestinal primary, especially with large bilateral ovarian masses [59].

INTERPRETATION OF MULTIPLE MARKERS

Pathologists are accustomed to using panels of immunohistochemical markers, partly because we are taught to be wary of single stains, in case of spurious results. The expected outcomes are usually presented in tabular format, as with Table 6.4. The datasets to be evaluated, however, are complex, comprising multiple quantitative and qualitative data points. Their assimilation and integration are equally complex, and are usually performed by a neural network – literally, within the pathologist's brain. It is often difficult, however, for the pathologist to describe exactly how the diagnosis was arrived at.

The development of diagnostic algorithms beyond tables, for example, decision trees, requires a more explicit process. As DeYoung and colleagues stated, 'The sequence of interpretation of a group of immunostains should be governed by their relative statistical values, moving from most specific to the least or from the highest positive predictive value to lowest' [20]. Clearly this requires that specificity, sensitivity and predictive values must be known for each marker [20]. All three parameters vary according to the population analysed, which must therefore be chosen carefully in any research study to represent the clinical scenario under consideration.

Note that, in Table 6.4, the figure given for each marker in its expected site is in fact the sensitivity (= true positive/true positive + false negative). The specificity is the inverse of the amount (i.e. lack) of staining for that marker in the 'other' tumours (= true negative/true negative + false positive). Thus PSA, which stains almost all prostatic carcinomas, but very few other tumours, is both specific and sensitive. So, when pathologists compare data with a table, they are in fact following the rules described above, but are generally unaware of formally doing so.

NEW HORIZONS

Clearly histopathology as a specialty is based on morphology and likely to remain so for the immediate future. The complementary role of immunohisto-chemistry, which is a form of molecular pathology since its target is protein, is well established and continues to move forward: it is the gold standard in lymphoma sub-typing and, as we have seen, the problem of categorising adeno-carcinomas by site is slowly being solved.

The future may hold new markers, new methods and new ways of thinking about tumours. New markers will emerge from candidate gene approaches and from large-scale mRNA profiling and proteomics [60]. A number of cDNA array and other mRNA expression studies have already addressed the clinical question of carcinoma and adenocarcinoma subtyping [61]–[63]. Whether these will lead to pathologists likewise undertaking high-tech methods of tumour analysis or whether individual markers will become established from the hundreds highlighted by such studies remains to be seen: the paradigm is the identification of new clinical subsets within histologically homogeneous diffuse large B-cell lymphomas [64], and distillation of the diagnostic criteria from hundreds of genes down to a few markers including bcl–6 and CD10.

As new chemotherapeutic regimens emerge, however, the main question may not be whether the tumour comes from the breast but whether it will behave clinically and respond to therapy as would a breast cancer. In that situation, ER-positivity may answer both questions. Elsewhere, other markers predictive of outcome and therapeutic sensitivity, such as thymidylate synthase or mismatch repair proteins in the colon, may become standard. Pathologists are ideally placed to undertake the translational studies required to bring such markers forward into routine clinical use.

CONCLUSION

Metastatic cancer of unknown origin is a common clinical problem. Pathological assessment is important for both confirmation of the diagnosis and for tumour sub-typing [11]. Most CUP patients have adenocarcinomas and identification of the primary site is becoming increasingly important with the emergence of more targeted therapies, even for the previously insensitive tumours. Pathology with immunohistochemistry is recognised as more useful and cost-effective in the search for a site of origin than an exhaustive and invasive clinical search. While immunohistochemistry remains a diagnostic adjunct, which should be interpreted only in the context of both morphology and clinical data [20], its application will help to solve the diagnostic dilemma of adenocarcinoma of unknown origin in most cases.

NOTE ADDED IN PROOF

A recent paper from our group with a diagnostic table and decision tree for the prediction of the primary site is:
Dennis JL, Hvidsten TR, Wit EC, *et al*. Markers of adenocarcinoma characteristic of the site of origin: development of a diagnostic algorithm. *Clin Cancer Res* 2005; **11**: 3766–72.

REFERENCES

1. Souhami R, Tobias J. Cancer from an unknown primary site. *Cancer and Its Management.* 4th edn. (Blackwell Science, Oxford, 2003), pp. 325–8.
2. Pavlidis N, Briasoulis E, Hainsworth J, Greco FA. Diagnostic and therapeutic management of cancer of an unknown primary. *Eur J Cancer* 2003; **39**: 1990–2005.
3. Hillen HF. Unknown primary tumours. *Postgrad Med J* 2000; **76**: 690–3.
4. Pavlidis N. Cancer of unknown primary: biological and clinical characteristics. *Ann Oncol* 2003; **14**(Suppl 3): iii 11–18.
5. Briasoulis E, Pavlidis N. Cancer of unknown primary origin. *Oncologist* 1997; **2**: 142–52.
6. Hainsworth JD, Greco FA. Treatment of patients with cancer of an unknown primary site. *N Engl J Med* 1993; **329**: 257–63.
7. Mintzer DM, Warhol M, Martin AM, Greene G. Cancer of unknown primary: changing approaches. A multidisciplinary case presentation from the Joan Karnell Cancer Center of Pennsylvania Hospital. *Oncologist* 2004; **9**: 330–8.
8. Bugat R, Bataillard A, Lesimple T *et al*. Summary of the standards, options and recommendations for the management of patients with carcinoma of unknown primary site (2002). *Br J Cancer* 2003; **89**(Suppl 1): S59–66.
9. Varadhachary GR, Abbruzzese JL, Lenzi R. Diagnostic strategies for unknown primary cancer. *Cancer* 2004; **100**: 1776–85.
10. Muir C. Cancer of unknown primary site. *Cancer* 1995; **75**: 353–6.
11. Lenzi R, Hess KR, Abbruzzese MC, Raber MN, Ordonez NG, Abbruzzese JL. Poorly differentiated carcinoma and poorly differentiated adenocarcinoma of unknown origin: favorable subsets of patients with unknown-primary carcinoma? *J Clin Oncol* 1997; **15**: 2056–66.
12. Nystrom JS, Weiner JM, Heffelfinger-Juttner J, Irwin LE, Bateman JR, Wolf RM. Metastatic and histologic presentations in unknown primary cancer. *Semin Oncol* 1977; **4**: 53–8.
13. van de Wouw AJ, Janssen-Heijnen ML, Coebergh JW, Hillen HF. Epidemiology of unknown primary tumours; incidence and population-based survival of 1285 patients in Southeast Netherlands, 1984–1992. *Eur J Cancer* 2002; **38**: 409–13.

14. Blaszyk H, Hartmann A, Bjornsson J. Cancer of unknown primary: clinicopathologic correlations. *Apmis* 2003; **111**: 1089–94.
15. Ayoub JP, Hess KR, Abbruzzese MC, Lenzi R, Raber MN, Abbruzzese JL. Unknown primary tumors metastatic to liver. *J Clin Oncol* 1998; **16**: 2105–12.
16. Hammar SP. Metastatic adenocarcinoma of unknown primary origin. *Hum Pathol* 1998; **29**: 1393–402.
17. Sheahan K, O'Keane JC, Abramowitz A *et al*. Metastatic adenocarcinoma of an unknown primary site. A comparison of the relative contributions of morphology, minimal essential clinical data and CEA immunostaining status. *Am J Clin Pathol* 1993; **99**: 729–35.
18. Dabbs DJ. *Diagnostic Immunohistochemistry.* (Churchill Livingstone, Edinburgh, 2002).
19. Jaffe ES. Hematopathology: integration of morphologic features and biologic markers for diagnosis. *Mod Pathol* 1999; **12**: 109–15.
20. DeYoung BR, Wick MR. Immunohistologic evaluation of metastatic carcinomas of unknown origin: an algorithmic approach. *Semin Diagn Pathol* 2000; **17**: 184–93.
21. Lagendijk JH, Mullink H, Van Diest PJ, Meijer GA, Meijer CJ. Tracing the origin of adenocarcinomas with unknown primary using immunohistochemistry: differential diagnosis between colonic and ovarian carcinomas as primary sites. *Hum Pathol* 1998; **29**: 491–7.
22. Lagendijk JH, Mullink H, van Diest PJ, Meijer GA, Meijer CJ. Immunohistochemical differentiation between primary adenocarcinomas of the ovary and ovarian metastases of colonic and breast origin. Comparison between a statistical and an intuitive approach. *J Clin Pathol* 1999; **52**: 283–90.
23. Perry A, Parisi JE, Kurtin PJ. Metastatic adenocarcinoma to the brain: an immunohistochemical approach. *Hum Pathol* 1997; **28**: 938–43.
24. Brown RW, Campagna LB, Dunn JK, Cagle PT. Immunohistochemical identification of tumor markers in metastatic adenocarcinoma. A diagnostic adjunct in the determination of primary site. *Am J Clin Pathol* 1997; **107**: 12–19.
25. Torenbeek R, Lagendijk JH, Van Diest PJ, Bril H, van de Molengraft FJ, Meijer CJ. Value of a panel of antibodies to identify the primary origin of adenocarcinomas presenting as bladder carcinoma. *Histopathology* 1998; **32**: 20–7.
26. Tot T. Cytokeratins 20 and 7 as biomarkers: usefulness in discriminating primary from metastatic adenocarcinoma. *Eur J Cancer* 2002; **38**: 758–63.
27. Tot T. Adenocarcinomas metastatic to the liver: the value of cytokeratins 20 and 7 in the search for unknown primary tumors. *Cancer* 1999; **85**: 171–7.
28. Zamecnik J, Kodet R. Value of thyroid transcription factor-1 and surfactant apoprotein A in the differential diagnosis of pulmonary carcinomas: a study of 109 cases. *Virchows Arch* 2002; **440**: 353–61.
29. Werling RW, Yaziji H, Bacchi CE, Gown AM. CDX2, a highly sensitive and specific marker of adenocarcinomas of intestinal origin: an immunohistochemical survey of 476 primary and metastatic carcinomas. *Am J Surg Pathol* 2003; **27**: 303–10.
30. Moskaluk CA, Zhang H, Powell SM, Cerilli LA, Hampton GM, Frierson HF, Jr. Cdx2 protein expression in normal and malignant human tissues: an immunohistochemical survey using tissue microarrays. *Mod Pathol* 2003; **16**: 913–19.
31. Ordonez NG. Application of mesothelin immunostaining in tumor diagnosis. *Am J Surg Pathol* 2003; **27**: 1418–28.
32. Kaufmann O, Dietel M. Thyroid transcription factor-1 is the superior immunohistochemical marker for pulmonary adenocarcinomas and large cell carcinomas compared to surfactant proteins A and B. *Histopathology* 2000; **36**: 8–16.
33. Kaufmann O, Deidesheimer T, Muehlenberg M, Deicke P, Dietel M. Immunohistochemical differentiation of metastatic breast carcinomas from metastatic adenocarcinomas of other common primary sites. *Histopathology* 1996; **29**: 233–40.
34. Frierson HF, Jr., Moskaluk CA, Powell SM *et al*. Large-scale molecular and tissue microarray analysis of mesothelin expression in common human carcinomas. *Hum Pathol* 2003; **34**: 605–9.
35. Wick MR, Lillemoe TJ, Copland GT, Swanson PE, Manivel JC, Kiang DT. Gross cystic disease fluid protein-15 as a marker for breast cancer: immunohistochemical analysis of 690 human neoplasms and comparison with alpha-lactalbumin. *Hum Pathol* 1989; **20**: 281–7.

36. Loy TS, Quesenberry JT, Sharp SC. Distribution of CA 125 in adenocarcinomas. An immunohistochemical study of 481 cases. *Am J Clin Pathol* 1992; **98**: 175−9.

37. Chu P, Wu E, Weiss LM. Cytokeratin 7 and cytokeratin 20 expression in epithelial neoplasms: a survey of 435 cases. *Mod Pathol* 2000; **13**: 962−72.

38. Park SY, Kim HS, Hong EK, Kim WH. Expression of cytokeratins 7 and 20 in primary carcinomas of the stomach and colorectum and their value in the differential diagnosis of metastatic carcinomas to the ovary. *Hum Pathol* 2002; **33**: 1078−85.

39. Stenhouse G, Fyfe N, King G, Chapman A, Kerr KM. Thyroid transcription factor 1 in pulmonary adenocarcinoma. *J Clin Pathol* 2004; **57**: 383−7.

40. Goldstein NS, Bassi D. Cytokeratins 7, 17, and 20 reactivity in pancreatic and ampulla of vater adenocarcinomas. Percentage of positivity and distribution is affected by the cut-point threshold. *Am J Clin Pathol* 2001; **115**: 695−702.

41. Swierczynski SL, Maitra A, Abraham SC *et al*. Analysis of novel tumor markers in pancreatic and biliary carcinomas using tissue microarrays. *Hum Pathol* 2004; **35**: 357−66.

42. Rosai J. *Rosai and Ackerman's Surgical Pathology*. 9th edn. (Mosby, Edinburgh, 2004).

43. Chu PG, Weiss LM. Keratin expression in human tissues and neoplasms. *Histopathology* 2002; **40**: 403−39.

44. Fan Z, van de Rijn M, Montgomery K, Rouse RV. Hep par 1 antibody stain for the differential diagnosis of hepatocellular carcinoma: 676 tumors tested using tissue microarrays and conventional tissue sections. *Mod Pathol* 2003; **16**: 137−44.

45. McCluggage WG. Recent advances in immunohistochemistry in the diagnosis of ovarian neoplasms. *J Clin Pathol* 2000; **53**: 327−34.

46. Tot T. The role of cytokeratins 20 and 7 and estrogen receptor analysis in separation of metastatic lobular carcinoma of the breast and metastatic signet ring cell carcinoma of the gastrointestinal tract. *Apmis* 2000; **108**: 467−72.

47. Chu PG, Weiss LM. Immunohistochemical characterization of signet-ring cell carcinomas of the stomach, breast, and colon. *Am J Clin Pathol* 2004; **121**: 884−92.

48. Semjonow A, Albrecht W, Bialk P *et al*. Tumour markers in prostate cancer − EGTM recommendations. *Anticancer Res* 1999; **19**: 2785−2820.

49. Pecciarini L, Giulia Cangi M, Doglioni C. Identifying the primary sites of metastatic carcinoma: the increasing role of immunohistochemistry. *Curr Diag Pathol* 2001; **7**: 168−75.

50. Abutaily AS, Addis BJ, Roche WR. Immunohistochemistry in the distinction between malignant mesothelioma and pulmonary adenocarcinoma: a critical evaluation of new antibodies. *J Clin Pathol* 2002; **55**: 662−8.

51. Bevitt DJ, Milton ID, Piggot N *et al*. New monoclonal antibodies to oestrogen and progesterone receptors effective for paraffin section immunohistochemistry. *J Pathol* 1997; **183**: 228−32.

52. Klapdor R, Aronsson A-C, Duffy MJ *et al*. Tumour markers in gastrointestinal cancers − EGTM recommendations. *Anticancer Res* 1999; **19**: 2785−2820.

53. Ordonez NG. The immunohistochemical diagnosis of mesothelioma: a comparative study of epithelioid mesothelioma and lung adenocarcinoma. *Am J Surg Pathol* 2003; **27**: 1031−51.

54. Kuusela P, Haglund C, Roberts PJ. Comparison of a new tumour marker CA 242 with CA 19−9, CA 50 and carcinoembryonic antigen (CEA) in digestive tract diseases. *Br J Cancer* 1991; **63**: 636−40.

55. Almeida R, Silva E, Santos-Silva F *et al*. Expression of intestine-specific transcription factors, CDX1 and CDX2, in intestinal metaplasia and gastric carcinomas. *J Pathol* 2003; **199**: 36−40.

56. Moll R, Lowe A, Laufer J, Franke WW. Cytokeratin 20 in human carcinomas. A new histodiagnostic marker detected by monoclonal antibodies. *Am J Pathol* 1992; **140**: 427−47.

57. Ellis IO, Hitchcock A. Tumour marker immunoreactivity in adenocarcinoma. *J Clin Pathol* 1988; **41**: 1064−7.

58. Tenti P, Aguzzi A, Riva C *et al*. Ovarian mucinous tumors frequently express markers of gastric, intestinal, and pancreatobiliary epithelial cells. *Cancer* 1992; **69**: 2131−42.

59. Seidman JD, Kurman RJ, Ronnett BM. Primary and metastatic mucinous adenocarcinomas in the ovaries: incidence in routine practice with a new approach to improve intraoperative diagnosis. *Am J Surg Pathol* 2003; **27**: 985−93.

60. Liotta LA, Petricoin E. Molecular profiling of human cancer. *Nature Reviews: Genetics* 2000; **1**: 48–56.
61. Su AI, Welsh JB, Sapinoso LM *et al*. Molecular classification of human carcinomas by use of gene expression signatures. *Cancer Res* 2001; **61**: 7388–93.
62. Ramaswamy S, Tamayo P, Rifkin R *et al*. Multiclass cancer diagnosis using tumor gene expression signatures. *Proc Natl Acad Sci USA* 2001; **98**: 15149–54.
63. Dennis JL, Vass JK, Wit EC, Keith WN, Oien KA. Identification from public data of molecular markers of adenocarcinoma characteristic of the site of origin. *Cancer Res* 2002; **62**: 5999–6005.
64. Alizadeh AA, Eisen MB, Davis RE *et al*. Distinct types of diffuse large B-cell lymphoma identified by gene expression profiling. *Nature* 2000; **403**: 503–11.

7

Immune responses to tumours: current concepts and applications

Elizabeth J. Soilleux

SCOPE AND IMPORTANCE OF TUMOUR IMMUNOLOGY

Tumour immunology encompasses the study of innate and adaptive immune responses to neoplastic cells [1]. Because an adaptive immune response is usually necessary to direct an innate response towards a tumour, most research has been directed towards understanding adaptive (antigen specific) anti-tumour immune responses [1]. This review provides an overview of adaptive immunity, of methods used in tumour antigen identification, of evidence demonstrating the importance of adaptive immunity in tumour biology, and of efforts being made to use such knowledge in tumour immunotherapy and prediction of prognosis.

EVIDENCE THAT TUMOUR IMMUNOLOGY IS IMPORTANT

The importance of immune responses in preventing or slowing tumour development may vary with tumour type. One way to anticipate tumour types in which immune responses play important preventive or 'braking' roles is to look for tumours occurring at a greater frequency in immunocompromised individuals than in the general population [2]. For example, individuals infected with human immunodeficiency virus/acquired immune deficiency syndrome (HIV/AIDS) are at higher risk of squamous neoplasia of the cervix and anal canal, and lymphoid malignancies (Table 7.1) [2]. Many neoplasms seen in HIV/AIDS are also seen in individuals immunocompromised for other reasons [2].

Tumours in the immunocompromised are frequently related to viral infection, such as human papillomavirus (HPV) in cervical and anal squamous neoplasms, Epstein–Barr virus (EBV) in many lymphoid and some epithelial

Progress in Pathology Volume 7, ed. Nigel Kirkham and Neil Shepherd. Published by Cambridge University Press. © Cambridge University Press 2007.

Table 7.1 Malignancies occurring at increased frequency in HIV/AIDS

Condition	Relative risk in HIV/AIDS	Pathogenesis
Kaposi's sarcoma [2]	97.5–202.7 [2]	HHV8 (KSHV) [2]
Non-Hodgkin's lymphoma [2]	37.4–54.6 [2]	EBV, HHV8 (KSHV) [2]
Hodgkin's lymphoma [2]	8–6.4 [2]	EBV [2]
Cervical (invasive) carcinoma [2]	9.1 [2]	HPV, smoking [2]
Carcinoma of the tongue [2]	1.8–7.1 [2]	HPV, EBV [2]
Carcinoma of the rectosigmoid/rectum/ anus [2]	3.3–3.0 [2]	HPV (anal carcinoma) [2]
Primary liver carcinoma [2]	5.1 [2]	HBV, HCV, alcohol [2]
Tracheal, bronchial and lung [2]	3.3–7.5 [2]	Smoking [2]
Brain and central nervous system (CNS) [2]	3.1–3.4 [2]	EBV (CNS lymphoma) [2]
Skin (excluding melanoma and Kaposi's sarcoma) [2]	20.8–7.5 [2]	Ultraviolet light, HPV [2]
Squamous cell carcinoma of the conjunctiva [104]	Not known	Ultraviolet light, HPV [104]
Leiomyosarcoma [105]	10 000 in children; much less in adults) [106]	Unknown

neoplasms, human herpes virus 8/Kaposi's sarcoma herpes virus (HHV-8/KSHV) in Kaposi's sarcoma and certain lymphomas, and hepatitis B virus (HBV) and hepatitis C virus (HCV) in hepatocellular carcinoma [2]. Immunocompetent individuals may also show some increase in risk of developing these malignancies in the setting of chronic infection with the relevant virus [2].

Several different routes may be involved in the development of infection-related neoplasia [2]. Neoplasia may be the result of recurrent immune stimulation in the case of lymphoid malignancy [3]. However, in many neoplasms, the sequelae of persistent infection are probably more important. Persistent infection may allow viral oncoproteins to alter cell function or may predispose to inflammatory or immune-mediated cellular injury. Cellular injury may lead to deoxyribonucleic acid (DNA) damage and other reactive changes [4]. Therefore, simple epidemiological considerations have given important clues to the aetiology of various neoplasms and the role of the immune system in preventing neoplastic development. Having established that a deficiency of adaptive immune response may be important in the pathogenesis of certain neoplasms, we will now consider the elements involved in adaptive immunity, and how these may become activated against neoplastic cells.

OVERVIEW OF THE IMMUNE RESPONSE

When an infectious agent enters the body, usually via an epithelial surface, the immune system must first recognise its presence, distinguishing it from

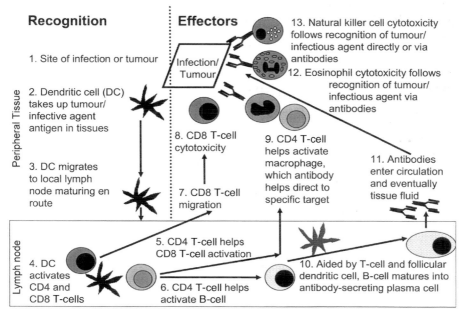

Recognition

1. Site of infection or tumour

Peripheral Tissue

2. Dendritic cell (DC) takes up tumour/ infective agent antigen in tissues

3. DC migrates to local lymph node maturing en route

Effectors

Infection/ Tumour

8. CD8 T-cell cytotoxicity

7. CD8 T-cell migration

9. CD4 T-cell helps activate macrophage, which antibody helps direct to specific target

13. Natural killer cell cytotoxicity follows recognition of tumour/ infectious agent directly or via antibodies

12. Eosinophil cytotoxicity follows recognition of tumour/ infectious agent via antibodies

11. Antibodies enter circulation and eventually tissue fluid

Lymph node

4. DC activates CD4 and CD8 T-cells

5. CD4 T-cell helps CD8 T-cell activation

6. CD4 T-cell helps activate B-cell

10. Aided by T-cell and follicular dendritic cell, B-cell matures into antibody-secreting plasma cell

Fig. 7.1 Overview of immune responses against tumours and infectious agents. Immune responses depend on recognition of an agent as foreign, followed by generation of effectors to combat that agent. Proteins or other molecules from the tumour or infectious agent are taken up by dendritic cells (DCs) and transported to a local lymph node (LN), although some molecules may reach the node in tissue fluid and be taken up by follicular dendritic cells, which are important in the generation of B-cell responses. T-lymphocytes, activated in the LN, may migrate to the site of infection/tumour. CD8 T-cells attack the infectious agent/tumour directly, while CD4 T-cells activate macrophages, which are then cytotoxic. Additionally, CD4 T-cells help B-cells CD8 T-cells to become activated in the LN. The majority of activated B-cells then become plasma cells, which may remain in the medulla of the LN secreting antibody, or may circulate to the site of the infectious agent/tumour. Eosinophils recognise antibody-coated infectious agents or tumours and secrete enzymes, reactive oxygen species and a variety of other toxic and pro-inflammatory agents in the direction of the stimulus. Natural killer cell (NK) mechanisms of cytotoxicity are similar to those of CD8 T-cells. They recognise infectious agents/tumours when coated with antibody, but can also recognise them by poorly understood, antibody-independent means [5].

part of the host. Second, an effective response must be generated [5]. This response must be of an appropriate phenotype and must be in the correct location, in order to maximise destruction of the infectious agent and to minimise collateral damage to host tissues [5]. Having expended time and energy determining that the organism is not self, a useful byproduct would be the generation of immunological memory, allowing a more rapid response to a future challenge from that particular agent [5]. Finally, immune responses must be controlled and downregulated, so that the risk of damage to host tissues is minimised, as soon as the threat of invasion by the infectious agent has ceased [5]. Faced with these challenges and limitations, it is remarkable that immune responses can be so effective and that immune-mediated disease is not more common.

Table 7.2 Principle functions and immunohistochemical markers of leucocytes

Cell type	Immunohistochemical markers	Major functions	Synonyms
Interstitial dendritic cell	CD68 (may be weak), S100, DC-SIGN, dectin, DEC-205, HLA-DR [8], [9], [23]	Antigen uptake in peripheral tissues, followed by antigen processing and transport to local lymph nodes [23]	Histiocytes
Langerhans cell	CD68+/−, S100, CD1a, Langerin, HLA-DR [8], [9], [23]	Antigen uptake in squamous epithelia, followed by antigen processing and transport to local lymph nodes [23]	
Interdigitating dendritic cell	CD68+/−, S100, CD80, CD83, CD86, DC-LAMP, HLA-DR [8], [9], [23]	Antigen presentation to T-lymphocytes in lymph nodes [23]	Histiocytes, DC1s are probably a subset of interdigitating DCs
Plasmacytoid dendritic cell	BDCA-2, BDCA-4, CD123, CD40, HLA-DR [8], [12] (plasmacytoid DCs are not detected in routine immunohistochemical practice)	Initiation of Th2 responses, induction of tolerance, production of anti-viral cytokines	DC2
CD4 T-lymphocyte	CD45, CD3, TCR$\alpha\beta$, CD4 [5]	Provision of 'help' to B-cells, macrophages and CD8 T-cells, in the form of cytokines and contact-dependent signals [5]	CD4 T-cell, helper T-cell
CD8 T-lymphocyte	CD45, CD3, TCR$\alpha\beta$/$\gamma\delta$, CD8 [5] ($\alpha\beta$ and $\gamma\delta$ sets are defined on the basis of TCR type; both have similar functions [5])	Cytotoxic lysis of target cells, some cytokine production [5]	CD8 T-cell, cytotoxic T-cell

Table 7.2 (*cont.*)

Cell type	Immunohistochemical markers	Major functions	Synonyms
Natural killer cell	CD45, CD16, CD56, KIRs, ILTs, certain subunits of CD3 may be present. Separate specialised uterine subset, besides peripheral blood subset [5], [14]	Cytotoxicity towards antibody-coated target (ADCC), recognition (by poorly understood means) and lysis of MHC-negative cells and some cytokine production [5], [14]	Killer cell, large granular lymphocyte
B-lymphocyte	CD45, CD19, CD20, CD22, CD79a, immunoglobulin, HLA-DR) [3], [5]	Differentiation into antibody-secreting plasma cells and memory B-cells [5]	B-cell
Plasma cell	CD45, CD79a, VS38C, CD138, immunoglobulin [3]	Terminally differentiated B-cell, specialised for antibody production [5]	
Follicular dendritic cell	CD21, CD23, CD35 HLA-DR [3], [5]	Unlike all other types of leucocytes described in this table, FDCs are not believed to be bone marrow derived [5]	
Macrophage	CD14, CD64, CD68, HLA-DR, macrophage mannose receptor [17], [18]	Phagocytosis, some ADCC [5]	Histiocyte
Eosinophil	CD15, CD23, eosinophilic cationic protein (ECP), major basic protein (MBP) [3], [5]	ADCC, anti-helminth responses, role in allergic disease [5]	
Neutrophil	CD11a/CD11b/CD11c, CD15, CD18, CD33, CD66b, myeloperoxidase [3], [5]	Phagocytosis, possibly some ADCC [5]	Polymorphonuclear leucocyte (PMN/PNL), polymorph
Mast cell/basophil	CD117, tryptase [20]	Initiation of inflammatory responses following local trauma, role in anti-helminth and allergic responses [5]	

It is not possible to consider the immune system in great detail here, and a number of standard textbooks on immunology may be consulted for further information [5]–[7]. However, the main arms of immunity involved in tackling neoplasms will be considered (Fig. 7.1, Table 7.2) [5]. Immune responses directed against tumours are analogous to those against infectious agents (Fig. 7.1) [5]. It can be seen from the figure that complex interactions between different cell types are of critical importance. These interactions and the roles of each cell are considered below.

DENDRITIC CELLS

Dendritic cells (DCs) are specialised antigen-presenting cells (APCs) that maximise their surface area for antigen uptake and contact with other cell types by means of their dendritic morphology. They take up both self and non-self antigen and process it into an appropriate form for recognition by T-cells. The processed antigen is then presented to T-cells, and any T-cells that can bind the antigen with reasonable affinity may also receive co-stimulatory signals from the DC, in order to overcome the T-cell's activation threshold [5], [8], [9]. However, if the antigen is deemed to be self antigen or is encountered by the DC in the absence of damage to the host ('danger signals' – see below), it is possible that the T-cell will receive no co-stimulatory signals from the DC and will therefore not become activated [9]. Additionally, few autoreactive T-cells should exist, as the majority are deleted during thymic maturation. These strategies contribute to the maintenance of immunological tolerance to self tissues [5]. It is believed that DCs are the only cell type able to activate a naive T-cell and therefore the only cell type able to initiate an immune response (Fig. 7.1) [5]. While many older books suggest that macrophages also initiate immune responses [10], this discrepancy is likely to be the result of difficulties in finding markers to discriminate between macrophages and DCs [8], [11].

While all DCs have broadly similar phenotypes and roles, specific subsets are found in different locations and may lead to phenotypically different immune responses [8], [9]. However, the initiating stimulus and conditions under which it was encountered are more likely to be important in determining the exact nature of the subsequent immune response [12]. Useful immunohistochemical markers for DCs are summarised in Table 7.2, including some of the markers of specific DC subsets [8], [9], [12] etc. Interstitial DCs are found in most tissues, except the testis and central nervous system (CNS). Langerhans cells (LCs) are found within squamous epithelia of skin, vulva, vagina, cervix, oropharynx and oesophagus [8]. Interstitial DCs and LCs migrate to local lymph nodes (LNs), entering via the cortical sinuses and moving into the paracortical T-cell areas, where their close contact with T-cells allows T-cell activation [9]. Within the paracortical T-cell areas, they are known as interdigitating DCs [9]. Plasmacytoid DCs lack the characteristic dendritic morphology, instead having a rounded, plasma cell-like appearance and characteristic immunophenotype (Table 7.2) [12]. They have been described at a variety of locations, particularly within specialised immune tissues, and have important roles in tolerance, generation of antibody responses and production of certain antiviral cytokines [12]. Follicular dendritic cells (FDCs) also demonstrate dendritic morphology, but, unlike other dendritic cells, are not bone-marrow derived. They express the markers CD21, CD23 and CD35 and are found within germinal centres, where they play important roles in B-cell responses [5].

CD4 T-CELLS (T-LYMPHOCYTES)

Lymphocytes are small round leucocytes with a long lifespan that spend much of their time associated with sites of specialised lymphoid tissue. They comprise T-lymphocytes (T-cells), B-lymphocytes (B-cells) and natural killer (NK) cells, the subsets differing in terms of their recognition and/or effector mechanisms and the sites at which they are found (Fig. 7.2) [5]. With the exception of NK-cells, all lymphocytes have very specific receptors. Each individual cell is able to recognise only a single antigen or a very narrow range of antigens with structural similarities [5]. An individual B- or T-lymphocyte gains the ability to recognise one or a few specific antigens, which the majority of other B- or T-lymphocytes will not recognise. This is achieved by means of a complex rearrangement process, during lymphocyte development [5]. Individual gene segments each encoding part of the antigen-binding region of the B- or T-cell receptors are spliced together in randomly varying combinations, giving each cell a virtually unique receptor [5]. Surface markers of various lymphocyte subsets are summarised in Table 7.2.

T-cells express a gene product of the rearranged T-cell receptor (TCR) locus and CD3 (Table 7.2) [5]. They may express either the CD4 or the CD8 molecule on their surface (Fig. 7.2, Table 7.2). CD4 T-cells (T_{helper}-cells) recognise antigen derived from the extracellular environment of the APC associated with the Class II major histocompatability complex molecule (MHC) (Fig. 7.3) and are important in helping other cells respond (Fig. 7.1) [5]. CD8 T-cells (cytotoxic T-cells) recognise antigen derived from inside the APC associated with Class I MHC (Fig. 7.3) [5]. If the APC is a DC, this results in activation of the CD8 T-cell, but poorly understood protective mechanisms exist to prevent destruction of the DC by the CD8 T-cell [13]. When antigen is presented to a T-cell by a cell other than a DC, the consequences are critically dependent on the activation state of the T-cell. If the T-cell has previously been activated by a DC, antigen presentation will increase the T-cell's level of activation, leading to either enhanced cytokine production (CD4 T-cells) or cytotoxicity (CD8 T-cells). However, if the T-cell has received no previous activation signal, no response will occur. This arrangement helps prevent the breakdown of immunological self tolerance [5].

CD4 T-cells have varying roles, with some aiding macrophage activation, while others are critically important in B-cell activation and clonal expansion (Fig. 7.1) [5]. Additionally, cytokine production by CD4 T-cells helps modulate the behaviour of a variety of other leucocytes [5]. CD4 T-cells important in macrophage activation are known as $T_{helper}1$ (Th1)-cells and tend to produce cytokines such as interferon-γ and interleukin(IL)-2, while $T_{helper}2$ (Th2)-cells

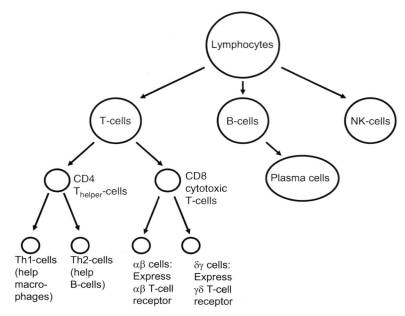

Fig. 7.2 Types of lymphocyte. Lymphocytes can be divided into three main groups, by the expression of surface receptors. T-lymphocytes express a surface protein encoded by a rearranged product of the TCR locus, in addition to expression of CD3, while B-lymphocytes express a surface protein encoded by a rearranged product of the B-cell receptor (BCR or immunoglobulin) locus [5]. Natural killer (NK) cells express neither of these receptors, but express high levels of CD56 and CD16 [5]. T-lymphocytes may express one of two co-receptors. CD4 expression signifies an ability to act as helpers of B-lymphocytes or macrophages, while CD8 expression signifies a cytotoxic function. CD4 T-cells may be further subclassified according to function, with $T_{helper}1$ (Th1) cells able to help macrophages and to produce cytokines such as interferon-γ and interleukin(IL)-2. $T_{helper}2$ (Th2) cells are important for B-cell activation and can produce the cytokines IL-4, IL-5, IL-10 and IL-13 [5]. CD8 T-cells generally use the α and β genetic loci to produce their TCR, but a small proportion of T-cells express a more evolutionarily primitive receptor type instead, which is the product of the γ and δ TCR loci [5]. Following activation, B-cells may differentiate into specialised antibody-producing cells, known as plasma cells [5].

are important for B-cell activation and produce cytokines such as IL-4, IL-5, IL-10 and IL-13 (Fig. 7.2) [5].

CD8 T-CELLS (T-LYMPHOCYTES)

As discussed above, CD8 T-cells require activation by a DC presenting a peptide/Class I MHC complex that the T-cell is able to bind (Figs. 7.1 and 7.2). Subsequent recognition of the same peptide/Class I MHC complex on the surface of a cell that is not a DC will lead to cytotoxicity (Fig. 7.1) [5]. Cytotoxicity occurs by means of directional release of substances from intracellular granules, including enzymes (known as granzymes), pore-forming molecules, such as perforin, and apoptosis-inducing cytokines in the direction of the target.

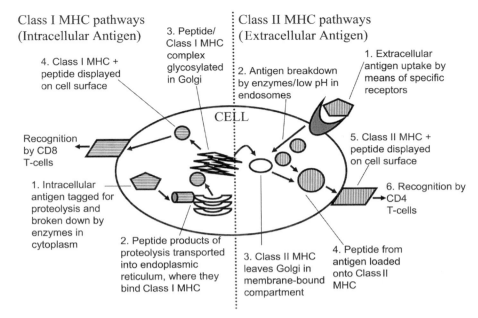

Class I MHC pathways
(Intracellular Antigen)

3. Peptide/
Class I MHC
complex
glycosylated
in Golgi

Class II MHC pathways
(Extracellular Antigen)

4. Class I MHC +
peptide displayed
on cell surface

2. Antigen breakdown
by enzymes/low pH in
endosomes

1. Extracellular
antigen uptake by
means of specific
receptors

CELL

Recognition
by CD8
T-cells

5. Class II MHC +
peptide displayed
on cell surface

1. Intracellular
antigen tagged for
proteolysis and
broken down by
enzymes in
cytoplasm

6. Recognition by
CD4
T-cells

2. Peptide products of
proteolysis transported
into endoplasmic
reticulum, where they
bind Class I MHC

3. Class II MHC
leaves Golgi in
membrane-bound
compartment

4. Peptide from
antigen loaded
onto Class II
MHC

Fig. 7.3 Processing of intracellular and extracellular antigen for presentation to T-lymphocytes with Class I and Class II major histocompatability complex (MHC) [5].

Additionally, expression of Fas ligand on the CD8 T-cell surface may interact with the death receptor Fas on the target cell surface, inducing apoptosis [5]. Most CD8 T-cells express a T-cell receptor (TCR) composed of an α and a β chain, but a small proportion express a TCR composed of a γ and a δ chain. $\gamma\delta$ T-cells are found in restricted locations and may recognise a narrower range of antigens, but otherwise have similar functions to $\alpha\beta$ T-cells) [5].

NATURAL KILLER (NK) CELLS

Natural killer (NK) cells are large granular lymphocytes that lack the B-cell (immunoglobulin) receptor, the TCR and the majority of subunits of CD3 (Table 7.2) [5]. They express CD56, CD16 and variable combinations of the immunoglobulin superfamily receptors, including the immunoglobulin-like transcripts (ILTs) and the killer inhibitory receptors (KIRs) [14]. NK-cell recognition mechanisms remain unclear, but variable complements of activating and inhibitory ILTs and KIRs allow semi-specific recognition of particular MHC alleles [14]. Additionally, CD16 and other Fc receptors for immunoglobulin allow recognition of immunoglobulin-coated targets (Fig. 7.1) [5]. Some effector mechanisms of NK-cells are analogous to those of CD8 T-cells, but they may additionally perform antibody-dependent cell-mediated cytotoxicity (ADCC), which involves liberation of a variety of cytotoxic mediators, including enzymes and reactive oxygen species in close proximity to their target [5].

B-CELLS (B-LYMPHOCYTES), PLASMA CELLS AND ANTIBODY

B-lymphocytes express the rearranged gene products of the immunoglobulin locus, both as a surface molecule (B-cell receptor (BCR)) and as a secreted protein product, in addition to markers such as CD19, CD20, CD21, CD22, CD23 and CD79a (Table 7.2) [3], [5]. Immunoglobulin (antibody) is used in the specific recognition of antigen that does not require previous enzymatic degradation [5]. Following activation, B-cells undergo rapid clonal proliferation, accompanied by somatic mutation of their immunoglobulin receptor (antibody), with follicular dendritic cell (FDC)-mediated selection for cells with BCRs demonstrating higher antigen affinity (Table 7.2) [5]. B-cells then differentiate into plasma cells, which are relatively short-lived cells specialised for the production of large quantities of immunoglobulin [5]. Plasma cells may remain in the medulla of LNs, secreting large quantities of immunoglobulin into the bloodstream, or they may migrate to the site of infection or tumour [5]. Plasma cells lose expression of CD19, CD20 and CD22, but generally retain CD79a expression and gain CD138 and VS38C expression (Table 7.2) [3].

EOSINOPHILS, MACROPHAGES AND OTHER CELLS OF THE INNATE IMMUNE SYSTEM

Eosinophils are granulocytes with characteristic histological appearance. They immunostain for myeloperoxidase, CD15 and CD23 (Table 7.2) [5]. Their main role in immunity is the recognition of antibody targets, particularly those that are too large for phagocytosis, such as helminthic parasites, against which they initiate antibody-dependent cell-mediated cytotoxicity (ADCC). Eosinophil-mediated ADCC is similar to NK-mediated killing, with the additional liberation of major basic protein, eosinophil-derived neurotoxin, leukotrienes and prostaglandins [5]. Eosinophils may be important in certain anti-tumour responses [15], [16].

Macrophages are phagocytic cells with a short lifespan that differentiate from blood monocytes [5]. They express a number of markers also expressed by DCs, including CD68 and HLA-DR, but, in addition, they express CD14, the macrophage mannose receptor and CD64 (Table 7.2) [8], [17], [18]. While they may perform ADCC under certain conditions, their expression of numerous receptors for antibody, complement and foreign carbohydrates makes them adept phagocytes [5]. While they can present antigen to previously activated CD4 T-lymphocytes in order to obtain cytokine-mediated and contact-dependent T-cell 'help', they are unable to activate naive T-cells (T-cells that have never previously been activated) [5].

Neutrophils are short-lived phagocytic granulocytes with characteristic morphology, which express CD11a/CD11b/CD11c, CD15, CD18, CD33 CD66b, and myeloperoxidase [3], [5]. They may perform some ADCC, in addition to phagocytosis [5]. Their main role is in acute inflammation following injury, infection, necrosis and other stimuli [10]. In neoplasia, neutrophils are most frequently seen where necrosis occurs [10]. They do not play a major part in initiating immune responses [5]. Mast cells are a rare tissue granulocyte, closely related to basophils, which circulate in blood [19]. Both express CD117 and tryptase [20]. Their anti-tumour roles appear be relatively limited [21].

ANTIGEN PRESENTATION

An antigen is a protein and/or carbohydrate that may be specifically recognised by the variable receptors on B-lymphocytes (immunoglobulin or BCR) or T-lymphocytes (TCR) [5]. B-cells recognise parts of intact protein and/or carbohydrate molecules, with no requirement for enzymatic degradation or presentation of the molecule [5]. Both CD4 and CD8 T-cells, however, recognise only processed peptides derived from protein antigens. Therefore, antigens containing no protein cannot elicit a T-cell response, although they may sometimes elicit a B-cell response [5]. Antigens are 'presented' to the T-cell associated with a specific protein, the major histocompatability (MHC) protein [5]. Extracellular antigen is taken up into APCs by means of various receptors including carbohydrate receptors, such as DC-SIGN, Langerin and the macrophage mannose receptor (Fig. 7.3) [22], [23]. These receptors are responsible for the process of pattern recognition, which allows the discrimination of relatively conserved features of pathogenic organisms that are absent from host tissues [22]. This process therefore contributes to self tolerance, because potentially pathogenic antigens are taken up and presented to the immune system in preference to self antigens. Following uptake, antigen of extracellular origin passes through a number of membrane-bound compartments in the cell, undergoing digestion to 10 to 34 amino acid peptides. Such peptides are then displayed with Class II MHC on the APC's surface for perusal by T-lymphocytes (Fig. 7.3) [5].

Intracellular antigens are frequently normal host proteins that are constituents of the cell. Much more rarely, these are viral proteins, or mutated host proteins [5]. Intracellular antigens, tagged with ubiquitin to label them for degradation, undergo proteolysis in the cytoplasm. Eight to nine amino acid peptides are transported into the endoplasmic reticulum (ER) in an ATP-dependent fashion. In the ER they form complexes with nascent Class I MHC molecules and traffic through the Golgi, where the MHC-peptide complexes undergo glycosylation, prior to display on the cell surface. Thus, peptides presented with Class I MHC provide a unique opportunity for CD8 T-lymphocytes to survey the contents of each cell for neoplastic change and viral infection [5].

Virtually all cells, except cells of the CNS and eye, germ cells and some muscle cells, express Class I MHC. Only relatively specialised immune cells express Class II MHC, including DCs, B-cells, macrophages and thymic epithelial cells, although Class II can be induced by inflammatory stimuli on other cell types [5]. In general, intracellular antigens are presented with Class I MHC, while extracellular antigens are presented with Class II MHC. However, DCs need to be able to initiate all types of immune response, including those directed against intracellular antigens. Because DCs do not become infected with every virus and do not express a wide range of tumour antigens, mechanisms exist to allow DCs to express antigens taken up from their extracellular environment with Class I MHC, leading to activation of CD8 T-cells [24].

Antigen presentation to T-lymphocytes does not always lead to an immune response. First, many host self antigens will be presented. All autoreactive T-cells capable of responding to these self antigens should already have been deleted during T-cell maturation in the thymus. Second, the environment in which the presentation takes place is of critical importance. Previously, immunologists suggested that the default response was the induction of an immune response, unless tolerance to a particular antigen had previously been induced [25]. However, since many harmless environmental antigens, which have never previously been encountered, fail to stimulate immune responses, it is now believed that the default response is for the immune system to do nothing unless it encounters specific signals. This concept forms the basis of Matzinger's 'Danger Model' [22]. In this model, danger signals induce expression of co-stimulatory molecules on DCs, thus ensuring that antigen presentation leads to an effective immune response, rather than induction of tolerance [22]. Danger signals include constituents of infectious agents, such as viral proteins and bacterial DNA, in addition to certain host molecules that are released during necrosis and infection [22].

Many infectious agents are recognised by the presence of conserved pathogen-associated molecular patterns (PAMPs), allowing preferential uptake of these antigens into DCs and macrophages and/or inducing specific signals in these cells [26]. Such signals may be transmitted via the recently discovered, evolutionarily conserved membrane-bound TLRs (toll-like receptors), which act as pattern recognition receptors (PRRs) for components of viruses, bacteria and fungi [22]. The various TLRs show overlapping specificity for molecules, including lipopolysaccharide (LPS), bacterial lipoproteins, the bacterial chaperone protein heat shock protein 60 (Hsp60) and DNA CpG sequences (found in all living creatures). In addition to binding pathogen-associated molecules, TLRs may also bind endogenous molecules transducing 'alarm signals', such as the human heat shock protein Hsp70, mammalian RNA and DNA, and extracellular breakdown products of hyaluron (produced when blood vessels are damaged) [22], [27]. Hsps are markers of cellular stress due to insults such as trauma, hypoxia and infection. In particular, cell death by necrosis liberates Hsps, while cell death by apoptosis does not, providing one explanation for the induction of inflammatory and immune responses by necrotic but not apoptotic cell death [28]. Given that under normal physiological conditions, only apoptosis occurs, this arrangement allows necrosis-inducing damage by infections or other extraneous agents to stimulate an immune response [10]. In addition to 'alarm signals' transduced via TLRs, various cytokines, including interferon-alpha (IFN-α), interleukin-1β, interleukin-12 and tumour necrosis factor-alpha (TNF-α) may alert the immune system to danger, again via effects on APCs [22]. Understanding the effects of danger signals on the phenotypes of immune responses is critical in finding ways to induce immune responses to tumours [29]. Prior to discussing the implications of the 'Danger Model' in the design of immunotherapeutic strategies, we need to consider which antigens may be important and what is known about naturally occurring anti-tumour immune responses.

OVERVIEW OF METHODS FOR DEFINING CANDIDATE TUMOUR ANTIGENS

GENETIC APPROACH TO DETERMINING ANTIGENS RECOGNISED BY CD8 T-CELLS (FIG. 7.4)

A cDNA library constructed from a tumour can be transfected into cells of an appropriate MHC type and the clones generated can be screened for their ability to stimulate CD8 T-cells from the patient and positive clones selected [30], [31]. CD8 T-cell stimulation may be determined by cell lysis or by measurement of cytokine production, either by use of the ELISPOT assay, intracellular cytokine analysis or quantitative real-time polymerase chain reaction (PCR) analysis of cytokine expression [31], [32]. In order to determine the exact peptide within the protein responsible for CD8 T-cell stimulation, DNA from positive clones is fragmented and subcloned, effectively forming a new cDNA library composed of fragments of proteins of interest. The peptide fragments from clones able to stimulate the patient's CD8 T-cells are sequenced and the identity of the full protein ascertained by comparison to database sequences [30], [31]. A specific motif, consisting of particular amino acids in an appropriately spaced conformation, is required to bind Class I MHC. Therefore, the cDNA sequence of positive clones may be used to predict the sequence of the encoded protein

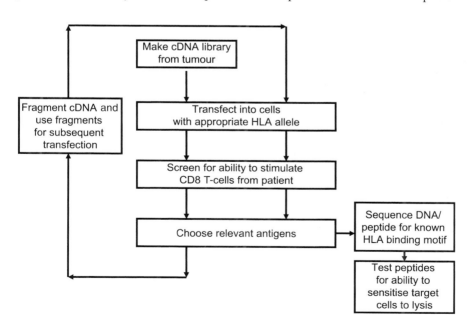

Fig. 7.4 Principles of genetic approaches to identification of antigens recognised by CD8 T-cells [30], [31].

and the ability of that protein to generate suitable peptides that can bind Class I MHC [33]. Finally, these predicted peptides can be synthesised, loaded onto cells expressing an appropriate Class I MHC type and tested for their ability to sensitise target cells to lysis by the patient's CD8 T-cells [30], [31].

cDNA MICROARRAY COMPARISON OF MALIGNANT AND CORRESPONDING NORMAL TISSUES

These and other subtractive hybridisation techniques have been used to determine the identity of proteins overexpressed or differentially expressed in tumours [34]. However, peptides from these antigens must still be screened for their ability to stimulate T-cells, as described below.

BIOCHEMICAL APPROACHES TO DETERMINING ANTIGENS RECOGNISED BY CD8 T-CELLS

These include the elution of peptides from Class I MHC molecules on the surface of tumour cells (Fig. 7.5) [1], [31]. These are fractionated by high-performance liquid chromatography (HPLC) and each fraction is tested for its ability to sensitise target cells to lysis by CD8 T-cells. Peptides from fractions sensitising to lysis are purified and sequenced [31]. These short sequences may be compared with database sequences to determine the protein of origin [31]. More recent methods, for example electrospray ionisation (ESI) mass spectro-photometry and matrix-associated laser desorption/ionisation (MALDI) mass spectrophotometry, have allowed detailed identification of peptides derived

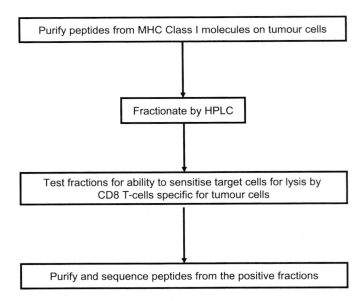

Fig. 7.5 Principles of biochemical approaches to identification of antigens recognised by CD8 T-cells. This method is particularly useful for the identification of antigens subject to post-translational modification [1], [31].

from the surface of tumour cells in association with Class I MHC [35]. However, these peptides must still be tested for their ability to stimulate T-cells.

FUNCTIONAL TESTING OF ANTIGENICITY

Candidate antigens identified genetically or biochemically can then be functionally tested for antigenicity (Fig. 7.6) [1], [31]. Molecular genetic and biochemical methods have demonstrated overexpression of certain proteins and mutation of various genes in tumours. Corresponding protein sequences may then be examined for MHC-binding motifs (as discussed above [33]) and relevant peptides predicted to bind MHC may be synthesised. These peptides can be loaded onto APCs and tested in vitro for their ability to stimulate lymphocytes from cancer patients [31]. Alternatively, these peptides may be refolded with appropriate MHC molecules to produce peptide-MHC multimers that can be used to assay for T-cell responses. The magnitude of T-cell responses can be assayed by means of the ELISPOT assay for cytokine production, by measurement of intracellular cytokine analysis, or by quantitative real-time polymerase chain reaction (PCR) analysis of cytokine RNA expression [32].

ANALYSIS OF ANTIBODY RESPONSES IN CANCER PATIENTS

Analysis by SEREX (serological analysis of tumour antigens by recombinant cDNA expression cloning) allows determination of which antigens can be recognised by host (patient) antibodies (Fig. 7.7) [36]. This method requires production of a cDNA library from fresh tumour cells, followed by enrichment for tumour-specific transcripts by subtraction of transcripts found in normal tissues [36].

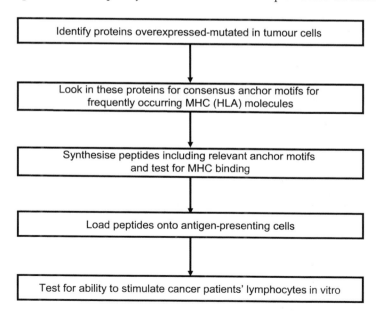

Fig. 7.6 Testing of genetically or biochemically identified candidate antigens for antigenicity [1], [31].

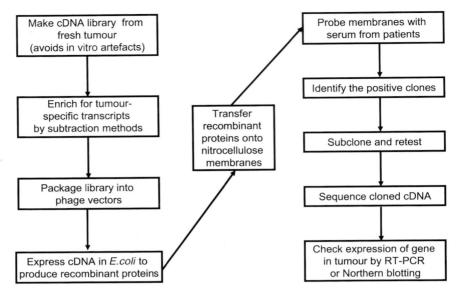

Fig. 7.7 Serological analysis of tumour antigens by recombinant cDNA expression cloning (SEREX). Because antigens are expressed in *E. coli*, this method rarely detects post-translationally modification epitopes. Nitrocellulose membranes are probed with patient serum and detected by means of enzymatically conjugated secondary antibody [1], [36].

Transcripts are expressed in *E. coli* and these clones are transferred onto nitro-cellulose membranes and probed with patient serum. Positive clones are picked and the process repeated, until a small number of clones that are recognised well by patient serum are identified [36]. cDNA from these clones is then sequenced and the DNA sequence compared with sequences in databases [36]. Many of these antigens will represent part or all of previously identified proteins, for example restin, which was shown to elicit an antibody response in Hodgkin's lymphoma (HL) [36]. However, some novel proteins may also be identified, for example HOM-HD-21, a novel galectin expressed in HL [36]. Some antigens identified by SEREX may also be recognised by CD8 T-lymphocytes [36]. Larger studies using serum from cancer patients may then be warranted to investigate the clinical significance of these antigens. Antibodies against various tumour antigens are detectable in 10–30% of cancer patients, but the presence of antibodies shows no correlation with tumour stage or tumour burden [36]. It remains to be determined whether the presence of antibodies correlates with expression of Class I or Class II MHC. It is likely that only antibodies recognising surface antigens could affect tumour progression [36].

TYPES OF TUMOUR ANTIGENS

A number of tumour antigens have been identified by the methods described above (summarised in Table 7.3). These can be separated into five major categories.

Table 7.3 Categories of tumour antigen

Category of tumour antigen	Definition	Examples
Tumour-specific shared antigens (cancer-testis antigens)	Normally silent genes may be expressed due to promoter demethylation as a component of genome-wide demethylation (or due to constitutive hypomethylation in the testis) [1]. Responses are restricted to individuals with particular MHC types [1]. Because germ cells are Class I MHC negative, responses to cancer-testis antigens are not normally induced [1]	MAGE-3 (melanoma, some sarcomas, neuroblastoma, normal germ cells) [107], NY-ESO-1 (oesophageal carcinoma) [1], BAGE and GAGE (melanoma and some carcinomas) [37]
Differentiation antigens	Antigens also expressed in normal differentiating cells [1]	Tyrosinase, gp100 and melan-A/MART-1 in melanoma [32], also expressed in normal melanocytes in skin and choroid [1]. Unique B-cell idiotypes associated with VJ/VDJ rearrangement (B-cell lymphoma) [1], [38], CD20 (B-cell lymphoma) and prostate specific antigen (prostatic carcinoma) [32]
Antigens resulting from mutations	Point mutations and translocations often contribute to oncogenesis [1]. Mutations are often unique to an individual tumour and therefore cannot be used in generic vaccines [1]	Point mutations in CDK4 (melanoma) [32], Ras (pancreatic carcinoma), p53 (many human cancers) [1], β-catenin (melanoma, bronchogenic carcinoma), CASP-8 (head and neck cancers) and MUM-3 (melanoma) [32]. Fusion proteins, e.g. bcr-abl (chronic myeloid leukaemia) [3]
Antigens overexpressed in tumours	Antigens are expressed at lower levels in normal tissues, but at higher levels of expression, they may be recognised by tumour infiltrating lymphocytes (TIL),	HER-2/neu (breast carcinoma) [1], p53 (many human cancers) [1], CD117 ((c-kit) gastrointestinal stromal tumours) [39], MUC-1

Table 7.3 (*cont.*)

Category of tumour antigen	Definition	Examples
	suggesting a threshold for CD8 T-cell activation [40]	(breast carcinoma) [108]
Viral antigens		Antigens from HTLV-1 (adult T-cell leukaemia/ lymphoma) [41], HPV (cervical carcinoma), EBV (Burkitt's lymphoma/ nasopharyngeal carcinoma) and hepatitis B or C (hepatocellular carcinoma) [108]

TUMOUR SPECIFIC SHARED (TUMOUR-TESTIS) ANTIGENS (TABLE 7.3)

Expression of these antigens is restricted almost entirely to tumours. They are known as 'shared antigens' because the ability to recognise them is shared by individuals with several different MHC types [1]. Other individuals have MHC types that cannot present any peptides from the antigen. Examples include the melanoma antigen, MAGE-3, recognised by individuals possessing Class I MHC types, HLA-A1, HLA-A2, HLA-B44 [1]. Although initially isolated from melanoma, MAGE-3 expression has also been reported in sarcomas, neuroblastoma and normal germ cells in testis. Further examples of shared antigens include the oesophageal cancer antigen, NY-ESO-1 [1] and BAGE and GAGE found in melanomas and some carcinomas [37]. In general, expression of shared antigens results from promoter demethylation that occurs as a component of genome-wide demethylation, during development of neoplasia. Demethylation switches on normally silent genes and may contribute to genomic instability [1]. Hypomethylation is constitutive in the testis, allowing expression of tumour-specific shared antigens [1]. However, the testis is an 'immunologically privileged' site because germ cells are Class I and II MHC negative, avoiding immune responses to tumour-specific shared antigens [1], [5].

DIFFERENTIATION ANTIGENS (TABLE 7.3)

Differentiation antigens are expressed in normal differentiating cells and in tumours of corresponding lineages. Tyrosinase, gp100 and melan-A/MART-1 are expressed in melanoma and in normal melanocytes in skin and choroid [1], [32]. A B-cell idiotype is a unique part of the BCR that a T- or B-lymphocyte can recognise. Because gene segment rearrangement during B-lymphocyte development produces a vast number of different receptors with different amino acid sequences, each B-lymphocyte is likely to possess one or more virtually unique idiotype(s). A B-cell lymphoma develops clonally from a single B-cell, and therefore all the tumour cells express the same unique idiotypes that may be recognised by T-cells [1], [38]. Other differentiation antigens include CD20 (B-cell lymphoma) and prostate specific antigen (prostatic carcinoma) [32].

ANTIGENS RESULTING FROM MUTATIONS (TABLE 7.3)

Point mutations and translocations in critical cell-cycle control proteins often contribute to oncogenesis. These mutated proteins may be recognised by the immune system [1]. The resulting mutated proteins are often specific both to the tumour and to the individual, preventing their generic use in tumour therapy [1]. Examples include point mutations in CDK4 [32] and ras (in pancreatic and gastrointestinal carcinomas) [1] and fusion proteins resulting from translocations, such as the bcr-abl gene product in chronic myeloid leukaemia [3].

ANTIGENS OVEREXPRESSED IN TUMOURS (TABLE 7.3)

Proteins expressed in normal tissues may be overexpressed, usually as a consequence of gene amplification. Examples include HER-2/neu and MUC-1 in breast carcinoma, p53 in many human cancers [1] and CD117 (c-kit) in gastrointestinal stromal tumours [39]. The fact that these overexpressed antigens can stimulate CD8 T-cell responses in vivo suggests a physiological threshold for CD8 T-cell activation [40].

VIRAL ANTIGENS (TABLE 7.3)

A number of malignancies are related to infection with specific viruses, and where part or all of the viral genome remains in the tumour cells, viral antigens may be considered to be tumour antigens, expression of which is usually more or less confined to the tumour. HTLV-1 antigens are found in virtually all cases of adult T-cell leukaemia/lymphoma (ATLL) [41], while HPV16 or 18 E7 is present in most cervical carcinomas. EBV antigens are expressed in Burkitt's lymphoma, some cases of Hodgkin's and non-Hodgkin's lymphoma and nasopharyngeal carcinoma [1]. HBV or HCV antigens are present in a proportion of cases of hepatocellular carcinoma [1].

EVIDENCE THAT ANTI-TUMOUR ADAPTIVE IMMUNE RESPONSES OCCUR

EVIDENCE FOR B-CELL/ANTIBODY RESPONSES

SEREX has demonstrated specific antibodies against a number of tumour components, as discussed above (Table 7.3) [1], [36]. These include antibodies against melanoma antigen (MAGE) in melanoma patients and NY-ESO-1 in patients with oesophageal carcinoma. Additionally, infiltrating, tumour antigen-specific B-cells/plasma cells have been demonstrated in bronchogenic carcinoma, medullary carcinoma of the breast and cervical carcinoma [42]–[44].

EVIDENCE FOR CD4 T-CELL RESPONSES

Appreciable numbers of CD4 T-cells have been demonstrated histologically infiltrating colorectal carcinoma [45], bronchogenic carcinoma [46], carcinoma of the breast [47] and many other tumours [48]. Tumour-specific infiltrating CD4 T-cells have been demonstrated in histological specimens from patients with testicular embryonal carcinoma [49], breast carcinoma, ovarian carcinoma [50], pancreatic carcinoma [51] and melanoma [52].

Depletion of CD4 T-cells in experimental animals causes a reduced response to tumour vaccines that would normally cause systemic immunity [5] and an enhanced susceptibility to virally induced neoplasia [53], but few studies provide convincing evidence of enhanced susceptibility to other neoplasms [54]. As discussed above, the majority of tumours occurring at an increased frequency in HIV/AIDS are related to viral infection [2]. CD4 T-cells may also play an important role in virally driven neoplasia in immunocompetent patients. CD4 T-cells from patients with cervical neoplasia, which is largely HPV-driven, show IL2 secretion in response to specific peptides from HPV16 E7, when presented with Class II MHC [55]. Interferon (IFN) and IFN receptor knockout mouse experiments have shown enhanced lymphoid and epithelial tumorigenesis [56]. However, the exact cell type responsible could not be easily determined in this system, as CD8 T-cell and NK-cell responses also involve IFN. CD4 T-cell adoptive transfer work in both human cancer patients and mice suggests that CD4 T-cells play a role in providing systemic immunity to tumours [57].

In conclusion, while CD4 T-cells appear to play two important anti-tumour roles, namely the production of cytokines aiding the initiation of CD8 responses and an antiviral role, results of depletion experiments suggest that CD4 T-cells are not the most important lymphocyte in anti-tumour responses [53]. This correlates with the fact that most tumour cells (like the majority of human tissue) are MHC Class II negative, thus avoiding CD4 T-cell activation [58]. Thus, human and animal studies support a role for CD4 T-cells in producing cytokines and other signals that help activate other cell types (Fig. 7.1) [5].

Regulatory CD25+ CD4 T-cells known to be important for the maintenance of self tolerance have also been described in many tumours [58]. Deletion of this subset has been shown to enhance responses both to endogenous tumour antigens and to vaccination with tumour antigens [58]. However, whether regulatory T-cell subset deletion may induce undesirable autoimmune responses remains to be determined.

EVIDENCE FOR CD8 T-CELL RESPONSES

There are many reports of tumour infiltration by activated CD8 T-lymphocytes and many studies have shown these CD8 T-cells to be capable of specific tumour cell lysis, both in primary neoplasms, for example melanoma and breast, ovarian and renal cell carcinoma [59]–[61], and in metastatic disease [62]. In syngeneic mouse experiments, the adoptive transfer of CD8 T-cells from immunised donors into tumour-bearing hosts enhances anti-tumour immunity [63]. Conversely, depletion of CD8 cells reduces anti-tumour immunity [64]. Additionally, most tumours are Class I MHC positive but Class II MHC negative, allowing effective presentation of peptides to CD8 T-cells previously activated by DCs (Fig. 7.1) [65]. Accordingly, in vitro lysis of tumour cells takes place in a Class I restricted manner [1]. Therefore, CD8 T-cells appear to play a critical role in anti-tumour responses. Additionally, the majority of $\gamma\delta$ T-cells express CD8 rather than CD4. Limited data suggest that $\gamma\delta$ T-cells can lyse tumour cells and/or produce cytokines upon challenge with tumour cells [66].

EVIDENCE FOR NK-CELL RESPONSES

NK-cell infiltration has been reported in various human tumours, including squamous cell carcinoma of the head and neck, carcinomas of the cervix, stomach, thyroid and colorectum, renal cell carcinoma and melanoma [67]–[74]. NK-cells can spontaneously lyse MHC Class I negative tumour cells in vitro and in vivo [14], besides being able to eliminate tumour cells from the rodent circulation [75]. Furthermore, NK-cell depletion in animal models suggests NK-cells protect against methylcholanthrene-induced tumours, most probably via the early detection and removal of transformed cells [76]. Therefore, NK-cells appear to play an important role in anti-tumour responses.

EVIDENCE FOR DC INVOLVEMENT IN TUMOUR BIOLOGY

Variable numbers of DCs have been reported in a range of carcinomas and sarcomas. These DCs often have a relatively immature phenotype that would induce a poor T-cell response, most likely as a consequence of the lack of danger signals within the tumour environment [77]. This protective mechanism against autoimmunity may prove one of the most significant barriers to immunotherapy [29]. Although DCs can be isolated from explanted tissue, no convincing data are available demonstrating their ability to sensitise either CD4 or CD8 T-cells to tumour antigens. However, this is mainly a consequence of technical difficulties [11]. In addition to immature DCs, plasmacytoid DCs have recently been observed in a number of tumours [78], [79]. Plasmacytoid DCs, in particular, often induce Th2 responses that are likely to be ineffective against tumours [78], although if appropriate danger signals are present, more effective anti-tumour responses may be induced [79].

It can, therefore, be argued that since DCs initiate the majority of immune responses via T-cell activation, our quest for effective immunotherapy should be focussed on DCs and the tolerogenic effect of the tumour environment. Before considering the strategies being employed to overcome these difficulties, we will briefly discuss whether consideration of the immune response in tumours is of prognostic significance.

TUMOURS IN WHICH CONSIDERATION OF THE IMMUNE RESPONSE IS CONSIDERED AN IMPORTANT PROGNOSTIC VARIABLE

Melanoma, breast cancer and colorectal carcinoma have been studied in most detail, with numbers of tumour-infiltrating lymphocytes (TIL) in melanoma showing the greatest prognostic significance (Table 7.4) [80]–[82]. In diagnostic practice, lymphocytic infiltration in melanoma is assessed by eye as brisk, non-brisk or absent, in order to satisfy the requirements of the Minimum Dataset drawn up by the Royal College of Pathologists [83]. It is likely that numbers of TIL are of genuine prognostic significance in a range of other tumours, in particular non-melanocytic skin tumours and carcinomas of the gastrointestinal system, prostate and urinary bladder (Table 7.4) [84]–[90]. Additionally, head and neck lymphoepitheliomas (undifferentiated carcinomas with a lymphoid stroma) have a significantly better prognosis than either keratinising or non-keratinising conventional squamous cell carcinomas [91], [92]. Meanwhile, the very small numbers of TIL in pancreatic carcinoma have been suggested as one reason for its very poor prognosis [93]. At present, it is difficult to justify inclusion of an assessment of lymphocytic infiltrate in the majority of Royal College of Pathologists' Minimum Datasets (Table 7.4). It should be remembered that while immunological events in the tumour may be of prognostic significance, immunological events in the draining lymph nodes are likely to be at least as important [94]. However, at present, histological or immunohistological interpretation of these events remains difficult.

CURRENT TRIALS AND TRIBULATIONS WITH IMMUNOTHERAPY

Tumour immunotherapy attempts to redirect or upregulate immunity to give an efficient response to one or more tumour antigen(s). Prophylactic vaccination is not strictly a form of immunotherapy, because it is given before the tumour develops [95]. Many prophylactic vaccination strategies have focused on the prevention of viral infection; for example, recent, increasingly successful efforts to prevent cervical neoplasia with a vaccine against human papillomavirus [96]. Tumour immunotherapy can be divided into approaches where antigen is administered to the patient, approaches where patient lymphocytes are briefly removed and stimulated in vitro, and approaches where adjuvants, but no antigen, are given [97]. Several of these methods can be combined.

Methods of antigen administration for in vivo induction of an immune response (vaccination) include: (i) administration of the protein ($+/-$ carbohydrate) antigen alone in a manner analogous to vaccination against infections; (ii) administration of naked or liposomal DNA encoding the antigen, in the expectation that some cells will take up and express the corresponding protein and present some of it in an antigenic form with MHC [98]; (iii) administration of DCs transfected with the DNA encoding the antigen. Antigen DNA

Table 7.4 Prognostic significance of immune parameters in malignant tumours

Neoplasm	Prognostic significance of tumour infiltrating lymphocytes (TIL)	Included in Royal College of Pathologists' Minimum Dataset?	Other parameters considered
Melanoma	Brisk TIL response in vertical growth phase melanoma gives 1.5 to 3 times longer survival than absence of lymphocytic response. Non-brisk response gives intermediate survival [80], [81]. More CD4, but not CD8 T-cells, are present in regressing than non-regressing tumours [84]	Yes	Lymph node metastases from melanomas classified as having brisk, non-brisk or absent TIL reponses predict survival in a similar fashion [94]
Squamous cell carcinoma, skin	More CD4 T-cells are present in keratoacanthomas, which are throught to be capable of regression, than in squamous cell carcinomas [84], [85]	No	CD4 T-cells infiltrating keratoacanthomas have a more activated phenotype than those infiltrating squamous cell carcinomas [85]
Basal cell carcinoma, skin	More CD4, but not CD8 T-cells are present in regressing than non-regressing tumours [84]	No	Infiltrating CD4 T-cells show an activated phenotype [84]
Squamous cell carcinoma, head and neck	Fewer infiltrating T lymphocytes where survival is poorer in many head and neck carcinomas [109], although peritumoral lymphocytic inflammation in carcinoma of the tongue has no prognostic significance [110]	No. Lymphoepithelioma is not included as a separate histological type	Lymphoepitheliomas (undifferentiated carcinomas with a lymphoid stroma) have a significantly better prognosis than either keratinising or non-keratinising conventional squamous cell carcinomas. However, these are rare in Western populations [91], [92]

Table 7.4 (cont.)

Neoplasm	Prognostic significance of tumour infiltrating lymphocytes (TIL)	Included in Royal College of Pathologists' Minimum Dataset?	Other parameters considered
Oesophageal carcinoma	A dense intratumoural T-cell infiltrate is associated with a better prognosis [86]	No	A correlation was also demonstrated between the number of dendritic cells and T-cells in each patient [86]
Gastric carcinoma	TIL numbers correlate with better outcome [87]	No	TIL numbers also correlate with higher levels of microsatellite instability [111]. There are reports of lymphoepithelioma-like gastric carcinomas with a better prognosis [112]
Pancreaticobiliary carcinoma	Very few TIL [93]	No	This has been suggested as one reason for the very poor prognosis of pancreatic carcinoma [93]
Hepatocellular carcinoma and intrahepatic cholangiocarcinoma	Increased numbers of TIL improves prognosis [113]	No Minimum Dataset is available at time of writing	Increased numbers of infiltrating dendritic cells also improve prognosis [113]
Colorectal carcinoma	Numbers of infiltrating CD8 T-cells and macrophages correlate with survival [88]. Number of activated (OX-40+) CD4 T-cells correlates with survival [45]	No	Increased numbers of peritumoral lymphocytes and the so-called Crohn's-like reaction are associated with higher levels of microsatellite instability and a proportion of these tumours are associated with hereditary nonpolyposis colorectal cancer, which generally have a better prognosis than conventional colorectal tumours [114]. Numbers of TIL are also independent

Cancer type		Minimum Dataset	
Bronchogenic carcinoma	CD8 T-cell infiltration has no significant impact on survival in non-small cell carcinoma [117], [118], although it is associated with poorer differentiation [117]. In the small number of operated cases of small cell carcinoma, numbers of TIL correlate with survival [119]	No	prognostic indicators in colorectal cancer stratified according to microsatellite instability status [115]. Intratumoral natural killer cell numbers correlate with survival [116] Numbers of tumour-infiltrating natural killer cells and dendritic cells may be important in determining prognosis in non-small cell carcinoma [120]–[123] Lymphoepithelioma-like carcinoma has a better prognosis than conventional small cell and non-small cell carcinomas [124]
Gestationa trophoblastic tumours	No data available	No Minimum Dataset is available at time of writing	
Ovarian carcinomas and germ cell tumours	Numbers of TIL correlate with better survival [125]. Few data are available on other types of ovarian tumours	No	
Endometrial carcinoma	Few data available, but no obvious correlation between TIL and survival [126]	No	
Cervical carcinoma	Increased numbers of TIL in early invasive carcinoma correlate with improved survival [127]	No	
Vaginal carcinoma	No data available	No	
Vulval carcinoma	Peritumoural lymphoplasmocytic infiltration appears to show	No	

Table 7.4 (*cont.*)

Neoplasm	Prognostic significance of tumour infiltrating lymphocytes (TIL)	Included in Royal College of Pathologists' Minimum Dataset?	Other parameters considered
	no correlation with prognosis [128]		
Testicular tumours	Classical seminoma TIL numbers do not show significant correlation with survival [129]	No	
Prostatic carcinoma	Increased numbers of TIL improves prognosis [89], [90]	No	
Renal cell carcinoma	Data regarding prognostic significance of TILs conflict, possibly due to a need for consideration by tumour subtype [130], [131]	No	
Transitional cell carcinoma of the bladder	Increased TIL numbers correlate with poorer prognosis in Ta-T1 tumours, but improved prognosis in T3 and T4 tumours [132]	No	
Breast carcinoma	A heavy infiltrate of B-lymphocytes in so-called 'medullary carcinoma' is believed to signify an improved prognosis [133]. B-cell and NK-cell,	No	Increased numbers of eosinophils in the tumour, but not in the blood, signify a better prognosis [136]. In poorer prognosis HER-2+ patients, increased numbers of TIL improve

		but not T-cell infiltration, shows correlation with survival [134], [135]	prognosis [137]. c-erbB2, int-2, and c-myc gene amplification correlates with increased numbers of TILs [138]
Lymphoma	No	Although T-cell infiltration is described in B-cell lymphomas, its correlation with prognosis remains unclear [3]	
Central nervous system tumours	No	Most studies on gliomas demonstrated no significant statistical correlation between numbers of lymphocytes or macrophages and survival [139]–[141]. Increased numbers of TIL may improve prognosis in glioblastoma [142], [143]	NK-cell presence in glioblastomas was unrelated to numbers of lymphocytes and to survival [144]

constructs in vaccinia or adenovirus allow DCs to express the antigen and present it with both Class I and Class II MHC, giving an immune response analogous to a naturally occurring response against an infectious agent. However, due to problematic immune responses to vaccinia or adenovirus antigens, efforts are now being being made to introduce naked DNA encoding antigens into DCs [98]; (iv) administration of DCs loaded with the protein [98]; (v) administration of DCs loaded just with the relevant peptide for presentation with MHC [98]; (vi) genetically engineered bacteria carrying tumour antigens induce potent immune responses, due to the intrinsic danger signals the bacteria provide. Species able to infect DCs, such as salmonella and mycobacteria, are of particular interest, as these would target tumour antigens to potent APCs, capable of presentation of tumour antigens with both Class I and Class II MHC [98]. An adjuvant can be given with any of these [98]. Adjuvants are defined as substances incorporated into or injected simultaneously with antigen, which potentiate the immune response [5]. They include extracts from infectious agents and cytokines, which may be given as proteins or encoded by a DNA construct in a DC [5], [98]. Clinical trials in this area are too numerous to summarise here, but some progress is being made. While DC vaccination with a single antigen (MAGE-3) in melanoma produced a strong measurable cytotoxic T-cell response but no clinical response, a separate trial vaccinating with four antigens (melan-A, tyrosinase, gp-100 and MAGE-3) caused some regression of metastases in stage IV melanoma patients [97].

Patient lymphocytes can be stimulated during a brief period of culture in vitro using broadly similar methods of antigen administration to those described above and then returned to the patient (adoptive cellular immunotherapy) [99]. Early attempts using TIL, amplified in vitro with IL-2, gave poor results, underlining the importance of stimulation with antigen rather than adjuvant alone [99].

Careful antigen selection is required in designing any immunotherapeutic regime [1]. An important consideration is the potential for immunopathology involving non-neoplastic cells. An antigen expressed at much higher levels or solely by the tumour would be preferred [1]. Furthermore, some antigens may be selected because they can be used in the production of generic vaccines applicable to large numbers of patients with similar tumours, e.g. vaccines against amplified genes such as HER-2/neu in breast cancer or p53 in a wider range of malignancies [1]. However, if the vaccine is designed against a protein carrying a particular mutation, it may be patient-specific, as tumours in other individuals are unlikely to harbour an identical mutation [1].

Administration of adjuvant alone (either to the patient or to patient lymphocytes in vitro) in order to upregulate existing immune responses has generally met with poor results [100]. One current success story is the instillation of BCG into the bladder for the treatment of transitional cell carcinoma. This method often eradicates residual tumour and prevents recurrence. The exact mechanism remains unclear, but it is believed to involve non-specific activation of most leucocyte types, with CD4 T-cells probably being the most important [101].

One further manipulation of the immune system in tumour therapy is the use of (relatively) tumour-specific monoclonal antibodies. Antibodies of certain immunoglobulin classes may be directly cytotoxic or they may be conjugated to particular toxins, which they deliver specifically and efficiently to the tumour. As above, there is a risk of collateral immunpathological damage to non-neoplastic cells expressing the same antigen. Examples include the cytotoxic antibody rituximab, an anti-CD20 antibody used as adjuvant therapy for B-cell lymphomas, anti-HER-2/neu used in breast and ovarian cancer, and anti-VEGF used in lung and renal cell carcinoma [102]. Monoclonal antibodies, including anti-CD33 (for use against acute myeloid leukaemia) and anti-CD25 (for use against lymphoid malignancies) have been coupled to cytotoxic agents [102]. Manipulations to make bi-specific antibodies, which bind a tumour antigen and a leucocyte surface molecule, in order to bring leucocytes into close proximity with the tumour, have met with limited success [102].

POTENTIAL PROBLEMS OF IMMUNOTHERAPY

A number of problems hamper tumour immunotherapy, some of which are alluded to above. Autoimmunity (discussed above) remains largely a theoretical rather than a clinical problem, possibly because there is a lower threshold for cancer regression than normal tissue destruction [103]. Although T-cell anti-tumour responses may be measurable in vitro, it is not clear how effective these T-cells are in vivo [58]. Additionally, little information is available regarding variation in antigen expression between tumours [58] and it would be impractical clinically to investigate this in every case. Darwinian selection processes (survival of the fittest cells) occur in tumours. Where an effective immune response is induced, subclones with specific antigen-loss may occur [58]. To an extent, this can be circumvented by simultaneous immunisation with several antigens. MHC-loss variants that fail to present antigens may evolve, although NK cells frequently lyse MHC-negative cells and may therefore prevent this [58]. Loss of functional death signalling pathways (e.g. the Fas pathway) has been reported in neoplastic cells, while the neoplastic cells may express Fas ligand and induce death of infiltrating immune cells [58]. Furthermore, CD4+ CD25+ suppressor T-cells may be found within neoplasms, in addition to immunosuppressive cytokines, such as IL-10 and TGF-β [58]. Most importantly, immune responses are critically dependent upon the environment in which they occur. Matzinger's 'Danger Model' predicts a lack of alarm signals in the tumour environment, leading to a lack of co-stimulatory molecule expression on APCs, and many of the failures of tumour immunotherapy can be ascribed to this [58]. Overcoming intrinsic mechanisms for the maintenance of self tolerance still presents many difficulties.

CONCLUSION

There have been many recent rapid advances in our understanding of tumour immunology, with an explosion of tumour antigen identification and an improved understanding of the reasons behind weak or ineffective anti-tumour responses. In particular, the application of Matzinger's 'Danger Model' to tumour immunity and the identification of regulatory T-cell subsets within tumours have provided some explanation of the observed difficulties with tumour immunotherapy. Descriptive data regarding numbers of TIL and other leucocytes have prognostic implications for many malignancies. At present, a rough assessment of numbers of TIL is carried out only for melanoma. Although we now have good working models for tumour immune responses, considerable work is still necessary to develop reliable and effective means of tumour immunotherapy for routine clinical use.

REFERENCES

1. Jager D, Jager E, Knuth A. Immune responses to tumour antigens: implications for antigen specific immunotherapy of cancer. *J Clin Pathol* 2001; **54**: 669−74.
2. Boshoff C, Weiss R. AIDS-related malignancies. *Nat Rev Cancer* 2002; **2**: 373−82.
3. Jaffe ES, International Agency for Research on Cancer. *Pathology and Genetics of Tumours of Haematopoietic and Lymphoid Tissues* (IARC Press, Lyon, 2001).
4. Venitt S. Mechanisms of spontaneous human cancers. *Environ Health Perspect* 1996; **104**(Suppl 3): 633−7.
5. Roitt IM, Delves PJ. *Roitt's Essential Immunology* (Blackwell Science, Malden, MA, 2001).
6. Goldsby RA. *Immunology* (Freeman, New York, 2003).
7. Parham P. *The Immune System* (Garland Publishing, New York, 2000).
8. Soilleux EJ. DC-SIGN (dendritic cell-specific ICAM-grabbing non-integrin) and DC-SIGN-related (DC-SIGNR): friend or foe? *Clin Sci (Lond)* 2003; **104**: 437−46.
9. Hart DN. Dendritic cells: unique leukocyte populations which control the primary immune response. *Blood* 1997; **90**: 3245−87.
10. Cotran RS, Kumar V, Collins T, Robbins SL. *Robbins Pathologic Basis of Disease* (Saunders, Philadelphia, 1999).
11. Coventry BJ, Austyn JM, Chryssidis S, Hankins D, Harris A. Identification and isolation of CD1a positive putative tumour infiltrating dendritic cells in human breast cancer. *Adv Exp Med Biol* 1997; **417**: 571−7.
12. Gilliet M, Liu YJ. Human plasmacytoid-derived dendritic cells and the induction of T-regulatory cells. *Hum Immunol* 2002; **63**: 1149−55.
13. Knight SC, Askonas BA, Macatonia SE. Dendritic cells as targets for cytotoxic T lymphocytes. *Adv Exp Med Biol* 1997; **417**: 389−94.
14. Cooper MA, Fehniger TA, Caligiuri MA. The biology of human natural killer-cell subsets. *Trends Immunol* 2001; **22**: 633−40.
15. Takanami I, Takeuchi K, Gika M. Immunohistochemical detection of eosinophilic infiltration in pulmonary adenocarcinoma. *Anticancer Res* 2002; **22**: 2391−6.
16. Hung K, Hayashi R, Lafond-Walker A *et al.* The central role of CD4(+) T-cells in the antitumor immune response. *J Exp Med* 1998; **188**: 2357−68.
17. Ancuta P, Weiss L, Haeffner-Cavaillon N. CD14+CD16++ cells derived in vitro from peripheral blood monocytes exhibit phenotypic and functional dendritic cell-like characteristics. *Eur J Immunol* 2000; **30**: 1872−83.
18. Linehan SA, Martinez-Pomares L, Stahl PD, Gordon S. Mannose receptor and its putative ligands in normal murine lymphoid and nonlymphoid organs: in situ expression of mannose receptor by selected macrophages, endothelial cells, perivascular microglia, and mesangial cells, but not dendritic cells. *J Exp Med* 1999; **189**: 1961−72.
19. Kawakami T, Galli SJ. Regulation of mast-cell and basophil function and survival by IgE. *Nat Rev Immunol* 2002; **2**: 773−86.
20. Hermes B, Feldmann-Boddeker I, Welker P *et al.* Altered expression of mast cell chymase and tryptase and of c-Kit in human cutaneous scar tissue. *J Invest Dermatol* 2000; **114**: 51−5.
21. Dimitriadou V, Koutsilieris M. Mast cell-tumor cell interactions: for or against tumour growth and metastasis? *Anticancer Res* 1997; **17**: 1541−9.
22. Matzinger P. The danger model: a renewed sense of self. *Science* 2002; **296**: 301−5.

23. Figdor CG, van Kooyk Y, Adema GJ. C-type lectin receptors on dendritic cells and Langerhans cells. *Nat Rev Immunol* 2002; **2**: 77–84.
24. Nguyen LT, Elford AR, Murakami K *et al.* Tumor growth enhances cross-presentation leading to limited T cell activation without tolerance. *J Exp Med* 2002; **195**: 423–35.
25. Janeway CA, Jr. The immune system evolved to discriminate infectious nonself from noninfectious self. *Immunol Today* 1992; **13**: 11–16.
26. Kirschning CJ, Schumann RR. TLR2: cellular sensor for microbial and endogenous molecular pattrns. *Curr Top Microbiol Immunol* 2002; **270**: 121–44.
27. Termeer C *et al.* Oligosaccharides of Hyaluronan activate dendritic cells via toll-like receptor 4. *J Exp Med* 2002; **195**: 99–111.
28. Basu S, Binder RJ, Suto R, Anderson KM, Srivastava PK. Necrotic but not apoptotic cell death releases heat shock proteins, which deliver a partial maturation signal to dendritic cells and activate the NF-kappa B pathway. *Int Immunol* 2000; **12**: 1539–46.
29. Fuchs EJ, Matzinger P. Is cancer dangerous to the immune system? *Semin Immunol* 1996; **8**: 271–80.
30. Sahin U, Tureci O, Schmitt H *et al.* Human neoplasms elicit multiple specific immune responses in the autologous host. *Proc Natl Acad Sci USA* 1995; **92**: 11810–13.
31. Rosenberg SA. Progress in the development of immunotherapy for the treatment of patients with cancer. *J Intern Med* 2001; **250**: 462–75.
32. Yee C, Greenberg P. Modulating T-cell immunity to tumours: new strategies for monitoring T-cell responses. *Nat Rev Cancer* 2002; **2**: 409–19.
33. Kiessling A, Schmitz M, Stevanovic S *et al.* Prostate stem cell antigen: identification of immunogenic peptides and assessment of reactive CD8+ T cells in prostate cancer patients. *Int J Cancer* 2002; **102**: 390–7.
34. Nelson PS. Identifying immunotherapeutic targets for prostate carcinoma through the analysis of gene expression profiles. *Ann NY Acad Sci* 2002; **975**: 232–46.
35. Bonner PL, Lill JR, Hill S, Creaser CS, Rees RC. Electrospray mass spectrometry for the identification of MHC class I-associated peptides expressed on cancer cells. *J Immunol Methods* 2002; **262**: 5–19.
36. Preuss KD, Zwick C, Bormann C, Neumann F, Pfreundschuh M. Analysis of the B-cell repertoire against antigens expressed by human neoplasms. *Immunol Rev* 2002; **188**: 43–50.
37. Mazzocchi A, Storkus WJ, Traversari C *et al.* Multiple melanoma-associated epitopes recognized by HLA-A3-restricted CTLs and shared by melanomas but not melanocytes. *J Immunol* 1996; **157**: 3030–8.
38. Ruffini PA, Neelapu SS, Kwak LW, Biragyn A. Idiotypic vaccination for B-cell malignancies as a model for therapeutic cancer vaccines: from prototype protein to second generation vaccines. *Haematologica* 2002; **87**: 989–1001.
39. Blanke CD, Eisenberg BL, Heinrich MC. Gastrointestinal stromal tumors. *Curr Treat Options Oncol* 2001; **2**: 485–91.
40. Eisenbach L, Bar-Haim E, El-Shami K. Antitumor vaccination using peptide based vaccines. *Immunol Lett* 2000; **74**: 27–34.
41. Rickinson AB. Immune intervention against virus-associated human cancers. *Ann Oncol* 1995; **6**(Suppl 1): 69–71.
42. Imahayashi S, Ichiyoshi Y, Yoshino I *et al.* Tumor-infiltrating B-cell-derived IgG recognizes tumor components in human lung cancer. *Cancer Invest* 2000; **18**: 530–6.
43. Coronella JA *et al.* Evidence for an antigen-driven humoral immune response in medullary ductal breast cancer. *Cancer Res* 2001; **61**: 7889–99.
44. O'Brien PM, Tsirimonaki E, Coomber DW *et al.* Immunoglobulin genes expressed by B-lymphocytes infiltrating cervical carcinomas show evidence of antigen-driven selection. *Cancer Immunol Immunother* 2001; **50**: 523–32.
45. Petty JK, He K, Corless CL, Vetto JT, Weinberg AD. Survival in human colorectal cancer correlates with expression of the T-cell costimulatory molecule OX-40 (CD134). *Am J Surg* 2002; **183**: 512–18.
46. Kuo SH, Chang DB, Lee YC, Lee YT, Luh KT. Tumour-infiltrating lymphocytes in non-small cell lung cancer are activated T lymphocytes. *Respirology* 1998; **3**: 55–9.

47. Gaffey MJ, Frierson HF Jr, Mills SE *et al*. Medullary carcinoma of the breast. Identification of lymphocyte subpopulations and their significance. *Mod Pathol* 1993; **6**: 721–8.

48. Yannelli JR *et al*. Growth of tumor-infiltrating lymphocytes from human solid cancers: summary of a 5-year experience. *Int J Cancer* 1996; **65**: 413–21.

49. Suekane S, Nakao M, Inoue M, Noda S, Itoh K. Histocompatibility leukocyte antigen-A2-restricted and tumor-specific cytotoxic T lymphocytes from tumor-infiltrating lymphocytes of patient with testicular embryonal cancer. *Jpn J Cancer Res* 1997; **88**: 1181–9.

50. Dadmarz RD, Ordoubadi A, Mixon A *et al*. Tumor-infiltrating lymphocytes from human ovarian cancer patients recognize autologous tumor in an MHC Class II-restricted fashion. *Cancer J Sci Am* 1996; **2**: 263.

51. Boon T, Cerottini JC, Van den Eynde B, van der Bruggen P, Van Pel A. Tumor antigens recognized by T lymphocytes. *Annu Rev Immunol* 1994; **12**: 337–65.

52. Topalian SL, Rivoltini L, Mancini M *et al*. Human CD4+ T-cells specifically recognize a shared melanoma-associated antigen encoded by the tyrosinase gene. *Proc Natl Acad Sci USA* 1994; **91**: 9461–5.

53. Hasenkrug KJ, Brooks DM, Dittmer U. Critical role for CD4(+) T-cells in controlling retrovirus replication and spread in persistently infected mice. *J Virol* 1998; **72**: 6559–64.

54. Dunn GP, Bruce AT, Ikeda H, Old LJ, Schreiber RD. Cancer immunoediting: from immunosurveillance to tumor escape. *Nat Immunol* 2002; **3**: 991–8.

55. Hohn H, Pilch H, Gunzel S *et al*. CD4+ tumor-infiltrating lymphocytes in cervical cancer recognize HLA-DR-restricted peptides provided by human papillomavirus-E7. *J Immunol* 1999; **163**: 5715–22.

56. Street SE, Trapani JA, MacGregor D, Smyth MJ. Suppression of lymphoma and epithelial malignancies effected by interferon gamma. *J Exp Med* 2002; **196**: 129–34.

57. Zeng G. MHC Class II-restricted tumor antigens recognized by CD4+ T cells: new strategies for cancer vaccine design. *J Immunother* 2001; **24**: 195–204.

58. Khong HT, Restifo NP. Natural selection of tumor variants in the generation of "tumor escape" phenotypes. *Nat Immunol* 2002; **3**: 999–1005.

59. Dionne SO, Smith MH, Marincola FM, Lake DF, Antigen presentation of a modified tumor-derived peptide by tumor infiltrating lymphocytes. *Cell Immunol* 2001; **214**: 139–44.

60. Kooi S, Zhang HZ, Patenia R *et al*. HLA class I expression on human ovarian carcinoma cells correlates with T-cell infiltration in vivo and T-cell expansion in vitro in low concentrations of recombinant interleukin-2. *Cell Immunol* 1996; **174**: 116–28.

61. Kuge S *et al*. Interleukin-12 augments the generation of autologous tumor-reactive CD8+ cytotoxic T lymphocytes from tumor-infiltrating lymphocytes. *Jpn J Cancer Res* 1995; **86**: 135–9.

62. Shimizu Y, Weidmann E, Iwatsuki S, Herberman RB, Whiteside TL. Characterization of human autotumor-reactive T-cell clones obtained from tumor-infiltrating lymphocytes in liver metastasis of gastric carcinoma. *Cancer Res* 1991; **51**: 6153–62.

63. Enomoto A, Kato K, Yagita H, Okumura K. Adoptive transfer of cytotoxic T lymphocytes induced by CD86-transfected tumor cells suppresses multi-organ metastases of C1300 neuroblastoma in mice. *Cancer Immunol Immunother* 1997; **44**: 204–10.

64. Kohda H, Sekiya C, Torimoto Y *et al*. Importance of cytotoxic T lymphocytes in the rejection of transplanted hepatocellular carcinoma. *J Gastroenterol* 1994; **29**: 282–8.

65. Rees RC, Mian S. Selective MHC expression in tumours modulates adaptive and innate antitumour responses. *Cancer Immunol Immunother* 1999; **48**: 374–81.

66. Ferrarini M, Ferrero E, Dagna L, Poggi A, Zocchi MR. Human gammadelta T cells: a nonredundant system in the immune-surveillance against cancer. *Trends Immunol* 2002; **23**: 14–18.

67. Schiltz PM, Beutel LD, Nayak SK, Dillman RO. Characterization of tumor-infiltrating lymphocytes derived from human tumors for use as adoptive immunotherapy of cancer. *J Immunother* 1997; **20**: 377–86.

68. Lee RS, Schlumberger M, Caillou B *et al*. Phenotypic and functional characterisation of tumour-infiltrating lymphocytes derived from thyroid tumours. *Eur J Cancer* 1996; **32A**: 1233–9.

69. Hald J, Rasmussen N, Claesson MH. Tumour-infiltrating lymphocytes mediate lysis of autologous squamous cell carcinomas of the head and neck. *Cancer Immunol Immunother* 1995; **41**: 243–50.

70. Hilders CG, Ras L, van Eendenburg JD, Nooyen Y, Fleuren GJ. Isolation and characterization of tumor-infiltrating lymphocytes from cervical carcinoma. *Int J Cancer* 1994; **57**: 805–13.

71. Nakashima M, Janiszewska M, Steplewski Z *et al*. Proliferation, phenotype, and cytotoxicity of human lymphocytes isolated from lymph nodes invaded by melanoma cells. *Hybridoma* 1994; **13**: 241–6.

72. Karimine N, Nanbara S, Arinaga S *et al*. Lymphokine-activated killer cell activity of peripheral blood, spleen, regional lymph node, and tumor infiltrating lymphocytes in gastric cancer patients. *J Surg Oncol* 1994; **55**: 179–85.

73. Ostenstad B, Lea T, Schlichting E, Harboe M. Human colorectal tumour infiltrating lymphocytes express activation markers and the CD45RO molecule, showing a primed population of lymphocytes in the tumour area. *Gut* 1994; **35**: 382–7.

74. Hayakawa K, Salmeron MA, Parkinson DR *et al*. Study of tumor-infiltrating lymphocytes for adoptive therapy of renal cell carcinoma (RCC) and metastatic melanoma: sequential proliferation of cytotoxic natural killer and noncytotoxic T-cells in RCC. *J Immunother* 1991; **10**: 313–25.

75. Ljunggren HG, Ohlen C, Hoglund P *et al*. Afferent and efferent cellular interactions in natural resistance directed against MHC class I deficient tumor grafts. *J Immunol* 1998; **140**: 671–8.

76. Mather GG, Talcott PA, Exon JH. Characterization of a chemically induced tumor model and the effects of natural killer cell depletion by antiasialo GM-1. *Immunobiology* 1994; **190**: 333–45.

77. Kusmartsev S, Gabrilovich DI. Immature myeloid cells and cancer-associated immune suppression. *Cancer Immunol Immunother* 2002; **51**: 293–8.

78. Zou W, Machelon V, Coulomb-L'Hermin A *et al*. Stromal-derived factor-1 in human tumors recruits and alters the function of plasmacytoid precursor dendritic cells. *Nat Med* 2001; **7**: 1339–46.

79. Salio M, Cella M, Vermi W *et al*. Plasmacytoid dendritic cells prime IFN-gamma-secreting melanoma-specific CD8 lymphocytes and are found in primary melanoma lesions. *Eur J Immunol* 2003; **33**: 1052–62.

80. Clark WH Jr, Elder DE, Guerry D 4th *et al*. Model predicting survival in stage I melanoma based on tumor progression. *J Natl Cancer Inst* 1989; **81**: 1893–904.

81. Clemente CG, Mihm MC Jr, Bufalino R *et al*. Prognostic value of tumor infiltrating lymphocytes in the vertical growth phase of primary cutaneous melanoma. *Cancer* 1996; **77**: 1303–10.

82. Menard S, Tomasic G, Casalini P *et al*. Lymphoid infiltration as a prognostic variable for early-onset breast carcinomas. *Clin Cancer Res* 1997; **3**: 817–19.

83. Branston LK, Greening S, Newcombe RG *et al*. The implementation of guidelines and computerised forms improves the completeness of cancer pathology reporting. The CROPS project: a randomised controlled trial in pathology. *Eur J Cancer* 2002; **38**: 764–72.

84. Halliday GM, Patel A, Hunt MJ, Tefany FJ, Barnetson RS. Spontaneous regression of human melanoma/nonmelanoma skin cancer: association with infiltrating CD4+ T-cells. *World J Surg* 1995; **19**: 352–8.

85. Patel A, Halliday GM, Cooke BE, Barnetson RS. Evidence that regression in keratoacanthoma is immunologically mediated: a comparison with squamous cell carcinoma. *Br J Dermatol* 1994; **131**: 789–98.

86. Furihata M, Ohtsuki Y, Sonobe H *et al*. Prognostic significance of simultaneous infiltration of HLA-DR-positive dendritic cells and tumor infiltrating lymphocytes into human esophageal carcinoma. *Tohoku J Exp Med* 1993; **169**: 187–95.

87. Ishigami S, Natsugoe S, Tokuda K *et al*. CD3-zetachain expression of intratumoral lymphocytes is closely related to survival in gastric carcinoma patients. *Cancer* 2002; **94**: 1437–42.

88. Funada Y, Noguchi T, Kikuchi R *et al*. Prognostic significance of CD8+ T cell and macrophage peritumoral infiltration in colorectal cancer. *Oncol Rep* 2003; **10**: 309–13.

89. Epstein NA, Fatti LP. Prostatic carcinoma: some morphological features affecting prognosis. *Cancer* 1976; **37**: 2455–65.
90. Vesalainen S, Lipponen P, Talja M, Syrjanen K. Histological grade, perineural infiltration, tumour-infiltrating lymphocytes and apoptosis as determinants of long-term prognosis in prostatic adenocarcinoma. *Eur J Cancer* 1994; **30A**, 1797–803.
91. Bansberg SF, Olsen KD, Gaffey TA. Lymphoepithelioma of the oropharynx. *Otolaryngol Head Neck Surg* 1989; **100**: 303–7.
92. Ahuja AT, Teo PM, To KF, King AD, Metreweli C. Palatal lymphoepitheliomas and a review of head and neck lymphoepitheliomas. *Clin Radiol* 1999; **54**: 289–93.
93. von Bernstorff W, Voss M, Freichel S. Systemic and local immunosuppression in pancreatic cancer patients. *Clin Cancer Res* 2001; **7**: 925s–32s.
94. Mihm MC Jr, Clemente CG, Cascinelli N. Tumor infiltrating lymphocytes in lymph node melanoma metastases: a histopathologic prognostic indicator and an expression of local immune response. *Lab Invest* 1996; **74**: 43–7.
95. Finn OJ, Forni G. Prophylactic cancer vaccines. *Curr Opin Immunol* 2002; **14**: 172–7.
96. Koutsky LA *et al*. A controlled trial of a human papillomavirus type 16 vaccine. *N Engl J Med* 2002; **347**: 1645–51.
97. Schuler G, Schuler-Thurner B, Steinman RM. The use of dendritic cells in cancer immunotherapy. *Curr Opin Immunol* 2003; **15**: 138–47.
98. Pardoll DM. Spinning molecular immunology into successful immunotherapy. *Nat Rev Immunol* 2002; **2**: 227–38.
99. Paul S, Calmels B, Acres RB. Improvement of adoptive cellular immunotherapy of human cancer using ex-vivo gene transfer. *Curr Gene Ther* 2002; **2**: 91–100.
100. Yu Z, Restifo NP. Cancer vaccines: progress reveals new complexities. *J Clin Invest* 2002; **110**: 289–94.
101. Schamhart DH, de Boer EC, de Reijke TM, Kurth K. Urinary cytokines reflecting the immunological response in the urinary bladder to biological response modifiers: their practical use. *Eur Urol* 2000; **37**(Suppl 3): 16–23.
102. Carter P. Improving the efficacy of antibody-based cancer therapies. *Nat Rev Cancer* 2001; **1**: 118–29.
103. Turk MJ, Wolchok JD, Guevara-Patino JA, Goldberg SM, Houghton AN. Multiple pathways to tumor immunity and concomitant autoimmunity. *Immunol Rev* 2002; **188**: 122–35.
104. Newton R, Ziegler J, Ateenyi-Agaba C *et al*. The epidemiology of conjunctival squamous cell carcinoma in Uganda. *Br J Cancer* 2002; **87**: 301–8.
105. Mbulaiteye SM, Parkin DM, Rabkin CS. Epidemiology of AIDS-related malignancies an international perspective. *Hematol Oncol Clin North Am* 2003; **17**: 673–96, v.
106. Goedert JJ. The epidemiology of acquired immunodeficiency syndrome malignancies. *Semin Oncol* 2000; **27**: 390–401.
107. Ishida H, Matsumura T, Salgaller ML *et al*. MAGE-1 and MAGE-3 or -6 expression in neuroblastoma-related pediatric solid tumors. *Int J Cancer* 1996; **69**: 375–80.
108. Jager E, Jager D, Knuth A. Clinical cancer vaccine trials. *Curr Opin Immunol* 2002; **14**: 178–82.
109. Reichert TE, Day R, Wagner EM, Whiteside TL. Absent or low expression of the zeta chain in T cells at the tumor site correlates with poor survival in patients with oral carcinoma. *Cancer Res* 1998; **58**: 5344–7.
110. Sarioglu T, Yilmaz T, Sungur A, Gursel B. The effect of lymphocytic infiltration on clinical survival in cancer of the tongue. *Eur Arch Otorhinolaryngol* 1994; **251**: 366–9.
111. Grogg KL, Lohse CM, Pankratz VS, Halling KC, Smyrk TC. Lymphocyte-rich gastric cancer: associations with Epstein–Barr virus, microsatellite instability, histology, and survival. *Mod Pathol* 2003; **16**: 641–51.
112. Wang HH, Wu MS, Shun CT *et al*. Lymphoepithelioma-like carcinoma of the stomach: a subset of gastric carcinoma with distinct clinicopathological features and high prevalence of Epstein–Barr virus infection. *Hepatogastroenterology* 1999; **46**: 1214–19.
113. Yin XY, Lu MD, Lai YR, Liang LJ, Huang JF. Prognostic significances of tumor-infiltrating S-100 positive dendritic cells and lymphocytes in patients with hepatocellular carcinoma. *Hepatogastroenterology* 2003 Sep–Oct; **50**(53): 1281–4.

114. Jass JR. Pathology of hereditary nonpolyposis colorectal cancer. *Ann NY Acad Sci* 2000; **910**: 62−73; discussion 73−4.
115. Michael-Robinson JM, Biemer-Huttmann A, Purdie DM *et al*. Tumour infiltrating lymphocytes and apoptosis are independent features in colorectal cancer stratified according to microsatellite instability status. *Gut* 2001; **48**: 360−6.
116. Coca S, Perez-Piqueras J, Martinez D *et al*. The prognostic significance of intratumoral natural killer cells in patients with colorectal carcinoma. *Cancer* 1997; **79**: 2320−8.
117. Mori M, Ohtani H, Naito Y *et al*. Infiltration of CD8+ T-cells in non-small cell lung cancer is associated with dedifferentiation of cancer cells, but not with prognosis. *Tohoku J Exp Med* 2000; **191**: 113−18.
118. Toomey D, Smyth G, Condron C *et al*. Infiltrating immune cells, but not tumour cells, express FasL in non-small cell lung cancer: no association with prognosis identified in 3-year follow-up. *Int J Cancer* 2003; **103**: 408−12.
119. Eerola AK, Soini Y, Paakko P. A high number of tumor-infiltrating lymphocytes are associated with a small tumor size, low tumor stage, and a favorable prognosis in operated small cell lung carcinoma. *Clin Cancer Res* 2000; **6**: 1875−81.
120. Villegas FR, Coca S, Villarrubia VG *et al*. Prognostic significance of tumor infiltrating natural killer cells subset CD57 in patients with squamous cell lung cancer. *Lung Cancer* 2002; **35**: 23−8.
121. Takanami I, Takeuchi K, Giga M. The prognostic value of natural killer cell infiltration in resected pulmonary adenocarcinoma. *J Thorac Cardiovasc Surg* 2001; **121**: 1058−63.
122. Eerola AK, Soini Y, Paakko P. Tumour infiltrating lymphocytes in relation to tumour angiogenesis, apoptosis and prognosis in patients with large cell lung carcinoma. *Lung Cancer* 1999; **26**: 73−83.
123. Zeid NA, Muller HK. S100 positive dendritic cells in human lung tumors associated with cell differentiation and enhanced survival. *Pathology* 1993; **25**: 338−43.
124. Han AJ, Xiong M, Gu YY, Lin SX. Lymphoepithelioma-like carcinoma of the lung with a better prognosis. A clinicopathologic study of 32 cases. *Am J Clin Pathol* 2001; **115**: 841−50.
125. Deligdisch L, Jacobs AJ, Cohen CJ. Histologic correlates of virulence in ovarian adenocarcinoma. II. Morphologic correlates of host response. *Am J Obstet Gynecol* 1982; **144**: 885−9.
126. Dundar E, Tel N, Ozalp SS *et al*. The significance of local cellular immune response of women 50 years of age and younger with endometrial carcinoma. *Eur J Gynaecol Oncol* 2002; **23**: 243−6.
127. Bethwaite PB, Holloway LJ, Thornton A, Delahunt B. Infiltration by immunocompetent cells in early stage invasive carcinoma of the uterine cervix: a prognostic study. *Pathology* 1996; **28**: 321−7.
128. Husseinzadeh N, Wesseler T, Schellhas H, Nahhas W. Significance of lymphoplasmocytic infiltration around tumor cell in the prediction of regional lymph node metastases in patients with invasive squamous cell carcinoma of the vulva: a clinicopathologic study. *Gynecol Oncol* 1989; **34**: 200−5.
129. Evensen JF, Fossa SD, Kjellevold K, Lien HH. Testicular seminoma: histological findings and their prognostic significance for stage II disease. *J Surg Oncol* 1987; **36**: 166−9.
130. Kolbeck PC, Kaveggia FF, Johansson SL, Grune MT, Taylor RJ. The relationships among tumor-infiltrating lymphocytes, histopathologic findings, and long-term clinical follow-up in renal cell carcinoma. *Mod Pathol* 1992; **5**: 420−5.
131. Tomita K, Okui N, Kimura A *et al*. Prognostic significance of histopathological findings (including lymphocyte infiltration) in renal cell carcinoma. *Hinyokika Kiyo* 1996; **42**: 925−30.
132. Lipponen PK, Eskelinen MJ, Jauhiainen K, Harju E, Terho R. Tumour infiltrating lymphocytes as an independent prognostic factor in transitional cell bladder cancer. *Eur J Cancer* 1992; **29A**: 69−75.
133. Nzula S, Going JJ, Stott DI. Antigen-driven clonal proliferation, somatic hypermutation, and selection of B lymphocytes infiltrating human ductal breast carcinomas. *Cancer Res* 2003; **63**: 3275−80.

134. Lawry J, Rogers K, Duncan JL, Potter CW. The identification of informative parameters in the flow cytometric analysis of breast carcinoma. *Eur J Cancer* 1993; **29A**: 719−23.

135. Lucin K, Iternicka Z, Jonjic N. Prognostic significance of T-cell infiltrates, expression of beta 2-microglobulin and HLA-DR antigens in breast carcinoma. *Pathol Res Pract* 1994; **190**: 1134−40.

136. Lowe D, Jorizzo J, Hutt MS. Tumour-associated eosinophilia: a review. *J Clin Pathol* 1981; **34**: 1343−8.

137. Menard S, Fortis S, Castiglioni F, Agresti R, Balsari A. HER2 as a prognostic factor in breast cancer. *Oncology* 2001; **61**(Suppl 2): 67−72.

138. Tang RP, Kacinski B, Validire P *et al*. Oncogene amplification correlates with dense lymphocyte infiltration in human breast cancers: a role for hematopoietic growth factor release by tumor cells? *J Cell Biochem* 1990; **44**: 189−98.

139. Rossi ML, Jones NR, Candy E *et al*. The mononuclear cell infiltrate compared with survival in high-grade astrocytomas. *Acta Neuropathol (Berl)* 1989; **78**: 189−93.

140. Mork SJ, Halvorsen TB, Lindegaard KF, Eide GE. Oligodendroglioma. Histologic evaluation and prognosis. *J Neuropathol Exp Neurol* 1986; **45**: 65−78.

141. Brooks WH, Markesbery WR, Gupta GD, Roszman TL. Relationship of lymphocyte invasion and survival of brain tumor patients. *Ann Neurol* 1978; **4**: 219−24.

142. Palma L, Di Lorenzo N, Guidetti B. Lymphocytic infiltrates in primary glioblastomas and recidivous gliomas. Incidence, fate, and relevance to prognosis in 228 operated cases. *J Neurosurg* 1978; **49**: 854−61.

143. Di Lorenzo N, Palma L, Nicole S. Lymphocytic infiltration in long-survival glioblastomas: possible host's resistance. *Acta Neurochir (Wien)* 1977; **39**: 27−33.

144. Vaquero J, Coca S, Oya S *et al*. Presence and significance of NK cells in glioblastomas. *J Neurosurg* 1989; **70**: 728−31.

8

Post-mortem imaging – an update

Richard Jones

INTRODUCTION

There have been huge advances in clinical imaging over the last 10 years that have resulted in an improvement in the visualisation of both morphological and functional pathology.

Imaging techniques have been used to identify bone injury ever since Roentgen produced the first radiograph in 1895. Most of us are familiar with the ongoing utility of X-rays in both paediatric and adult pathology, particularly in a medico-legal context. Skeletal surveys are used to identify fractures in cases of suspected child abuse and to demonstrate bone trauma associated with bullets and other missiles.

In the second half of the 20th Century, more sophisticated imaging techniques were introduced. Computed Axial Tomography (CAT) scans (now Computed Tomography (CT) scans) were introduced in the early 1970s, followed by magnetic resonance imaging (MRI), nuclear medicine and positron emission tomography (PET). Each modality is used in different ways in clinical medicine, maximising their respective strengths and cost-effectiveness.

Autopsy rates, already in decline in England and Wales and elsewhere since the 1950s, further plummeted in the wake of the Alder Hey and Bristol tissue and organ 'scandals' of the late 1990s [1]–[3].

There has been an increased interest in the application of clinical imaging techniques to post-mortem diagnoses, either as an adjunct to, or as a replacement of the autopsy [4], [5].

Some of this research has been prompted by certain religious communities, whose attitudes to autopsy have previously been explored in detail [6], [7].

This chapter will provide an overview of the potential utility of post-mortem CT and MRI in the fields of paediatric/perinatal pathology, sudden adult death and forensic casework, and introduce the reader to developments in the field of three dimensional (3D) image reconstruction and micro-imaging.

199

Progress in Pathology Volume 7, ed. Nigel Kirkham and Neil Shepherd. Published by Cambridge University Press. © Cambridge University Press 2007.

POST-MORTEM CT AND MRI

In the late 1990s pathology in the UK was rocked by widely publicised alleged 'organ scandals', notably those involving the Royal Liverpool Children's Hospital — 'Alder Hey' (Redfern Report [8]) and the Bristol Royal Infirmary (Kennedy Report [9]). Request or 'hospital' autopsies have declined spectacularly. The majority of autopsies carried out in the UK are carried out on behalf of the Coroner or Procurator Fiscal [3].

The Government stated its interest in minimally invasive examinations, and in particular in the use of imaging techniques as an alternative to traditional autopsies. Sir Liam Donaldson, then Chief Medical Officer for England, commissioned a report on this issue following publication of the report 'The Removal, Retention and Use of Human Organs and Tissue from Post Mortem Examination' [10]. It was suggested that MRI and other less-invasive techniques could provide the benefits of conventional post-mortem examination without the need for dissection or the removal of organs, providing advantages to some religious communities.

The commissioned report favoured an MR imaging approach to autopsy to other 'less-invasive techniques' such as laparoscopic examination, but acknowledged that the evidence base for MRI autopsy was limited both in terms of numbers and a direct comparison with post-mortem dissection [11], [12].

In the recent position paper on the reform of the death certification process and in particular the role of the Coroner [13], the Government indicated that they wished there to be 'better use of post-mortem examinations', in agreement with the findings of the Fundamental Review of the Coroner's Service (Luce Report [14]) and of Dame Janet Smith in the Shipman Inquiry 3rd Report [15]. Where autopsies were considered necessary, they wished authorities to consider the 'minimum level of invasiveness' to establish the cause of death.

The Department of Health advertised an invitation to tender for a research programme into the 'less-invasive autopsy' in April 2004 — a contract worth £750,000, and designed to trial MRI versus autopsy in children and adults [16].

Benbow and Roberts [17] outline the pros and cons of the limited autopsy in the form of needle biopsy targeted examinations, examinations limited for example to a particular body cavity or organ system, 'endoscopic' autopsies and the use of cytology. Post-mortem angiography has also been described, and this technique has been used largely on an experimental basis to image the coronary arteries, vertebral arteries and vessels within the brain (including studying bridging vein ruptures) [18]–[20].

POST-MORTEM IMAGING IN PAEDIATRIC PATHOLOGY

Much of the original research into the use of post-mortem imaging has been in the paediatric field, and in particular, as a motion-sensitive technique, MRI is well-suited to the study of dead subjects. Intrauterine fetal anomalies were investigated in the early 1990s, but post-mortem CT scanning has not had a significant impact on this area of research [21].

Despite the extensive research into the utility of MRI, it has only been more recently that any attempt has been made to compare the outcome of perinatal post-mortem imaging results with the 'gold standard' of autopsy. There have been relatively few published papers covering this topic [22]–[24].

Brookes *et al.* [22] examined 20 stillborn, miscarried or aborted fetuses by MRI followed by autopsy, and found that MRI had equivalent or better diagnostic sensitivity than autopsy in 60% of cases and that the results of the examinations were similar in 90%.

MRI was particularly sensitive to central nervous system (CNS) abnormalities, which account for 20% of fatal congenital abnormalities, and highlighted conditions such as ventriculomegaly and intra-ventricular haemorrhage that were not picked up at autopsy. In addition, MRI was of benefit in diagnosing body space fluid abnormalities, where autopsy was not always successful.

Abnormalities of the musculoskeletal system were also demonstrated, and MRI gave an accurate diagnosis of acetabular dysplasia. MRI was not good at identifying cardiovascular anomalies, that account for approximately 4% of fatal congenital anomalies and technical problems surrounding spatial resolution were thought to be partly responsible. Fig. 8.1 illustrates a case of diaphragmatic hernia.

Woodward *et al.* [23] studied 26 fetuses using MRI followed by autopsy and grouped malformations into 'major' and 'minor'. They found that all examining

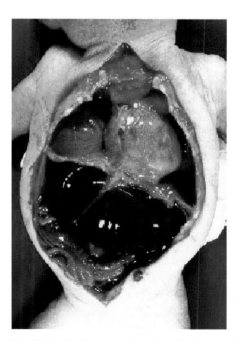 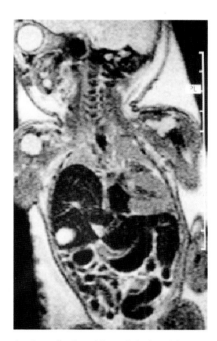

Fig. 8.1 Left: Necropsy showing diaphragmatic hernia, liver displaced into right hemithorax, deviating heart to left compressing and obliterating lungs. Right: T2-weighted MRI scan shows right diaphragmatic hernia and its contents; the stomach and bowel are filled with gas (seen as a signal void, i.e. black), which suggests presence of tracheo-oesophageal fistula. Reprinted with permission from Elsevier (*The Lancet*, 1996; **348**: 1139–41).

radiologists identified 79% of the 'major' malformations, with one radiologist identifying 91%. 'Minor' anomalies were poorly identified. In common with Brookes *et al.*, CNS malformations were well identified by MRI, and it was concluded that in situations where consent for autopsy was not forthcoming, MRI examination could present an excellent alternative, particularly where CNS anomalies were involved.

The selection processes in both the Woodward *et al.* and Brookes *et al.* studies were heavily slanted towards fetuses with congenital malformations, and Alderliesten *et al.* [24] studied 56 consecutive perinatal deaths in a non-selected obstetric population, of which 26 had both MRI and autopsy examinations.

MRI examinations post-mortem detected 56% of 'major' malformations subsequently identified at autopsy, and the team was disappointed by the inability of MRI to identify omphalocele, myelomeningocele, tracheo-oesophageal fistula or aortic coarctation, for example. Because the radiologists were blinded to clinical findings, and could not carry out an external examination, it is argued that some of these malformations would not ordinarily have been missed. The effects of maceration were also noted to be a complicating factor in the interpretation of MRI images.

The authors quoted a positive predictive value of MRI for detecting malformations (compared to the 'gold standard' of autopsy) as being 80% with a 65% negative predictive value. They concluded that a normal MRI examination did not necessarily equate to a normal fetus, and that parents refusing consent to autopsy should be counselled on the limitations of such an examination.

Further studies agreed that post-mortem MRI examination was sensitive to the evaluation of CNS anomalies allowing the neuroanatomy to be studied *in situ*. Cardiac anatomy was poorly demonstrated due to a combination of the lack of haemodynamic information and post-mortem changes, particularly thrombus formation [25]–[27].

All published studies to date involve small numbers of cases, some of which are subject to selection bias. All seem to suggest that there is broad agreement between MRI and autopsy findings, but that there are areas in which MRI is superior (CNS) whilst in others autopsy is superior (cardiac anomalies) (Table 8.1). A lack of experience in post-mortem image interpretation also occurs as a common theme.

The Royal College of Paediatrics and Child Health (RCPCH) concludes that:

'There is little evidence that there are valid alternatives to conventional autopsy. MRI might be the choice to examine brain morphology in a stillborn infant...If limited biopsy or MRI directed biopsy are to be advocated at all, then the working group believes it should only be after careful, prospective studies'. (Ref. [28], Appendix 2.)

POST-MORTEM IMAGING IN ADULTS

There have been very few published studies comparing post-mortem imaging of adults compared to autopsy [12].

Table 8.1 Post-mortem MRI in paediatric pathology

What is MRI good at?	What is MRI not good at?
• CNS evaluation – including spinal cord • Abnormal body cavity accumulations (ascites, pleural/pericardial effusions, haemothorax) • Structural abnormalities (diaphragmatic herniae, hydrops fetalis, dysplastic kidneys, renal ageesis, bladder dilatation, ureteral stenosis)	• Cardiac anomalies (VSD/ASD/coarctation) • Metabolic disease • Infection • Post-mortem decomposition • Artefacts/maceration • Pulmonary hypoplasia • Some structural anomalies (e.g. tracheo-oesophageal fistula)

Ros *et al.* [29] described their initial experiences comparing post-mortem MRI with autopsy in a mixed paediatric and adult population. They examined only six patients, and concluded that MRI was superior to autopsy in the detection of air and fluid in potential spaces, but inferior in the detection of small abnormalities. MRI examination failed to identify a subarachnoid haemorrhage, coronary artery atherosclerosis and a lung abscess.

Bisset *et al.* [6] described the operation of an MRI post-mortem examination 'service' in Manchester, UK that was established in 1997 with the support of the local Coroner. 53 bodies had been examined in three private MRI scanners, paid for by the local Jewish community.

The Coroner accepted the cause of death based on the clinical history and the results of the MRI scan in 47 cases (87%), whereas six cases proceeded to autopsy. All cases examined were adult sudden deaths, but in which there were no suspicious circumstances. The deaths had been reported to the Coroner because the hospital doctor or primary care physician could not issue a death certificate.

The results of those cases receiving both an MRI examination and autopsy were interesting in that all but one were found at autopsy to have died from ischaemic heart disease. MRI examination was able to identify pulmonary oedema, effusions and pulmonary consolidation and cardiomegaly, but could not identify the most common cause of sudden death in the UK and the western world [30], [31]. Those suffering from metabolic disease were excluded from MRI examination, as were those suffering from '... other pathology unlikely to cause macroscopic changes in anatomy'.

Bisset *et al.* [6] went on to explain that deaths certified by doctors were only 31–75% accurate, and that the causes of death given following a review of the medical records and an MRI post-mortem examination were 'at least as accurate'.

Publication of this paper resulted in a lively debate in the *British Medical Journal*, including comments that imaging provided information about modes of death rather than causes [32], doubts about the legality of accepting 'confident causes of death' based upon imaging alone [33], the limited numbers of cases receiving MRI examination and autopsy [34], a general lack of detail, particularly relating to ischaemic heart disease, and conditions resulting in an exclusion from the MRI examination, notably those conditions unlikely to result in any macroscopic changes in anatomy [35].

There was also concern about advocating MRI post-mortem examinations of the dead whilst the waiting lists for the living were already too long [32], [36].

Building upon this study, Roberts *et al.* [37] compared post-mortem MRI examination with autopsy in 10 Coronial cases, where suspicious, violent or drug-related deaths were excluded. In the study MRI images were reported blind by four radiologists, two of whom had experience of interpreting such images. The radiologists and pathologists were given access to the summary of circumstances of death provided by the reporting police officer, and the radiologists were asked to state how confident they were about each diagnosis given.

In only one case were all radiologists in full agreement about the 'definite' cause of death: disseminated bronchial carcinoma. An abnormality relating to the cause of death (but not necessarily the cause of death) was identified by at least one radiologist in eight cases; for example, left ventricular failure in a person found at autopsy to have ischaemic heart disease.

A 'correct' cause of death was identified by:

- one radiologist in three cases
- two radiologists in one case
- three radiologists in one case, and
- four radiologists in one case

MRI demonstrated free air in the abdomen, but was not able to locate the site of the perforated viscus, and the presence of pulmonary oedema and left ventricular abnormalities were interpreted as evidence of ischaemic heart disease. Severe coronary artery atheroma was not demonstrated by MRI examination, and left ventricular failure was interpreted indirectly based upon left ventricular and pulmonary venous dilatation and pulmonary oedema.

The effects of post-mortem decomposition, such as gas within the central hepatic vessels and bile ducts [38] and autolysis, caused difficulties in radiological interpretation. An old cerebral infarct was interpreted as an acute infarct, and a postmortem clot interpreted as antemortem thrombus.

Interestingly, other researchers [39] have been able to distinguish these two entities, commenting on a 'streaming clot surrounded by serum' and a lack of fibrin or haemosiderin susceptibility-induced effect being noted in fast field echo (FFE) or Spectral Presaturation Inversion Recovery (SPIR) sequences.

Surprisingly, there was seemingly no benefit in having radiological experience in interpreting post-mortem images, and MRI did not appear to be any more sensitive than autopsy at identifying minor brain lesions, such as cortical lacunar infarcts. Figs 8.2, 8.3 and 8.4 illustrate post-mortem decomposition in the liver and soft tissues.

Patriquin *et al.* [39] compared post-mortem MRI with autopsy in a further eight cases, and similarly found that MRI was good at identifying gross

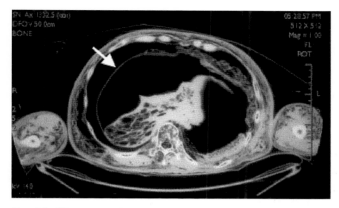

Fig. 8.2 CT cross-section through the liver shows gaseous swelling with a large subcapsular gas bubble (arrow). Reprinted from *Forens Sci Int*, **134**(1): 109–17 © 2003 Elsevier Ireland Ltd.

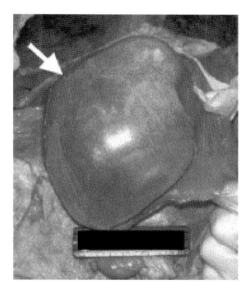

Fig. 8.3 Autopsy picture of decomposed liver with large gas bubble below the surface. Reprinted from *Forens Sci Int*, **134**(1): 109–17 © 2003 Elsevier Ireland Ltd.

pulmonary lesions, including Adult Respiratory Distress Syndrome (ARDS), but not severe coronary artery stenosis or a left anterior descending coronary artery bypass graft occlusion. Diffuse oedema in cadaveric lungs was confusing to radiologists more accustomed to the lung parenchyma of live patients, and the presence of fluid was found to obscure underlying pathology only discerned at autopsy.

In addition MR imaging missed an acute anterior wall myocardial infarction. However, only six cases had a full autopsy following imaging, the others having a limited dissection or 'biopsy autopsy'. Overall, they found that there were discrepancies between the determined causes of death by autopsy and by MRI in five of eight cases.

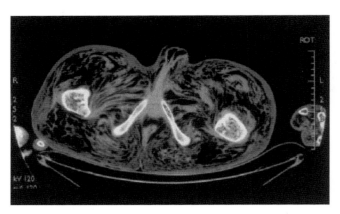

Fig. 8.4 Typical radiological signs of soft tissue decomposition in the CT cross-sectional image through the pelvic floor. Reprinted from *Forens Sci Int*, **134**(1): 109–17 © 2003 Elsevier Ireland Ltd.

Bronge *et al.* [40] investigated the utility of MRI versus autopsy on the brains of Alzheimer's disease patients. They found a good deal of correlation between the two methods, confirming the utility of MRI in the evaluation of adult CNS disease as in the paediatric field, but that pathological examination identified more extensive areas of involvement.

Post-mortem MRI has also been described as a useful tool for the investigation of cerebral micro bleeds, which are generally small and inconspicuous in routine histological sections [41]. The post-mortem MR imaging of formalin fixed brains to illustrate traumatic injury in a less 'gruesome, inflammatory and prejudicial' manner in court settings has previously been described by Harris [42].

Hsu *et al.* [43] have examined formalin fixed hearts using MRI compared to gross pathological and microscopic examination, and found that the T1 and T2 values for infarcted tissues are significantly different to non-infarcted tissues, and thus it is at least theoretically possible to identify such tissue, and even give a 3D volume to that area of myocardium involved using post-scanning rendering techniques. Table 8.2 compares the post-mortem MRI and autopsy for identifying a range of diseases or conditions in adults.

POST-MORTEM IMAGING IN FORENSIC CASES

The papers described in the previous section all investigated post-mortem MRI in sudden adult deaths, but specifically excluded those cases in which there were any suspicious features.

CT was first used in forensic medicine to image a gunshot wound to the head [18], and was used to examine mummies, but has not gained much interest in forensic science. An earlier report in the literature described the utility of radiography, CT and MRI in judicial hangings compared to autopsy findings [44].

Table 8.2 Post-mortem MRI in adults

What is MRI good at?	What is MRI not good at?
• CNS evaluation • Abnormal fluid/air collections, e.g. effusions, ascites, pneumothorax, air in mesenteric vessels, subcutaneous emphysema • Cardiovascular disease, e.g. major vascular abnormalities including aneurysms, IVC engorgement and left ventricular failure (indirectly) • Soft tissue lesions/tumours • Pulmonary lesions, e.g. pneumonia, ARDS, *pneumocystis carinii*, pneumonia with cyst formation • Perforation of viscus (but not necessarily the site) • Solid organ lesions, e.g. hepatic and splenic infarcts • Upper gastrointestinal tract pathology	• Metabolic disease • Cardiac disease, e.g. coronary artery definition, ischaemic heart disease, arrhythmias, atherosclerosis, conduction abnormalities • Thrombo-embolus versus post-mortem clot • Effects of decomposition, e.g. hepatic and portal tract gas formation • Oedema versus exudates • Lower gastrointestinal tract pathology

Donchin *et al.* [45] compared post-mortem CT with autopsy in trauma victims in Israel, and found CT to be more sensitive at identifying bone trauma, whilst autopsy was superior at determining soft tissue trauma. They concluded that post-mortem CT was a useful adjunct to autopsy, but where an autopsy was not possible; imaging could still yield important information as to the mechanism of traumatic deaths.

Cranial CT is frequently used to detect intracranial trauma in the living, and has also been of use in the interpretation of the mechanism of injury in those who subsequently died [46]. The use of MRI in documenting traumatic injuries to the head is also well-established, and Gentry *et al.* found MR imaging to be superior to CT, particularly in the detection of non-haemorrhagic lesions and some secondary forms of injury [47]. However, autopsy confirmation of the lesions identified was possible in only 1 out of their 40 patients.

Post-mortem cranial MRI has been described in a study of suspected child abuse, with subsequent autopsy correlation, where it was noted that MRI findings were useful in directing the autopsy and brain cut, but that autopsy was superior in detecting subarachnoid haemorrhage, suture separation, extracranial injuries and very small subdural haematomas [48]. MRI demonstrated cerebral oedema, contusion, shearing injury, ischaemia and infarction well.

A large active centre in Berne, Switzerland, has studied the utility of imaging modalities in the examination of sudden and suspicious deaths, and compared the findings with forensic autopsies. The 'Virtopsy project' was created in 2000.

The group has produced an impressive number of research papers covering the examination findings in a series of 40 sudden deaths [49], the examination of charred bodies [50], decomposed bodies [51] and a victim of a scuba diving accident [52].

A particularly fruitful area of research has been the use of post-mortem imaging in the examination of penetrating injuries, such as gunshots and other missiles (Figs 8.5–8.9). The group has investigated the utility of Multi-Slice CT (MSCT) and MRI in gunshot victims and found the imaging of fracture patterns and wound tracks to be superior to autopsy alone, and have performed a whole body examination in 60 s [53], [54].

2D multi-planar reformation and 3D shaded-surface display reconstruction allows the gunshot created complex of skull fractures, for example, and the associated brain injuries including the wound track to be documented and displayed in 3D, allowing targeted autopsy, preservation of evidence, presentation of evidence in court and future auditing of the findings.

In the largest series to date, Thali *et al.* used both Multislice CT (MSCT) and MRI to examine 18 cases of blunt trauma, eight cases involving gunshot wounds, two involving knife wounds, two drownings and two strangulations, as well as one involving electrocution (and a single case of sudden infant death syndrome) [49].

The findings are of interest not only in the forensic field, but also add to the weight of evidence available for sudden deaths in adults from natural disease. For example, myocardial infarction was visible on MRI in two of six cardiac deaths, whilst plaque rupture and thrombosis were not visible. In addition, inferior vena cava engorgement similar to that seen in right heart failure was identified in cases of drowning. Post-mortem hypostasis was distinguished from pulmonary contusion, as well as aspiration of stomach contents and blood. The ability of post-mortem MRI to identify abnormal fluid collections was also confirmed. The presence of neurotrauma and intracranial and intercerebral bleeds were well documented, and the utility of MRI and MSCT for demonstrating soft tissue and bone trauma was confirmed.

Unfortunately, imaging was not so good at identifying trauma of internal organs, where death had been too rapid for there to have been time for haematomas to develop.

A potential limiting factor for the examination of gunshot victims by CT is metal artefact, although reduction algorithms are becoming increasingly sophisticated. MRI examination of gunshot wounds can also be problematic where the bullet causes artefact, or worse, is attracted to the magnetic field. Metal artefacts may also assist in the identification of metal missile fragments, some of which may not be localised by traditional autopsy [55].

Oncology radiation therapy planning tools have also been used to good effect to determine the angle of a gunshot, based on the 3D localisation of bone fragments and the bullet, and the application of mathematical principles [56].

Researchers in Israel carried out post-mortem CT examinations in military personnel killed by penetrating injuries, particularly those caused by shrapnel from 'claymore' mines and artillery shells [55]. They confirmed the utility of CT for the detection of air/fluid in potential body spaces, and in particular at identifying tension haemopneumothorax. CT was particularly useful in

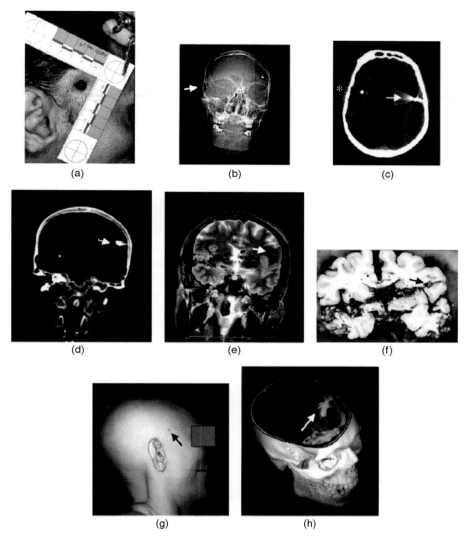

(a)   (b)   (c)

(d)   (e)   (f)

(g)   (h)

Fig. 8.5 Autopsy, CT and MRI data of a gunshot victim. (a) Photograph of entrance wound.
(b) Classical CT scout view. This projectional overview is obtained in the CT scanner for
planning the range of cross-sectional scanning. Note the small bullet fragments in the area of
the entrance wound (arrow), and the projectile located on the victim's left. (c) Cross-sectional
CT image showing air and bleeding in the entrance area (*, skull entrance wound not visible in
this section) and the projectile with streak artefacts (arrow). (d) Bone window of coronal CT
reformation showing the projectile from another view angle. The metal artefacts from the
projectile are still present (arrow). (e) MRI cross-section corresponding to (d). MRI tissue
details surpass CT: anatomy of the brain layers and the bullet track become visible. Due to
metal-induced artefacts the projectile is not visible (arrow). (f) Autopsy finding corresponding
to (d) and (e): bullet track and projectile (arrow). (g) 3D CT surface reconstruction of the face:
small entrance wound on the right temple (arrow, corresponding to (a)). For purposes of
maintaining victim anonymity, some parts of the digitally reconstructed face are obscured.
(h) 3D CT reconstruction of the skull after virtual removal of the top of the skull: entrance
wound area and the projectile with streak artefacts (arrow). Reprinted from *Forens Sci Int*,
138(1–3): 8–16 © 2003 Elsevier Ireland Ltd.

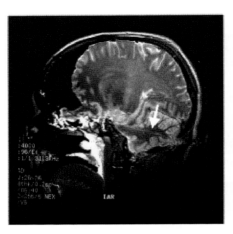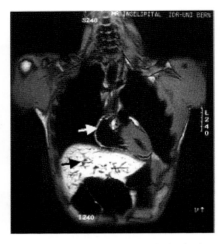

Fig. 8.6 Left: MR cross-section of cross-section of gunshot wound track through the brain stem and the cerebellum (arrow). Right: Coronal MR cross-section shows pathological air collections in the heart and liver vessels (arrows). Reprinted from *Forens Sci Int*, **138**(1–3): 8–16 © 2003 Elsevier Ireland Ltd.

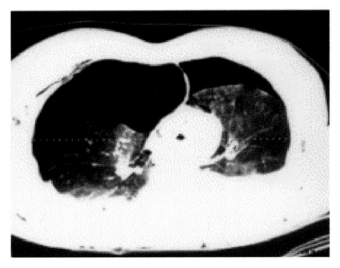

Fig. 8.7 Gunshot-induced pneumothorax in the CT cross-section of the chest. Reprinted from *Forens Sci Int*, **138**(1–3): 8–16 © 2003 Elsevier Ireland Ltd.

locating metal fragments, but was not able to image surface injuries, including abrasions and burns.

Imaging was able to identify bilateral lung consolidation, but was not capable of distinguishing whether this was due to aspiration of blood, contusion or pulmonary blast injury. They concluded that in the military context, autopsy was superior to post-mortem CT imaging alone, in that the size of ammunition

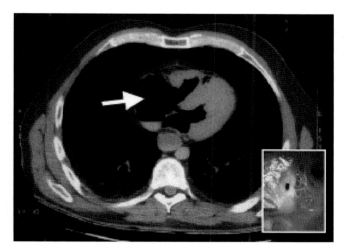

Fig. 8.8 CT cross-section with air embolism (arrow) in the right- and left-sided cavities of the heart, due to an open foramen ovale (photograph at lower right corner). Reprinted from *Forens Sci Int*, **138**(1–3): 8–16 © 2003 Elsevier Ireland Ltd.

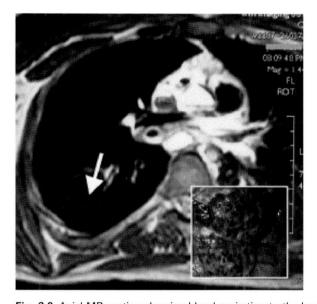

Fig. 8.9 Axial MR section showing blood aspiration to the lung (arrow). Corresponding autopsy finding at the right lower corner. Reprinted from *Forens Sci Int*, **138**(1–3): 8–16 © 2003 Elsevier Ireland Ltd.

fragments, their track within the body and the effectiveness of protective equipment could not be fully assessed.

A potential limiting factor to undertaking whole body imaging on cadavers is the lack of radiology support and resources available to the living, let alone the dead. However, this problem is not insurmountable, and may be tackled in innovative ways, such as the use of portable scanners located next to the

Table 8.3 Post-mortem imaging in forensic cases

- Bone trauma/fracture patterns
- Penetrating missile wounds/tracks/fragments, e.g. gunshot or shrapnel wounds
- Pathologic gas/fluid collections, e.g. air embolism, tension pneumothorax, hyperbaric trauma, subcutaneous emphysema, decomposition effects (MSCT)
- Soft tissue injury
- Neurotrauma, including shear trauma effects, concussive injuries and intra-cranial and intercerebral bleeds
- Lung contusions vs hypostasis
- Myocardial infarction
- Fire deaths/charred bodies
- Detecting packets of drugs in the gastrointestinal tract (a drugs 'mule')
- Judicial hanging

mortuary, or by agreeing service plans with radiology departments, funded by the local Coroner. Indeed, Rutty and Swift [57] have agreed access to the Leicester Royal Infirmary, UK, CT scanner at 1 hour's notice, 24 hours per day, 7 days a week.

The range of situations in which post-mortem imaging (MRI and MSCT) has been of use in forensic casework is given in Table 8.3.

DIGITAL IMAGE POST-PROCESSING AND 3D MODELLING

Developments in software have allowed sophisticated 'post-processing' of the digital images captured during a CT scan, which for example allows the reconstruction of two-dimensional images into three-dimensional 'models' of the imaged object.

The University of Berne Institute of Forensic Medicine team describe the 2D multi-planar reformation and 3D shaded surface display reconstruction of MSCT and MRI images of gunshot wounds (Figs 8.10 and 8.11), as well as the use of forensic 3D/CAD supported photogrammetry [53], [58], [59].

This technique is used to record physical wound details on a body surface at autopsy, and render 'virtual models' of the injury. The same process is undertaken for an object, and the two 'virtual models' can be manipulated and superimposed in virtual space in order to determine whether they match. Gun muzzle imprints [60] and tyre track impressions [61] have been illustrated and these techniques can be supplemented by surface colouring techniques (Figs 8.12—8.14) [62].

Oliver *et al.* describe their recreation of CT data from thumbnail hardcopy images, allowing the analysis of patterned surface injuries and bone trauma in the Rodney King case [63]. In the future, they hope that CT and MRI datasets can be combined to realise the benefits in trauma reconstruction using the strengths of each modality. In addition, they foresee the incorporation of imaging

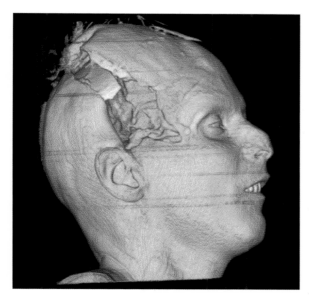

Fig. 8.10 Gunshot injury to the head and 3D-visualisation of soft tissues. Reprinted from *Forens Sci Int*, Thali and Dirnhofer, Forensic Radiology in German-Speaking Area, published online June 25, 2004; DOI: 10.1016/j.forsciint.2004.04.058 © with permission from Elsevier.

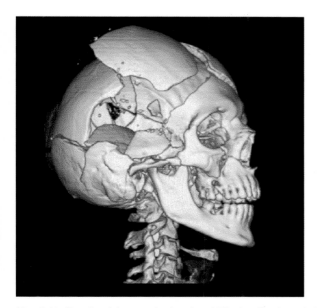

Fig. 8.11 Gunshot injury to the head and 3D-visualisation of skull. Reprinted from *Forens Sci Int*, Thali and Dirnhofer, Forensic Radiology in German-Speaking Area, published online June 25, 2004; DOI: 10.1016/j.forsciint.2004.04.058 © with permission from Elsevier.

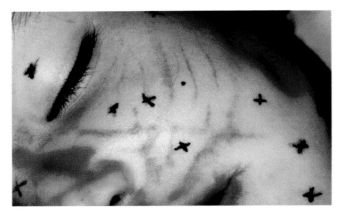

Fig. 8.12 Distinctive injury pattern (bruising) on the face looks like the tracks of a car tire. Reprinted from Forens Sci Int **113**(1–3): 281–7 © Elsevier Ireland Ltd.

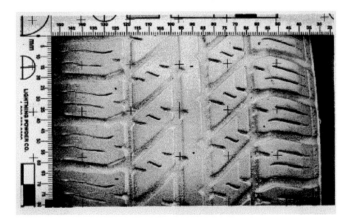

Fig. 8.13 Tire tread of the suspect vehicle. Reprinted from *Forens Sci Int* **113**(1–3): 281–7 © Elsevier Ireland Ltd.

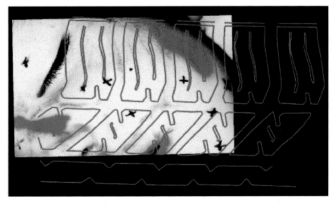

Fig. 8.14 Perfect match between multiple bruises on the head, and the tire tread. Reprinted from *Forens Sci Int* **113**(1–3): 281–7 © Elsevier Ireland Ltd.

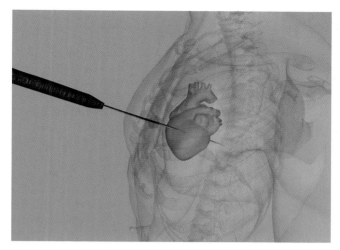

Fig. 8.15 Suicidal stab wound through the body. Reprinted with permission Mr Damian Schofield, Nottingham University, UK [64].

techniques with 'virtual reality' technology, allowing for the virtual manipulation of the body, coupled with biomechanical modelling of mechanisms of wounding and the body's response to that insult.

Developments in the field of 3D computer animation graphics and body modelling software are already finding their way into forensic science, including vehicular accident reconstruction and the reconstruction of knife wounds. March and Schofield and colleagues [64] have been at the forefront of research in the UK into the graphical and 3D representation of pathological data, in co-operation with the Medico-legal Centre in Sheffield (Fig. 8.15).

The use of Poser™ 3D body modelling software (www.curiouslabs.com), coupled with the overlaying of wound and injury images using Adobe® PhotoShop® (www.adobe.com), for example, has now become widespread in forensic medical practice, in order to present images to Courts that are considered to be less 'prejudicial' to a defendant, and less harrowing for juries.

FUTURE DEVELOPMENTS

We are a long way off from being able to do away with the traditional preparation and staining of tissues, but the resolution of microscopic anatomy is improving. Indeed, Rosai has said that:

'...there is hardly a procedure in the whole armamentarium of medicine that gives so much information so quickly and at such a little cost as the H&E technique despite the obdurate criticisms it had to endure over the years.' [65]

Micro-CT has been used to image retinal haemorrhages and electrical injury to skin [18], whilst research into magnetic resonance histology has included toxicological effects in vivo and developmental biological imaging [66], [67].

The first MR image of a cell was reported in 1987, and Ciobanu *et al.* describe their research into improving resolution to approximately $3.7\,\mu m \times 3.3\,\mu m \times 3.3\,\mu m$ [68]. Theoretical predictions by Blank *et al.* increase this resolution using electron spin resonance microscopy to $1 \times 1 \times 10\,\mu m$ [69]. Acquisition time, however, is still a considerable hurdle, being in the order of hours for each image.

MR spectroscopy is an area receiving much interest, being used to document pre-terminal and post-mortem metabolite concentrations in laboratory animal tissues, and in toxicological studies [18], [70], [71].

Developments in clinical imaging will also undoubtedly have further knock-on effects on the utility of post-mortem imaging. For example, detection tools for coronary arteries are being developed for multi-slice CT scanning protocols, and coronary artery plaques and the degree of stenoses are also being researched using MRI [72], [73].

CONCLUSIONS

This chapter has explored the utility of post-mortem imaging as an adjunct to, or as a replacement of traditional autopsy. Research has identified the benefits of post-mortem MRI in the identification of particularly fetal and paediatric CNS anomalies or injury, and the documentation of soft tissue trauma. Post-mortem multi-slice CT has similarly been shown to be superior to autopsy in the documentation and 3D reconstruction of fracture patterns in forensic cases. Gaps exist in the evidence base for the main causes of sudden adult death, but current research into the imaging of coronary arteries and areas of ischaemic myocardial damage may in turn prove to be useful in post-mortem imaging.

A significant hurdle to the introduction of widespread post-mortem imaging into routine practice appears to be one of resources, and there does not seem to be a straightforward answer to this. The Department of Forensic Pathology at Leicester University Medical School, UK appears to have access to a scanner at any time, but elsewhere such access is unheard of.

The time taken to perform a whole body scan has reduced substantially from 2 h in 1990 [29] to 60 s [54], but the resources required to interpret the images are still lacking. The interpretation of radiological images by pathologists raises interesting clinical governance issues, and there is perhaps some scope for training pathology Registrars in post-mortem image interpretation now.

By being present at the imaging examination, the pathologist can discuss findings with the radiologist, and assist in the interpretation of suspected artefacts due to decomposition, etc., or take additional precautions when opening the body, such as opening the heart under water. Additional health and safety precautions may be required, for example where imaging has indicated the presence of metal fragments within a body cavity, etc [57].

In the age of evidence-based medicine, we do not yet have a secure base upon which to abandon the traditional autopsy in favour of post-mortem imaging. However, research has shown that imaging techniques can be used as an adjunct to autopsy, and create a record of the pathological findings capable of being stored long-term, digitally manipulated to give 3D information and presented to others in the form of evidence in court or for peer review or audit. Perhaps the time has come to embrace post-mortem imaging and set the agenda for the future of autopsy, rather than find the role of post-mortem interpretation passed over to the radiologists?

REFERENCES

1. Start RD, Cotton DWK. The current status of the autopsy. In *Progress in Pathology 3*. Kirkham N, Lemoine NR (Eds.) (Churchill Livingstone, Edinburgh 1997) pp. 179–88.

2. Rutty GN, Duerdon RM, Carter N *et al*. Are coroners' necropsies necessary? A prospective study examining whether a 'view and grant' system of death certification could be introduced into England and Wales. *J Clin Pathol* 2001; **54**: 279–84.

3. Burton JL, Underwood JCE. Necropsy practice after the 'organ retention scandal': requests, performance, and tissue retention. *J Clin Patho* 2003; **56**: 537–41.

4. Handley R. Postmortem imaging: a viable alternative to autopsy . . . or just a dead end? *Adv Imaging* April 2001; 10–11.

5. Eustace SJ, Nelson E. Whole body magnetic resonance imaging — a valuable adjunct to clinical examination. *BMJ* 2004; **328**: 1387–8.

6. Bisset RAL, Thomas NB, Turnbull IW *et al*. Postmortem examinations using magnetic resonance imaging: four year review of a working service. *BMJ* 2002; **324**: 1423–4.

7. Geller SA. Religious attitudes and the autopsy. *Arch Pathol Lab Med* 1984; **108**: 494–6.

8. Redfern M. The Royal Liverpool Children's Hospital Inquiry, 2000, www.rlcinquiry.org.uk.

9. Kennedy I. Learning from Bristol. Inquiry into the Management of Care of Children Receiving Complex Heart Surgery at the Bristol Royal Infirmary, 2001, www.bristol-inquiry.org.uk/final_report/.

10. Department of Health. The Removal, Retention and Use of Human Organs and Tissue from Post-Mortem Examinations: Advice from the Chief Medical Officer, 2001, The Stationery Office, London UK.

11. Parker A. Less invasive autopsy — the place of magnetic resonance imaging, 2004, www.publications.doh.gov.uk/cmo/progress/organretention/mri-report.pdf.

12. Department of Health. Policy Research Programme Invitation to Tender — Less Invasive Autopsy. Calls for proposals document available on-line, 2004, www.dh.gov.uk/ProcurementAndProposals/RDCallsForProposals/fs/en.

13. Home Office. Reforming the Coroner and Death Certification Service — A Position Paper, Cm 6159, The Stationery Office, London, March 2004.

14. Luce T. Death Certification and Investigation in England, Wales and Northern Ireland — The Report of a Fundamental Review. Cm 58 2003, The Stationery Office, www.official-documents.co.uk/document/cm58/5831/5831.htm.

15. Smith J. The Shipman Inquiry — Third Report: Death Certification and the investigation of Deaths by Coroners, 2003, www.the-shipman-inquiry.org.uk/thirdreport.asp.

16. Department of Health. Policy Research Programme Invitation to Tender — Less Invasive Autopsy. Advert in *BMJ Careers* 3/4/04 p. a3.

17. Benbow EW, Roberts ISD. The autopsy: complete or not complete? *Histopathol* 2003; **42**: 417–23.

18. Thali MJ, Vock P. Role and techniques in forensic imaging. In *Forensic Medicine — Clinical and Pathological Aspects*. Payne-James JJ, Bussuttil A, Smock W (Eds.) (Greenwich Medical Media, London, 2003) 731–47.

19. Ehrlich E, Maxeiner H, Lange J. Postmortem radiological investigation of bridging vein ruptures. *Leg Med* 2003; **5**: S225–S7.

20. Prahlow JA, Scharling ES, Lantz P. Postmortem coronary subtraction angiography. *Am J Foren Med Pathol* 1996; **17**: 225–30.

21. Garden AS, Weindling AM, Griffiths RD *et al*. Fast-scan magnetic resonance imaging of fetal anomalies. *Am J Obstet Gynaecol* 1991; **166**: 1217–22.

22. Brookes JAS, Hall-Craggs MA, Sama VR *et al.* Non-invasive perinatal necropsy by magnetic resonance imaging. *Lancet* 1996; **348**: 1139–41.

23. Woodward PJ, Sohaey R, Harris DP *et al.* Postmortem fetal MR imaging: comparison with findings at autopsy. *AJR* 1997; **168**: 41–6.

24. Alderliesten ME, Peringa J, van der Hulst VPM *et al.* Perinatal mortality: clinical value of postmortem magnetic resonance imaging compared with autopsy in routine obstetric practice. *BJ Obs Gyn* 2003; **110**: 378–82.

25. Guo WY, Chang CY, Ho DM *et al.* A comparative MRI and pathological study on CNS disorders. *Child Nerv Sys* 2003; **17**: 512–18.

26. Huisman TAGM, Wisser J, Stallmach T *et al.* MR autopsy in fetuses. *Fet Diag Ther* 2002; **17**: 58–64.

27. Griffiths PD, Variend D, Evans M *et al.* Postmortem MR imaging of the fetal and stillborn central nervous system. *Am J Neuroradiol* 2003; **24**: 22–7.

28. Royal College of Paediatrics and Child Health. The Future of Paediatric Pathology Services, 2002, www.rcpch.ac.uk/publications/recent_publications/Pathol.pdf.

29. Ros PR, Li KC, Vo P *et al.* Pre-autopsy magnetic resonance imaging: initial experience. *Magnet Res Imag* 1990; **8**: 303–8.

30. Sheppard MN. Sudden adult death and the heart. In *Progress in Pathology 6.* Kirkham N., Shepherd N (Eds.) (Greenwich Medical Media, London, 2003) pp. 185–202.

31. Sheppard MN. The autopsy. Letter to editor, *Histopathol* 2004; **44**: 82–3.

32. Swift B. Postmortem radiology is useful but no substitute for necropsy. Letter to editor. *BMJ* 2002; **325**: 549.

33. Jarmulowicz MR. MRI postmortems – no validation. bmj.com rapid responses for Bisset *et al.* 2002; **324** (7351): 1423–4, available on-line 17/6/02 www.bmj.bmjjournals.com/cgi/eletters/324/7351/1423.

34. Bell JE, Ironside JW, Smith C. Letter in response to Bisset *et al.*, bmj.com rapid responses for Bisset *et al.* 2002; **324** (7351): 1423–4, available on-line 4/7/02 www.bmj.bmjjournals.com/cgi/eletters/324/7351/1423.

35. Leadbeatter S, James R, Davison A *et al.* Many more questions than answers. bmj.com rapid responses for Bisset *et al.* 2002; **324** (7351): 1423–4, available on-line 5/7/02 www.bmj.bmjjournals.com/cgi/eletters/324/7351/1423.

36. Salmon D. It is a mad, mad world, my masters. bmj.com rapid responses for Bisset *et al.* 2002; **324** (7351): 1423–4, available on-line 14/6/02 www.bmj.bmjjournals.com/cgi/eletters/324/7351/1423.

37. Roberts ISD, Benbow EW, Bisset R *et al.* Accuracy of magnetic resonance imaging in determining cause of sudden death in adults: comparison with conventional autopsy. *Histopathol* 2003; **42**: 424–30.

38. Yamazaki K, Shiotani S, Ohashi N *et al.* Hepatic portal venous gas and hyper-dense aortic wall as postmortem computed tomography finding. *Leg Med* 2003; **5**: S338–41.

39. Patriquin L, Kassarjian A, O'Brien M *et al.* Postmortem whole-body magnetic resonance imaging as an adjunct to autopsy: preliminary clinical experience. *J Magnet Res Imag* 2001; **13**: 277–87.

40. Bronge L, Bogdanovic N, Wahlund LO. Postmortem MRI and histopathology of white matter changes in Alzheimer brains. A quantitative, comparative study. *Dement Geria Cog Dis* 2002; **13**: 205–12.

41. Messori A, Salvolini U. Postmortem MRI as a useful tool for investigation of cerebral microbleeds. Letter to Editor, *Stroke* 2003; **34**: 376–7.

42. Harris LS. Postmortem magnetic resonance images of the injured brain: effective evidence in the courtroom. *Forens Sci Int* 1991; **50**: 179–85.

43. Hsu JCM, Johnson A, Smith WM *et al.* Magnetic resonance imaging of chronic myocardial infarcts in formalin-fixed human autopsy hearts. *Circulation* 1994; **89**: 2133–40.

44. Wallace SK, Cohen WA, Stern EJ *et al.* Judicial hanging: postmortem radiographic, CT, and MR imaging features with autopsy confirmation. *Radiology* 1994; **193**: 263–7.

45. Donchin Y, Rivkind AI, Bar-Ziv J, Hiss J *et al.* Utility of postmortem computed tomography in trauma victims. *J Trauma* 1994; **37**: 552–6.

46. Bauer M, Polzin S, Patzelt D. The use of clinical CCT images in the forensic examination of closed head injuries. *J Clin Forens Med* 2004; **11**: 65–70.

47. Gentry LR, Godersky JC, Thompson B. MR imaging of head trauma: review of the distribution and radiopathologic features of traumatic lesions. *AJR* 1988; **150**: 663–72.

48. Hart B, Dudley M, Zumwalt RE. Postmortem cranial MRI and autopsy correlation in suspected child abuse. *Am J Forens Med Pathol* 1996; **17**: 217–24.

49. Thali MJ, Yen K, Schweitzer W *et al.* Virtopsy, a new imaging horizon in forensic pathology: virtual autopsy by postmortem multislice computed tomography (MSCT) and magnetic resonance imaging (MRI) – a feasibility study. *J Foren Sci* 2003; **48**: 386–483.

50. Thali MJ, Yen K, Plattner T *et al.* Charred body: virtual autopsy with multi-slice computed tomography and magnetic resonance imaging. *J Forens Sci* 2002; **47**: 1326–31.

51. Thali MJ, Yen K, Schweitzer W *et al.* Into the decomposed body – forensic digital autopsy using multislice-computed tomography. *Forens Sci Int* 2003; **134**: 109–17.

52. Plattner T, Thali MJ, Yen K *et al.* Virtopsy – Postmortem Multislice Computed Tomography (MSCT) and Magnetic Resonance Imaging (MRI) in a fatal scuba diving incident. *J Forens Sci* 2003; **48**: 1347–55.

53. Thali MJ, Yen K, Vock P *et al.* Image-guided virtual autopsy findings of gunshot victims performed with multi-slice computed tomography (MSCT) and magnetic resonance imaging (MRI) and subsequent correlation between radiology and autopsy findings. *Forens Sci Int* 2003; **138**: 8–16.

54. Thali MJ, Schweitzer W, Yen K *et al.* New horizons in forensic radiology: the 60-second digital autopsy – full-body examination of a gunshot victim by Multi-slice Computed Tomography. *Am J Forens Med Pathol* 2003; **24**: 22–7.

55. Farkash U, Scope A, Lynn M *et al.* Preliminary experience with postmortem computed tomography in military penetrating trauma. *J Trauma: Inj, Inf Crit Care* 2000; **48**: 303–8.

56. Marchetti D, Tartaglione T, Mattiu G *et al.* Reconstruction of the angle of shot by using computed radiography of the head. *Am J Forens Med Pathol* 2003; **24**: 155–9.

57. Rutty GN, Swift B. Correspondence to 'accuracy of magnetic resonance imaging in determining cause of sudden death in adults': comparison with conventional autopsy. *Histopathol* 2004; **44**: 187–9.

58. Bruschweiler W, Braun M, Dirnhofer R *et al.* Analysis of patterned injuries and injury-causing instruments with forensic 3D/CAD supported photogrammetry (FPHG): an instruction manual for the documentation process. *Forens Sci Int* 2003; **132**: 130–8.

59. Thali MJ, Braun M, Dirnhofer R. Optical 3D surface digitising in forensic medicine: 3D documentation of skin and bone injuries. *Forens Sci Int* 2003; **137**: 203–8.

60. Thali MJ, Braun M, Brueschweiler W *et al.* Morphological imprint: determination of the injury-causing weapon from the wound morphology using forensic 3D/CAD supported photogrammetry. *Forens Sci Int* 2003; **132**: 177–81.

61. Thali MJ, Braun M, Bruschweiler W *et al.* Matching tyre tracks on the head using forensic photogrammetry. *Forens Sci Int* 2000; **113**: 281–7.

62. Subke J, Haase S, Wehner H-D *et al.* Computer aided shot reconstructions by means of individualised animated three-dimensional victim models. *Forens Sci Int* 2002; **125**: 245–9.

63. Oliver WR, Boxwala A, Rosenman J *et al.* Three-dimensional visualisation and image processing in the evaluation of patterned injuries: The AFIP/UNC experience in the Rodney King case. *Am J Forens Med Pathol* 1997; **18**: 1–10.

64. March J, Schofield D, Evison M *et al.* Three-dimensional computer visualisation of forensic pathology data. *Am J Forens Med Pathol* 2003; **25**: 60–70.

65. Rosai J. *Rosai and Ackerman's Surgical Pathology.* 9th edn, Vol. 1 (Mosby, Philadelphia, 2004); p. 37.

66. MRPath Incorporated. Magnetic Resonance Histology, 2001, www.mrpath.com/rd/tech/tech.html

67. Johnson GA, Benveniste H, Black RD *et al.* Histology by magnetic resonance microscopy. *Magnet Res Quart* 1993; **9**: 1–30.

68. Ciobanu L, Seeber DA, Pennington CH. 3D MR microscopy with resolution 3.7 μm by 3.3 μm by 3.3 μm. *J Magnet Res* 2002; **158**: 178–82.

69. Blank A, Dunnam CR, Borbat PP *et al.* High resolution electron spin resonance microscopy. *J Magnet Res* 2003; **165**: 116–27.

70. Emch B, Singer T, Rudin M *et al.* Magnetic resonance imaging (MRI) – a new diagnostic modality in toxicological studies. *Toxicol Let* 1996; **88**: 47.

71. Ith M, Bigler P, Scheurer E *et al*. Observation and identification of metabolites emerging during postmortem decomposition of brain tissue by means of in-situ 1H-Magnetic Resonance Spectroscopy. *Magnet Res Med* 2002; **48**: 915–20.

72. Dewey M. Multislice CT coronary angiography: evaluation of an automatic vessel detection tool. *Rofo Fortschr Geb Rontgenstr Neuen Bildgeb Verfahr* 2004; **176**: 478–83.

73. CORDA (The Heart Charity). CORDA Asymptomatic Subject Plaque Assessment Research – The CASPAR Project, www.rbh-cmr.org/caspar.htm accessed 22/6/04.

9

Understanding the Human Tissue Act 2004

Victoria Elliot and Adrian C. Bateman

'Beauty is momentary in the mind —
The fitful tracing of a portal;
But in the flesh it is immortal.
The body dies; the body's beauty lives.'

Wallace Stevens, 1879–1955 (American poet)

INTRODUCTION

The Human Tissue Act [1] gained Royal Assent on 15 November 2004 and its regulations have been in force since September 2006. It is a complex legal document which has been shrouded in controversy and a degree of confusion since its creation. Countless hours have been spent consulting on and finalising the details of the legislation that regulates comprehensively the storage, removal and use of human tissue from both the living and the dead. The principle issue underpinning the Act is one of patient consent.

Human tissue forms the foundation of pathologists' clinical work, research, audit and education. It must be stressed, however, that pathologists are not the only individuals who will have to work within these new laws; anatomists, transplant clinicians, geneticists and even museum curators are among many others who will need to abide by its rulings. Some of the difficulties encountered in the formation of this legislation stem from the diverse nature of the essential activities performed using human tissues. This is contributed to by the fact that the intricacies of much of this work are little known by those outside the respective fields (Fig. 9.1), and therefore there has been the need for considerable consultation.

The depth of emotion surrounding human tissue should not be underestimated. Ultimately the Human Tissue Act aims to restore public confidence, particularly following events in the UK at Bristol Royal Infirmary [2], the

Progress in Pathology Volume 7, ed. Nigel Kirkham and Neil Shepherd. Published by Cambridge University Press. © Cambridge University Press 2007.

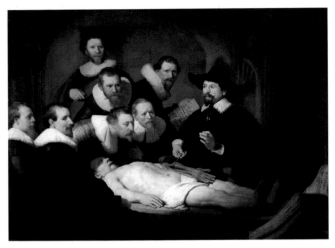

Fig. 9.1 Dr Nicolaas Tulp, the anatomist, famously depicted in Rembrandt's 'The Anatomy Lesson' (1632).

Royal Liverpool Children's Hospital (Alder Hey) [3] and after the findings of the Isaacs Report [4], [5] involving retention of adult brains. These have all had significant consequences in terms of the public's perception of the medical profession and, in particular, the activities of pathologists. The journey towards restoration of trust will no doubt be lengthy but, once achieved, will be of enormous benefit to the profession as a whole.

The impact of the Human Tissue Act 2004 will certainly be far reaching. To ensure its successful implementation within medical frameworks, the involvement and education of staff in all disciplines will be essential. Understanding of this legislation must not begin and end at the doors to the pathology department.

This chapter seeks merely to outline the key areas of the Act and highlight the most relevant aspects of the legislation from a pathologist's viewpoint.

HISTORICAL ASPECTS

The Human Tissue Act 2004 replaces the Human Tissue Act 1961, the Anatomy Act 1984 and the Human Organs Transplant Act 1989 in England and Wales. After investigations at Alder Hey and Bristol, legal review demonstrated that tissue and organ retention laws were inadequate and legislation regarding anatomical display and transplantation also needed amendment. After public consultation, the Government began to proceed with reforms to reflect advances in good practice [6].

In Northern Ireland, the new Act replaces The Human Tissue Act (Northern Ireland) 1962, the Human Organ Transplants (Northern Ireland) Order 1989 and the Anatomy (Northern Ireland) Order 1992. Scotland has its own legislation, The Human Tissue (Scotland) Act 2006.

THE STRUCTURE OF THE ACT

The Act is subdivided into three main sections:

Part 1 Outlines the activities that will require *consent* and from whom it should be obtained.

Part 2 Details the methods of *regulation*.

Part 3 Covers *supplementary* issues.

PART 1: THE SCHEDULED PURPOSES AND ACTIVITIES REQUIRING CONSENT

The key component of Part 1 of the Act is the listing of twelve 'scheduled purposes' which will require 'appropriate consent'. These are the various activities that the Act will regulate. A sound knowledge of the points included greatly assists the smooth navigation of the rest of the Act. The scheduled purposes are also subdivided into two parts, based on whether the individual from whom the tissue has come is alive or dead.

Utilisation of human tissue from both *the living and the dead for the following purposes will require appropriate consent:*

1. Anatomical examination — *which means macroscopic examination by dissection for the purposes of teaching, studying or researching into the gross structure of the human body*
2. Determining the cause of death — **except** *where an autopsy is ordered by the coroner*
3. Establishing after a person's death the efficacy of any drug or other treatment administered to him — *perhaps as part of a hospital request autopsy for example*
4. Obtaining scientific or medical information about a living or deceased person which may be relevant to any other person (including a future person) — *such information may be discovered fortuitously during the diagnostic process and this fundamental problem has been highlighted by the Royal College of Pathologists*
5. Public display
6. Research in connection with disorders, or the functioning, of the human body — *although in certain circumstances specific consent will not be required*
7. Transplantation

Utilisation of human tissue from the dead, but not *from the living, for the following purposes will require appropriate consent:*

8. Clinical audit
9. Education or training related to human health
10. Performance assessment
11. Public health monitoring
12. Quality assurance

Table 9.1 Lawful activities *if* appropriate consent is obtained. Note that appropriate consent varies according to the activity, e.g. for public display and anatomical examination written consent is required

Removal	Storage	Use
• Relevant material from a deceased body for use for purposes 1–12	• A deceased body for use for purposes 2–12 • A deceased body for use for purpose 1 plus death certificate • Relevant material from a deceased body for purposes 8–12 • Relevant material from a human body for purposes 1–7	• A deceased body for purposes 2–12 • A deceased body for purpose 1 plus registration of death • Relevant material from a deceased body for purposes 8–12 • Relevant material from a human body for purposes 1–7

Consent for many of these activities may be incorporated into consent for a hospital-request autopsy, or in certain circumstances, a coroner's autopsy.

For each of these twelve 'scheduled purposes', the handling of human tissue (or relevant material — see later) will fall into three main activities, which are each considered separately within the Act. These are:

- *Removal* of human tissue for a scheduled purpose
- *Storage* of human tissue for a scheduled purpose
- *Use* of human tissue for a scheduled purpose

If appropriate consent has been obtained (see later), then Table 9.1 outlines the lawful activities for scheduled purposes 1 to 12. Exceptions include bodies or relevant material from them, which are either imported or over 100 years old when the Act was enforced.

'Relevant material' from a human body is defined in the Act as any material consisting of, or including human cells, with the exception of gametes, embryos outside the body and hair and nail from a living person. Cell lines are also excluded, as is any other human material created outside the human body.

In summary, this means that in the case of a *deceased* individual, appropriate consent is required for removal, storage or use of relevant material from the body for all the 12 listed scheduled purposes. In the *living*, appropriate consent is needed for storage and use of any relevant bodily material for scheduled purposes 1 to 7 but not for purposes 8 to 12 (clinical audit, education and training, performance assessment, public health monitoring and quality assurance).

There are certain exemptions that are of particular relevance to pathology services:

- Work carried out for the functions of the coroner or under his authority is exempt from the requirements of Part 1 of the Act. However, it should be appreciated that once the coroner's role is completed, e.g. the inquest is over and the case is closed, any body/bodily material will once more fall under the legislation of the Act

- For material from a living person to be lawfully stored and used for purposes 8–12, further appropriate consent is not required
- Consent is *not required* for the use of *residual* (e.g. archival) material in research provided that a research ethics committee has approved the project and that the researcher cannot link the identity of individual patients to the research data, i.e. that the data are fully anonymised
- *Further* consent is not required for the use of lawfully banked material provided that a research ethics committee has approved the project and that the researcher cannot link the identity of individual patients to the research data, i.e. that the data are fully anonymised (consent will have been required for the initial removal and storage of this material)
- The storage and use, for scheduled purposes, of existing holdings of human tissue (e.g. archives of blocks and slides) is lawful, without further consent, up to the date upon which the Act took effect. 'Existing holdings' means the body of a deceased person or any relevant material that comes from a human body (living or deceased) held immediately before the day on which the Act came into force. This exemption does not apply where the existing holding is a body or a 'separated part' of a body, as these are considered as existing anatomical specimens. The exact nature of 'separated parts' is not defined any further by the Act but we interpret this as likely to include whole organs or major parts of limbs, for example
- With regard to *existing* anatomical specimens; where the person died in the three years immediately before the Act was enforced, the storage and use of the person's body or separate parts for anatomical examination is under the authorisation of the Anatomy Act 1984. The Anatomy Act 1984 also covers any ongoing anatomical examinations which were not concluded when the Act was enforced as long as they are within three years of the person's death. Any new storage after September 2006 of a person's body or use of that body or body parts as an anatomical specimen requires the necessary appropriate consent

CONSENT – THE CORNERSTONE OF THE ACT

Consent underpins the new Human Tissue Act and this critical issue is addressed particularly in Part 1. To review the basic issues surrounding consent, the Royal College have published 'A Brief Guide on Consent for Pathologists' and the advice given here is based on that document [7].

A dictionary definition of consent is 'to express willingness, to give permission or to agree' [8]. However, consent must demonstrate validity, which depends on:

- Provision of accurate information
- The patient's understanding of the information
- Appreciation of the consequences of a course of action
- Competency to give consent
- Lack of duress or manipulation

Consent will only be valid if these criteria have been fulfilled. Informed consent *implies* that the consent is valid; however, this is currently a poorly defined area.

The means by which consent is obtained is important, although this is unrelated to its validity. In simple, low-risk procedures such as taking blood, consent tends to be implied or oral. Riskier and more complicated interventions demand explicit, specific and, frequently, written consent.

The Human Tissue Act uses the term 'appropriate consent'; however, this phrase simply encompasses details about who is able to give consent in the various situations listed *rather than how* it is to be obtained. The content and level of the information that should be supplied to those giving consent and recommendations as to the approach to obtaining consent are not discussed within the body of the Act. However, guidelines on such matters have been issued by the Department of Health in recent years and versions of them should be available widely [9]. From the viewpoint of the law, once given correctly, another person cannot veto consent.

The Act subdivides that which is appropriate consent for adults from that which is appropriate consent for children (considered in the Act to be under 18 years old) in addition to whether the individual is alive or dead.

If an adult is living and competent (i.e. able to give informed consent), appropriate consent means his or her own consent.

Lack of capacity in adults is discussed in the Act, and under certain circumstances it is deemed that consent has been given. These situations are anticipated to be:

- When it is in the best interests of that person
- To allow for clinical research in line with the Clinical Trials Regulations 2004
- To allow for storage and research use of tissue from incapacitated persons within the boundaries of the Mental Capacity Bill

If an adult is deceased, any decision relating to the Act made by the individual during life should be upheld, provided that it was known immediately prior to their death. Storage or use of relevant material for public display or anatomical examination requires written consent signed by the adult concerned, or at their direction in the presence of at least one witness. Alternatively, consent for this may be contained within their will. Another adult individual (a 'nominated representative') may be appointed by an adult to deal with issues of consent relating to the Act. This appointment can be made orally or in writing but must take place in the presence of at least two witnesses contemporaneously. In the absence of these, a person in a 'qualifying relationship' with the adult concerned immediately prior to death may give consent. Qualifying relationships are listed in the Act in a hierarchical fashion (Table 9.2).

If a child is living and considered to be competent, then the requirements are similar to those of an adult. In children, the term 'Gillick competence' is applied in medicine. This term originates from the case of Victoria Gillick, who argued in a court of law that she wanted authority to be informed if her daughters sought contraceptive treatment [10]. The courts ruled against her and stated that if a doctor deems a child under the age of 16 capable, then they can consent to their

Rank*	Relationship
1	Spouse or partner
2	Parent or child
3	Sibling
4	Grandparent or grandchild
5	Niece or nephew
6	Stepfather or stepmother
7	Half sibling
8	Friend of longstanding

Table 9.2 Qualifying relationships for issues of consent

*Ranks are given in descending order

treatment without parental knowledge. These criteria are not fixed and the circumstances depend on the child and clinical situation. For example, a parent or guardian may give consent (apart from for anatomical examination or public display — see later) for someone aged less than 18 years even if the individual refuses consent. In practice, however, it is always best to take the child's views into account.

If a child is alive but a decision on consent has not been made, either because the child concerned is not competent or because the issue of consent has not been addressed, then appropriate consent is the consent of a person who has parental responsibility for that child. Mothers have parental responsibility although biological fathers do not necessarily. Married couples share parental responsibility.

If a child is deceased, any decision relating to the Act made by the child during life should be upheld, provided that they were considered competent and that this decision was known immediately prior to their death. In the absence of these, the consent of a person with parental responsibility for the child prior to death or, failing that, another person in a qualifying relationship with the child immediately prior to their death, may give consent.

To obtain appropriate consent for storage and use for public display or anatomical examination of relevant material from a deceased child there must be *additional* input. The consent must be in writing and signed by the child or by a person at the direction of the child in the presence of at least one witness.

POWERS TO DISPENSE WITH THE NEED FOR CONSENT

If the Human Tissue Authority (see later) is satisfied that the relevant material is from a living person, that it is not possible to trace that person (the donor), and that it is desirable in the interests of another individual (or future individual) that the material be used for the purposes of obtaining scientific or medical information about the person (the donor), then consent for use of such material is considered granted. There must be no reason to believe that the person concerned is dead, would not consent to such an activity or lacks capacity. In special circumstances (e.g. where there is an overwhelming public interest), the Secretary of State may make an order deeming there to be appropriate consent for the removal, storage and use of material for health-related research.

COMMITTING AN OFFENCE

A person has committed an offence if, without appropriate consent, as outlined above:

- They perform any activity for which consent is required as outlined in the scheduled purposes in Part 1 of the Act. However, if the person reasonably believes that they are carrying out the activity with appropriate consent or they believe that consent does not apply to the activity, then an offence has not been committed
- They falsely represent to a person performing any activity that there is appropriate consent when they know this to be is false or they do not believe it. An offence has also occurred if a person falsely informs an individual performing such an activity that it does not require appropriate consent when they know that to be false or do not believe it
- If a body is stored for use for the purposes of an anatomical examination if a death certificate has not been signed. However, if the individual concerned believes a certificate has been signed or they think that the activity they are performing does not require such steps, then an offence has not been committed
- If a body is used for the purposes of an anatomical examination if the death of the person concerned has not been registered. Again, if the person performing this activity either believes that the register has been signed or that the activity concerned does not require this, then an offence has not occurred

A person guilty of any offence as detailed above shall be liable to a fine on summary conviction and on conviction on indictment to imprisonment (not exceeding three years) or a fine, or both.

Further new offences include trafficking in human tissue for transplantation, carrying out licensable activities without holding a licence (see later) and having human tissue with the intent of analysing its DNA without the consent of the individual concerned, except for the purposes of criminal investigations.

Offences can be committed with respect to donated material (bodies or relevant material from a human body which is the subject of donation); these include storage or use of donated material for an unqualified purpose (Table 9.3).

Table 9.3 Qualifying uses of donated material (i.e. uses of donated material that are considered lawful under the Act)

Any scheduled purpose
Medical diagnosis or treatment
Decent disposal
Purposes specified by the Secretary of State

PART 2: REGULATION

Part 2 of the Act outlines the regulation of the new legislation. The main body that will advise and oversee matters relating to the Act is The Human Tissue Authority, which recently appointed Shirley Harrison (a previous lay member) as an interim chair. The Authority began licensing in April 2006 and its general functions include; providing general oversight and guidance as appropriate, ensuring compliance with Part 1 of the Act and the codes of practice, providing information and advice to professionals and the public, monitoring developments and advising the various Government departments accordingly. The Human Tissue Authority currently has a guaranteed lifespan of only three years, after which it is planned that it will merge with the Human Fertilization and Embryology Authority (HFEA) to form a new body; the Regulatory Authority for Tissue and Embryology (RATE).

The remit of the HTA includes:

- *Removal* from a human body of any relevant material for use for a scheduled purpose
- *Storage* of anatomical specimens, dead bodies or relevant material from them for use for a scheduled purpose
- *Import* of a human body or relevant material for use for a scheduled purpose
- *Disposal* of a dead body imported/stored for use/used for a scheduled purpose
- *Disposal* of relevant human material used for treatment purposes, anatomical examination, post-mortem, imported from a living person or imported from a dead body

Licenses are required for:

- The purposes of carrying out an anatomical examination
- The making of a post-mortem examination
- The removal from a body of relevant material (other than in the course of an anatomical examination or post-mortem) for a scheduled purpose other than transplantation
- The storage of an anatomical specimen
- The storage of the body of a deceased person or a relevant material from a human body for a scheduled purpose
- The use for a purpose of public display of a deceased person or relevant material which has come from the body of a deceased person

Licenses are held by 'designated individuals'. The duty of the individual license holder is to ensure that:

- The persons to whom the licence applies are suitable persons to participate in performing a licensed activity
- That suitable practices are used during the carrying out of any such activity
- That the conditions of the license are complied with

Any person who performs a license-requiring activity without one has committed an offence, unless they reasonably believe that whatever they are doing does not require one or that they reasonably believe that they are acting under the authority of a licence. Offenders are liable to a fine and/or prison sentence.

CODES OF PRACTICE

The Authority has six initial Codes of Practice offering guidance on the following areas:

- Consent
- Donation of organs, tissues and cells for transplantation
- Post-mortem examination
- Anatomical examination
- Removal, storage and disposal of human organs and tissues
- Donation of allogenic bone marrow and peripheral blood stem cells for transplant

The Human Tissue Authority will be responsible for the regular review and amendment of the codes of practice where required. Interim guidelines have also been published by the Royal College of Pathologists [11], [12].

FURTHER ASPECTS OF PART 2

Part 2 of the Act also contains legislation on transplantation, organ trafficking, and religious relics. These will not be considered in any further detail here.

PART 3 OF THE ACT

Part 3 is subdivided into miscellaneous and general sections. The general section consists mostly of definitions and administrative details. The miscellaneous section contains some points worthy of further attention. It details permission to use the least invasive procedure available, to allow temporary preservation of body organs in individuals who may be suitable organ donors. For example, cold perfusion procedures whilst discussions with relatives/next of kin are taking place regarding organ donation. However, if consent is not given then this period of permission ceases. Details on surplus tissue are also listed here. It is defined as any material which consists of or contains human cells which have come from a person's body in the course of their medical treatment, diagnostic investigations or their participation in research and has ceased to be used or stored for use for any scheduled purposes. Surplus tissue may be treated as waste.

Non-consensual use of DNA is discussed in this section; an offence has been committed if a person has any bodily material upon which they intend to analyse human DNA without qualifying consent, and that the results of any such analysis are used for purposes other than those scheduled in Part 1 of the Act. We interpret this as relating to 'DNA theft' for non-scheduled purposes, and that research may be performed using DNA extracted from residual material without specific consent, as long as a research ethics committee has approved the project and the data are fully anonymised. Penalties are in line with those outlined in the other areas of the Act. Exceptions to this ruling are if the material concerned is from a person who died at least 100 years before the date of the enforcement of the Act, if the material is from an existing holding and the researcher does not have access to the individual's personal details, and finally if the material originates from an embryo outside the human body. For the purposes of the Act it should be noted that material created outside the human body is not regarded as being from the human body.

AN OVERVIEW OF THE CORONERS (AMENDMENT) RULES 2005

Given the importance of the post-mortem in general coronial work, it is essential that the legislation brought in by the Human Tissue Act 2004 be mirrored in the Coroners Rules. Appropriate changes to create compatibility between the two were completed on 28 February 2005 and the Coroners (Amendment) Rules 2005 [13] came into force on 1 June 2005. They consist of a number of adjustments to the principal rules drawn up in 1984, of which many reflect the themes of the updated Human Tissue Act.

In summary, changes are as follows:

- In Rule 2 there is now recognition of the term 'partner' (meaning two individuals of the same or different sex who live together in an enduring family relationship)
- In Rules 9 and 12 regarding retention of material from post-mortem examinations and special examinations (e.g. histological examination); an individual (in many cases a pathologist) may preserve material that in their opinion bears upon the cause of death or identification of the deceased. When doing so they must notify the coroner in writing of the identity of the material being preserved, why this is required, and the time period for which the pathologist believes the material should be preserved. The coroner will then respond to the pathologist and outline the time periods for preservation that they feel are appropriate given the circumstances. They will also similarly notify the next of kin/representatives of the deceased and inform them of the options for dealing with the material once this period of time has expired. These options include giving consent for the material to be retained by the pathologist (e.g. for teaching and research purposes), requesting return of the material to the family or requesting lawful disposal by the pathologist. When the period of time has expired, records must be made of the means of disposal and these records must be maintained. In the event of a person being charged with an offence in relation to a particular case, the police must be

notified of preservation periods, as must the chairperson of any public inquiries that may result

- Rule 5 details individuals entitled to examine witnesses at an inquest. This list of people now includes a partner of the deceased
- Rule 6 adds new notification processes to the original Rule 57 which sets out entitlements of properly interested parties to inspect and supply copies of relevant documents/material
- Lastly, Rule 7 changes the post-mortem report form, so that when detailing the outcome of the examination the pathologist must state whether any organs or tissues were removed, and if so, who retains them and for how long

CONCLUSIONS

The Act is now law and those individuals who require a license should have obtained one via the Human Tissue Authority (www.hta.gov.uk). The Coroners (Amendment) Rules 2005 have also come into force, and departments have now amended their protocols in line with the new requirements.

In addition to the amended Rules, major reforms to the Coronial system are currently under parliamentary discussion. In particular, the Draft Coroner Reform Bill for England and Wales proposes a new role of Chief Coroner and a set of national standards. However, The Royal College of Pathologists have highlighted a number of concerns over the Bill and further discussions continue.

The issue of consent forms the key principle within the Act and the processes that surround consent are already firmly integrated in the daily running of pathology departments – autopsy work, tissue banking and ancillary molecular testing to name but a few such situations. The recommendations of the General Medical Council state that it is the responsibility of the doctor providing treatment or undertaking an investigation to obtain consent. If this is not practical, then the person to whom the task is delegated must be suitably trained and qualified with sufficient knowledge and a comprehensive understanding of the proposed intervention [17]. Pathologists usually rely on consent being obtained by an individual who in many instances will be unfamiliar to the pathologist, as will the pathologist be to them. Although well known to the bereaved family, the consent-taker may not be fully aware of the processes involved in, for example, a post-mortem and the additional investigations that may follow. Can we rely on this slightly distant consent process or does it expose an area of weakness in the system and ultimately increase the vulnerability of the pathologist to the harsher penalties of the Act? On this point alone it would seem prudent to optimise communication channels and accessibility between clinicians and pathologists, to ensure there is absolute clarity in the consent process. Ideally, all staff involved, at whatever level, should be aware of the Human Tissue Act, its penalties and the responsibility they have to ensure appropriate consent is correctly obtained.

The Human Tissue Act 2004, like many legal documents, is difficult to read and fully understand. Despite a basic understanding of its principles, translating them into practical changes to everyday activities in any pathology department remains a tortuous activity. The codes of practice are there to provide the step-by-step guidance necessary to allow pathologists to carry out work with human tissue, confident that they are acting safely within the law.

With all of these new changes there has been little focus on additional resources. Fulfilling the legal requirements of both the Human Tissue Act 2004 and the Coroners (Amendment) Rules 2005 is a sizeable task, and as yet there is no funding for the likely additional administration. Pathology nurses have already been successfully implemented in some NHS Trusts fortunate enough to secure trial periods of financial support, and they represent a useful bridge between pathology departments and the public.

With the Human Tissue Act 2004 and the Coroner's (Amendment) Rules 2005 in place, the pathology community faces a period of significant adjustment. However, the creation of this new legislation in part reflects flaws in past practices. Respect for the principles that underpin the Act must provide each of us with the momentum and commitment to see through this challenging metamorphosis.

REFERENCES

1. The Human Tissue Act 2004. ISBN 0 10 543004 8 (The Stationery Office Limited, London, 2004).
2. Learning from Bristol: The Report into Children's Heart Surgery at Bristol Royal Infirmary, July 2001.
3. The Royal Liverpool Children's Inquiry: Report, January 2001, HC12-II.
4. The Investigation of Events that Followed the Death of Cyril Mark Isaacs. (Department of Health, May 2003.)
5. Isaacs Report Response. (Department of Health, July 2003.)
6. The Human Tissue Act 2004. New Legislation on Human Organs and Tissue. (Department of Health, March 2005.)
7. Colvin B. A Brief Guideline on Consent for Pathologists. (The Royal College of Pathologists, January 2005.)
8. *The Concise Oxford Dictionary of Current English*. 8th edn. Allen RE. ed. (Clarendon Press, Oxford, 2004).
9. Families and Post mortems: a Code of Practice. (Department of Health, April 2003.)
10. Gillick v West Norfolk and Wisbech Area Health Authority, 1985, 3 All ER 402 (HL).
11. The Retention and Storage of Pathological Records and Archives, 3rd edn. (The Royal College of Pathologists, March 2005.)
12. Interim Guidance on the Use of Clinical Samples Retained in the Pathology Laboratory. (The Royal College of Pathologists, January 2005.)
13. The Coroners (Amendment) Rules 2005. ISBN 0110723503, (The Stationery Office Limited, London, 2005).
14. Underwood J. Letter to the Home Secretary. (The Royal College of Pathologists, May 2005.)
15. Hasleton P. Reforming the coroner and death certification service. *Curr Diag Pathol* 2004; **10**: 453–63.
16. Shipman Inquiry Third Report: Death Certification and Investigation of Deaths by Coroners. HMS0, Cm 5854, 2003.
17. Seeking Patients' Consent: the Ethical Considerations. (The General Medical Council, November 1998.)

10

The Multidisciplinary Team (MDT) meeting and the role of pathology

Sanjiv Manek and Bryan F. Warren

INTRODUCTION

National plans for cancer management in England are based currently on regional cancer networks. Within the cancer networks, Tumour Site Specific Groups (TSSGs) have been established for individual cancer sites in the body, and within individual trusts, multidisciplinary teams in a regular multidisciplinary team meeting decide cancer management. This chapter describes the structure and function of the multidisciplinary team meeting in the context of the multidisciplinary team (MDT) and its relationship to the relevant TSSG within the cancer network. There is little peer-reviewed published scientific literature on the effectiveness of this approach, so this chapter focuses on the practical issues of running a multidisciplinary team meeting, based on our personal experiences.

TUMOUR SITE SPECIFIC GROUPS

The purpose of TSSGs is to share good practice and to attempt to achieve consistency in investigation and management of cancer across each region. Each TSSG is comprised of a clinician from each trust in the network, and a clinician from each specialty involved in the investigation and management of cancer at that site within the body, and a primary care physician. A patient representative will also be present, along with a member of each of the professions allied to medicine who are important for that cancer site. The lead clinician for the cancer network and some of the cancer network managers and cancer intelligence gatherers and specialist nurses will be present also.

Meetings of the TSSG are chaired by a chairman elected from the group for a three-year term of office. Representatives of each major speciality form part of

235

Progress in Pathology Volume 7, ed. Nigel Kirkham and Neil Shepherd. Published by Cambridge University Press. © Cambridge University Press 2007.

the TSSG, and many of the other clinicians present will usually be the chairs of the MDT meeting from each individual trust. Meetings will usually occur four times a year, they are held during working hours and at different times, on different days and at different sites within the network. These variations are very important, so that the same clinicians' clinics and operating/endoscopy lists/outpatients clinics are not disrupted or used as a reason for irregular or non-attendance. A programme of work will be decided upon and distributed amongst TSSG members according to their speciality. The TSSG is supportive to MDTs in preparation for peer review assessments of cancer investigation and treatment. The chairman will usually take on the role of writing letters to trusts where a special problem of inequality of opportunity for treatment and/or investigation has been identified. This may include having to object to the closing of specialist wards or beds even as a temporary measure. It may include having to comment upon centres continuing to treat particular cancers when the population served is below that recommended in the Improving Outcomes Guidance (IOG) guidelines. The role of chairman is often not to be the bearer of good news. However, when audits are completed or new patient leaflets are designed and produced, the chairman's job is a little more rewarding.

MULTIDISCIPLINARY TEAMS

The multidisciplinary team within each trust is responsible for an individual cancer site. Clinicians treating cancers from a particular site must be a functional part of the relevant multidisciplinary team and attend the trust's multidisciplinary team meeting on a regular basis. The exception to this is the provision of emergency treatment by a general surgical or medical team. A patient with cancer treated by an on-call non-specialist team will then be referred to a member of the multidisciplinary team for discussion at the next available multidisciplinary team meeting. A record is kept of attendance and of patients discussed and decisions made on patient management.

The multidisciplinary team meeting is an essential part of cancer management planning. These meetings have evolved within individual NHS Trusts and have slightly different roles for the pathologist, and in this chapter we report our experience of our four MDT meetings in gynaecological malignancy, upper gastrointestinal malignancy, lower gastrointestinal malignancy and hepatobiliary malignancy.

The MDT meeting needs to be held at a time when all participants can attend, i.e. before work, after work or at lunchtime. This is now increasingly difficult with modern working practices, which demand that all activities are conducted within paid sessional times. If held at lunchtime, to encourage attendance, one needs to get some industry support and supply sandwiches and drinks, otherwise people will not be regular attendees. Equipment is improving all the time but the funding available to purchase it is not. We think it important to have a good quality digital projector and a versatile radiological demonstration medium.

REQUIREMENTS FOR MDT MEETINGS

Since the publication of the IOG guidelines for best clinical practice in individual cancer sites, the multidisciplinary team meetings have become a requirement for discussion of patient management, not only between individuals of different disciplines, but also between several individuals of the same discipline. Patients are now aware that such discussions occur and wait anxiously for the results of the next MDT meeting in which their care is discussed. Within each region there is a TSSG for each malignant site, which attempts to get consistent management between these various MDTs within the hospitals within the region. The personnel recommended for each MDT meeting will vary slightly from site to site, but in principle will include surgeons, physicians, oncologists, radiotherapists, pathologists, radiologists, specialist nurses, palliative care team representatives, and primary care physician and physicians with an interest, along with several other team members with special techniques such as endoscopic ultrasound or cytology. A register is kept, which will be scrutinised at peer-review meetings. All patients with malignancy should be discussed at an MDT meeting. It is usual for the patient to be discussed at the diagnostic stage, with biopsy pathology or cytology and radiology, to discuss a management plan. After a major resection, if relevant, it is then usual to re-discuss the pathological stage and future adjuvant therapy. Patients will also be discussed later if they show signs of recurrence.

ASSEMBLING LISTS OF PATIENTS TO BE DISCUSSED AT AN MDT MEETING

It is helpful to have a list of patients in the pre-operative state, the post-operative state and others/recurrences. Such lists are emailed to all team members using a password-protected file. It is often difficult to assemble a complete list of patients. This has been aided by the appointment of MDT coordinators who can gather the information from all hospital specialists and who can also check if the relevant investigations will be available for the meeting, since worthwhile discussion of patient management cannot occur without all relevant investigations. Getting help in this way from an MDT coordinator is crucial to the smooth running and appropriate function of the meeting. In some specialities it is appropriate for the pathologist to create the list and act as a gatekeeper to ensure almost complete patient listing. Referred cases from within the network can be added to the list by the pathologists and radiologist also. In other specialities this is much less straightforward. In gastrointestinal cancers, detection may be by a variety of practitioners, and some such as pancreatic cancer may not have biopsies, and it is here that the MDT coordinator's job becomes crucial.

DATA COLLECTION FORM

The data collection form needs the patient's name, hospital number and date of birth. It is crucial to ensure you are discussing the correct patient in these meetings. The list needs to have the start and finish time of the meeting, the location and the attending consultants. It may also form a useful audit record in pathology, and it is useful to have a column indicate whether the histopathology report is adequate, borderline or inadequate (Fig. 10.1). If pathologists hold a premeeting to discuss the slides, it is useful to record a further audit of consistency in reporting. An alternative method is for two pathologists to see the material at the time of reporting, and to record this fact on the report. A column for the reason for the patient being brought to the meeting is important. Other data, such as the patient's waiting time, may be incorporated into this document. While these may be filed away in a box file afterwards, it is more useful to enter the data on a computer, preferably by the MDT coordinator at the meeting on a laptop. Transfer of data may result in repeated inaccuracy. Data may be collected electronically onto a central hospital server. This may then go onto a locally agreed database, from which nationally required data may be taken, or may be entered directly onto a national database such as the Clatterbridge colorectal cancer database.

LOWER GI MDT MEETING
Consultant Surgeons' Names
Date, Time and Place of meeting

Name	Histology no.	Hospital no.	D.O.B.	Days elapsed on pathway	Specimen type	*A	*B	*I	Comments	Particular scans/films required	Specific question for MDT	Consultant surgeon
Post-operative patients												
Pre-operative patients												
Other patients												

* "Tick box" internal audit of whether pathology report was adequate, borderline, or inadequate

Fig. 10.1 MDT meeting record sheet.

PURPOSE OF DISCUSSING THE PATIENT IN THE MEETING

This needs to be clearly addressed and a decision needs to be made by the team on the next phase of the patient's management, before discussion of that patient is finished with and the discussion of the next patient begins. It is all too easy to discuss one patient then another without reaching a firm agreed conclusion on the next phase of management in the previous patient, and this defeats the whole purpose of the meeting. It is also useful to record the MDT's management decision in the notes in some way as well as on the central database. The final tumour stage may be entered in the notes and signed. It is consequently important to have the case notes available at the meeting.

CHAIRMAN OF THE MEETING

The chairman is preferably not a radiologist or pathologist who has to show images during the meeting, since chairing the meeting as well is too much work. The chairman needs to keep careful track of the time and to be clear about the management decision made by the team on each patient before the next patient is discussed. The chairman also needs to ensure that the MDT coordinator or data collection clerk has an accurate record of the management decision or the patient's tumour stage. It is useful to project on the wall a management decision and the tumour stage as it is typed in, if this is possible. The chairman needs to be a skilled manager of people and of strong character to ensure the smooth running of the meeting and the timely discussion of the patients.

MDT MEETING ROOM AND EQUIPMENT

Rooms suitable for MDT meetings need to be free from extraneous noise and interruption. The acoustic properties of the room need to be adequate for case discussion by MDT members sat at any point within the room. Some larger rooms may need a microphone system. There should room for comfortable seating for all team members, and the teams may be quite large. In large MDT meetings where images need to be viewed, it is clearly advantageous to have all the seats facing the front. Images from radiology and pathology need only be projected one at a time, so one screen is usually all that is necessary. One cannot study more than one image at once.

The equipment required in the room needs care in its selection and installation. Some MDTs have been lucky enough to gain funding from local charities or teaching grants to equip or re-equip their room. For ease of use, health and safety considerations and reliability, it is useful to rid the room of miles of wire and 13 Amp extension leads filling the front quarter of the room's floor area. This may provide considerable hazards for the mobile presenters in a semi-dark room. Ideally, the equipment and room lights on dimmer switches should all be controllable from behind one control desk, from which the presenters of X-rays, pathology, etc, should be able to show all their images. Ideally, the chairman should sit somewhere else at the front of the room at approximately 90° to the presenters' control desk, the screen and to the audience. Since only one image can be viewed at any one time, it is useful to present all images through a computer and digital projector. It is sensible to mount the digital projector on the ceiling. This has two advantages: one is to reduce the ease of theft, and the second is to not have the image interrupted by people walking in front of the projector.

In most MDT meetings it is necessary to present radiological images, endoscopic or operative still pictures or videos, and pathology images of macroscopic appearances and microscopic appearances of specimens. Radiological images may be available as radiographs, photographs of ultrasound investigations or digital images, either on computer disk or available from a central hospital computer server. The link between the hospital server and the MDT room computer will provide some of these images. Radiographs and photographs may be shown on an image viewing box designed for the purpose (Fig. 10.2) and linked to the main MDT room computer and digital projector. This viewing box again should be within reach of the radiologist seated at the control desk (Fig. 10.3). The image viewing box should also double up as an epidiascope (Fig. 10.4) for prints and diagrams, and pages from the patients' notes occasionally. For the present time it is still useful to have a 2×2 slide projector and a video machine (Fig. 10.5) connected into the control desk to present their images through the digital projector. These two 'antique items' will not be necessary in the future.

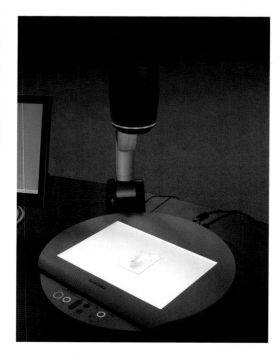

Fig. 10.2 Image viewing box.

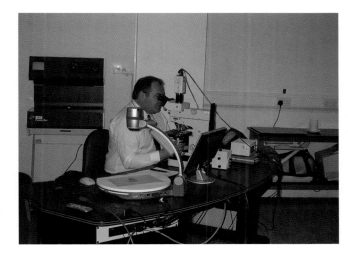

Fig. 10.3 MDT 'control desk'.

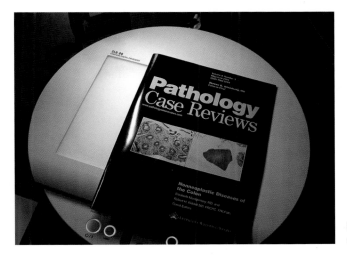

Fig. 10.4 Viewing box used as an epidiascope.

Macroscopic pathology images are best stored on a central server and called up on the MDT room computer as required. It is very difficult to comply with health and safety laws and show macroscopic specimens either fresh or fixed in an MDT meeting room. Also, with modern adequate dissection techniques, most specimens are sliced and sampled to such an extent that meaningful demonstration of tissue, which remains in the bucket, is not usually appropriate. Other ways to demonstrate the macroscopic appearances are by a video of the macroscopic appearances and dissected appearances, or by still computerised digital images stored on a computer or CD-rom disk. These methods are less satisfactory. If a 2×2 image of a macroscopic appearance of an older specimen is to be reviewed, it can be demonstrated on the 2×2 projector if available. If not

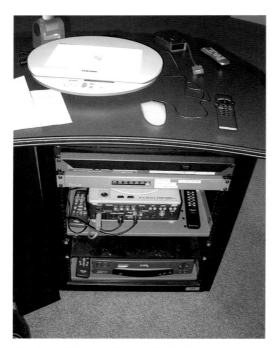

Fig. 10.5 Video machine and 2×2 slide projector built into MDT 'control desk' to project their images through the MDT room computer and digital projector.

available, a reasonable image may be obtained by putting it on the sub-stage lens of the microscope with the condenser in position and a low-power objective lens in place (Fig. 10.6). While microscopy can be demonstrated clearly using the microscope and digital projector, clear slide labelling with a non-permanent felt pen (red is a good visible colour in a semi-darkened room), and careful slide selection may make the process a good deal slicker and more professional. If large blocks of tumours are used to demonstrate T-stage and excision margins, they may be demonstrated to best effect by using the X-ray viewing box. Again it is useful to annotate them with the red felt pen. The tumour stage can be written on the glass slide. This is a good safeguard for accurate transcription of the tumour stage by MDT co-ordinators, specialist nurses and data collectors.

For MDT meetings, which deal with uncommon tumours, i.e. endocrine tumours or eye tumours, it may be sufficient to take digital images of radiology, macroscopic and microscopic pathology and prepare a seamless presentation in sequence on a computer. Such preparation is impractical for large MDT meetings for common tumours. It also removes the ability to have a spontaneous discussion of features of the histology and radiology, which have not been selected for demonstration prior to the meeting. Having the 'raw material' of slides and X-rays for the meetings allows discussion of several other important aspects of the patient, but for large-volume tumour sites, such as gastrointestinal or gynaecological sites, it is impractical to do this.

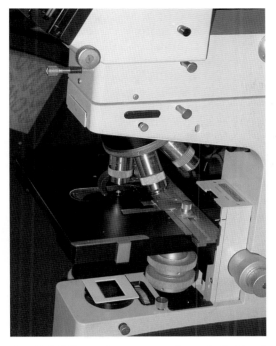

Fig. 10.6 Using a microscope to view a 2×2 slide of a macroscopic view of an older specimen.

VIDEO CONFERENCING

It is difficult to find funding for equipping rooms for MDT meetings, although some funding has been available for video conferencing, which has helped to take the MDT meeting to other sites from which patients will be referred to a centre for management. This is particularly important with specialisation within centres for tumours such as the cervix and vulva and the pancreas, where a population of two million is served by one centre, and some of the centres sending in patients may be a considerable distance from the main centre. Video conferencing is a new communication skill for most pathologists. A slick presentation requires some experience and practice.

PATHOLOGICAL INPUT INTO THE MDT MEETING

The role of the pathologist is twofold. It is to present the diagnostic biopsy or cytology preparation when the patient is first discussed at the MDT meeting, and to present the pathological stage in those patients who have proceeded to have surgery. At this point the patient is discussed and the pathological stage will usually contribute to decision making for follow-up and selection for consideration for adjuvant therapy.

It is crucial that the pathologist stands his ground and establishes whether there is truly a diagnostic biopsy to confirm the malignancy at the start of treatment planning. If there is not, further material will usually be obtained, although in some relatively inaccessible sites such as the pancreas, it is acceptable to begin treatment without a diagnostic biopsy. (See *British Society of Gastroenterology Guidelines for Pancreatic Cancer* [1].)

The pathologist also has an important role in comparing current with previous malignancies to determine whether or not there has been recurrence of the previous tumour or development of a new primary tumour.

AUDIT OF PATHOLOGY IN THE MDT MEETING

The pathologist presenting the cases at the MDT meeting need not have reported them originally. Indeed if he has not, this activity represents a useful form of audit of accuracy and consistency in pathology reporting. It is sometimes helpful for all pathologists within a discipline to meet before the MDT meeting and review the slides for each case. This may not be practical or easy in large-volume specialities. The MDT meeting presents a very useful way of auditing the quality of pathological reporting, and viewing surgical resection margins to assess the quality of the surgical excision. Macroscopic photographs are useful in most cancers, particularly colorectal, and these can be very useful to assess the quality of the surgical excision margin [2]. The quality of both the surgery and the pathology may be assessed by recording the numbers of lymph nodes, which are harvested (colorectal)[3]. It is useful to correlate the findings on the slides with the histopathology report for accuracy. Audit of the histopathology report for spelling and accuracy may also take place, and for whether or not the details of the minimum data sets are included in the report. The record sheet of the MDT meeting should record the adequacy of the histopathology report. We have a simple column for 'adequate', 'inadequate' or 'borderline' reports, and a column for comments as to why the report was not adequate and whether or not a supplementary report was issued. This in itself is an important audit record.

THE EXTENDED ROLE OF THE PATHOLOGIST IN THE MDT

Education of non-medical team members who have to see patients is very important. The clinical nurse specialist will often be questioned by patients about cancer staging and prognosis. They are also asked when the biopsy result or the pathological staging will be complete. We have found that small impromptu tutorials at the end of the MDT meeting when the teaching can be related to individual patients is valuable. We have lectured on local and national courses for clinical nurse specialists concerning the practicalities of pathology, turn around times and staging systems in relation to prognosis and treatment. We have also found benefit in spending time with some specialist nurses in our cut-up room to see the process at first hand.

PATIENT CONSULTATION

We have also been asked to demonstrate pathological findings and tumour stage to the patient on several occasions. We are both very pleased to be able to help in this way. Our practice is to see the patient outside of the MDT meeting, but usually in the MDT meeting room, to show them where the decisions have been discussed about their treatment. Some patients will wish to see images of the macrosocopic specimen, others only slides, and others may wish to talk to us without seeing any material. It is very important to allow sufficient time in an undisturbed setting for these consultations. It is also important to have a third party present such as a clinical nurse specialist, ward nurse, surgeon, etc. This is sometimes essential for chaperone purposes, but is crucial for communication. The patient may ask questions at a later date, and three people then know clearly what the patient has been shown and what the patient has been told. It is equally important to record this in the notes. We tend to do this as a letter to the surgeon to be filed in the notes. The letter will include statements about who met and what we have been asked to demonstrate or answer, what was shown and what was said.

NATIONAL MDT TRAINING

The training of MDT personnel as a whole team has started in colorectal cancer with a two-day course at the Pelican Centre in Basingstoke, which all colorectal MDT members are expected to attend. It is likely that other tumour sites will follow. The purpose is to ensure consistency of treatment throughout the country.

CONCLUSIONS

Pathologists vary in their level of involvement in the MDT meeting. Some wish to show no pathology. This is unfortunate in our view, since accurate, consistent patient management depends heavily on the discussion in these meetings. The training of junior pathologists, junior surgeons, junior physicians and junior oncologists is aided by a well-run, interestingly presented multidisciplinary team meeting. It is surprising to many pathologists how much pathology is expected of candidates for examinations in oncology, surgery and medicine and the opportunity for these juniors to learn their pathology really rests with the pathologist in the MDT meeting. This is an important role, which is often belittled or decried. In our view, the pathologist attending the MDT meeting has the opportunity to show his ability to communicate his subject to non-pathologists in an understandable, clinically appropriate and useful way. Sadly, this opportunity is lost in many institutions by many colleagues who are not at all keen to play a proper enthusiastic part in the running of the

Sanjiv Manek and Bryan F. Warren

MDT meeting. We hope this chapter has given some insight into the way that we conduct and enjoy our MDT meetings in Oxford, and we would be happy for any pathologist reading this to visit our MDT meetings if they wish to see them at first hand.

REFERENCES

1. British Society for Gastroenterology. *Guidelines for Pancreatic Cancer* (BSG, London), 2004.
2. Birbeck K, Macklin CP, Tiffin NJ *et al.* Rates of circumferential resection margin involvement vary between surgeons and predict outcomes in rectal cancer surgery. *Ann Surg* 2002; **235**: 449–57.
3. Shepherd NA, Quirke P. Colorectal cancer reporting: are we failing the patient? *J Clin Pathol* 1997; **50**: 266–7.

11

Drug induced liver injury

Susan E. Davies and Clare Craig

INTRODUCTION AND INCIDENCE

This chapter provides an extensive but not completely exhaustive overview of drug induced liver injury, with key concepts illustrated by examples of individual drugs. It also considers the problems associated with making a diagnosis of drug induced liver injury (DILI).

Our society has a massive desire for the consumption of active compounds; the drug industry is worth billions of pounds – many more billions being derived from the sale of over-the-counter preparations and the ever-growing market for complementary and alternative medicines (CAM).

The annual budget for prescription drugs in the UK is staggering; over £8 billion being spent in England alone in 2004 [1]. This corresponds to over 40 million prescription items being written every month in England. Undesirable effects of some drugs have become a major clinical problem: in a 6-month period in northern England, 6.5% of all cases admitted to hospital were associated with an Adverse Drug Reaction (ADR), many were related to GI haemorrhage and many probably avoidable [2]. Previously this rate was closer to 2%, although this may reflect the way information had been gathered, being dependent upon published data [3]. Certain groups of people appear to be more at risk of drug induced injury: a Norwegian study has implicated an ADR contributing to nearly 20% of hospital deaths in elderly patients, particularly in those with more than one illness and receiving multiple medications [4]. Major drug culprits were cardiovascular, anti-thrombotic and sympathomimetic. Post-mortem examination and drug analysis were pivotal in correctly identifying ADR as cause of death.

Hepatotoxicity is not the most common manifestation of an ADR, although it is the most common reason for withdrawal of a drug from the market, and an accurate incidence of DILI is difficult to determine [5], [6]. Proving causality can be difficult (this will be discussed later), and definitions of injury and aspects of record keeping are problematic. It is probable, however, that there

Progress in Pathology Volume 7, ed. Nigel Kirkham and Neil Shepherd. Published by Cambridge University Press. © Cambridge University Press 2007.

is underreporting. A prospective French study analysing the incidence of liver injury concluded there were 14 incidences per 100 000 [7]. The majority of these cases with apparent DILI were dealt with in the community, but 20% did need hospital care and the overall mortality rate was 6%. Extrapolating these figures to the recorded national French numbers suggests a 16-fold under-reporting. A lower estimated incidence has been reported in the UK, approximately 2.4 per 100 000 per year, but this figure was based on primary care physician computer records, and dependent on a clinical assessment of need for referral to hospital [8]. Under-reporting by some 6-fold has been described in UK inpatients, when nearly 10% of abnormal LFTs were retrospectively considered to be DILI [9]. A Spanish prospective study found an incidence of severe DILI of 7.4 per million per year, with increasing incidence with age and with an overall 12% mortality [10].

The incidence rises to 1 in 1000 patients taking certain drugs, e.g. chlorpromazine, azathioprine and sulfasalazine [8]. Certain groups of drugs are repeatedly implicated, usually common preparations, used in huge numbers including NSAIDs and anti-infectives, particularly antibacterials [7], [10].

WHY IS THE LIVER AT RISK?

METABOLISM

The liver is at risk of injury due to its key role within the metabolism of virtually all drugs and xenobiotics (foreign agents). Hepatocytes are adaptable and highly efficient in eliminating foreign compounds, although the regulation of the pathways used to achieve this is poorly understood. Initial bioactivation of a drug is by oxidation or reduction pathways, predominantly by the cytochrome p450 enzymes (CYPs) but also by mixed function oxidase systems. These enzymes are found predominantly within zone 3 hepatocytes. Frequently, metabolites are more active than their parent compound; they also need to be made hydrophilic before being able to be excreted in the bile or urine. This is primarily by conjugation to a gluronide, sulphate, acetate or glutathione form. If there is inadequate detoxification, the reactive metabolites can bind covalently to cellular macromolecules, usually proteins, leading to direct cellular damage, or indirectly by hypersensitivity mechanisms or interference with key cellular functions, particularly mitochondrial function. Apoptotic or necrotic pathways may be triggered, or there may be induction of a cytokine response leading to cell death.

Less than 10% of all the CYPs account for over 90% of the oxidation of all drugs: following exposure to some drugs the activities of these proteins may increase 5-fold with transcripts of their genes changing 50-fold [11]. The cellular pumps that involve uptake of drugs from the blood can also be regulated by drugs. Several protein families of ATP-binding transporters eject drugs from hepatocytes. These are present on the canalicular membrane and are involved in the end stages of bilirubin and bile salt excretion. Drugs may result in cholestasis due to interference with the overall membrane expression of one or more of these export pumps. They can also compete for the transporter [12].

Inherited defects in these systems can lead to drug accumulation and toxicity and can also be altered in pregnancy [6].

Several regulatory nuclear receptors for cytochrome p450s genes have been identified; these can bind naturally occurring compounds and xenobiotics [13]. Gene activation and expression follows conformational change occurring after ligand binding of compounds to these proteins. This is a rapidly expanding field of knowledge, but such receptors include the Pregnane X Receptor (PXR) which appears to have a major role within the liver, with effects upon the CYP3A genes and which can be activated by steroids and rifampicin. Another is the Constitutive Androstene Receptor (CAR), which has some overlap of activity with PXR but is triggered by phenobarbital and other similar behaving drugs. In addition to the genes involved in the CYPs, these nuclear receptors also affect the genes involved in the regulation of the drug export pumps.

MECHANISMS OF INJURY

Traditionally the mechanisms of DILI are divided into 'idiosyncratic' and 'intrinsic'. Intrinsic agents cause predictable, dose-dependent injury for which animal models can be utilised: as such they can be readily detected early in the development of any new drug and tend to be abandoned. As long as the therapeutic dose is not exceeded, intrinsic injury is rare, related to deliberate attempts at self-harm or unintentional misrecognition of a toxin.

Idiosyncratic reactions are unpredictable with only a very small proportion of people exposed to a drug developing an ADR. There are poor animal models, despite the various species used; this could reflect genetic sensitivities, immunological responses, modification by disease as well as idiosyncratic reasons. Onset is often seemingly dose independent and can occur at a markedly variable time after exposure. The low frequency of idiosyncratic reactions is due to the requirement for the occurrence of multiple discrete events, each of fairly low probability. These may include formation of reactive metabolites, pharmacokinetic interactions, type of exposure, environmental factors, including nutritional status and genetic factors [14]. There are several examples where the frequency of drug hypersensitivity is increased in the presence of a viral infection, particularly in HIV infection [15]. These may reflect the role of the immune system in seeing a hapten, neoantigen, formed as a 'dangerous' molecule. Coinfection with hepatitis C and B viruses (Fig. 11.1) and HIV appears to increase the risk of hepatotoxicity even further [16].

It appears to be immune mediated occurring in genetically susceptible individuals [17]. The serum contains antibodies that react with halothane-induced liver antigens. These neoantigens are formed by the covalent interaction of the reactive oxidative trifluoroacetylate metabolite of halothane with liver microsomal proteins [18]. A switch in use to the other volatile anaesthetics enflurane and isoflurane has led to significant reduction in this form of hepatotoxicity. Oxidative metabolism by cytochrome p450 of these compounds also produces similar immunoreactive microsomal protein adducts which cross-sensitise [18], [19]. The potential for hepatotoxicity appears directly related to the extent of their oxidative metabolism; approximately 20% of halothane is metabolised, compared with only 2% of enflurane and 0.2% of isoflurane. The occurrence

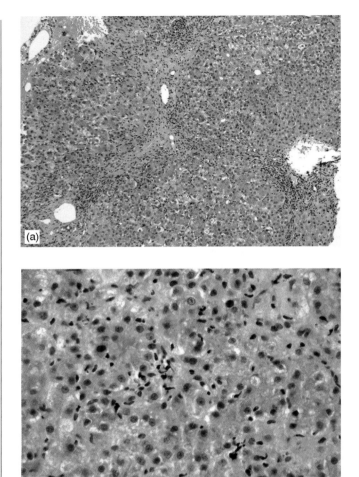

Fig. 11.1 A 23-year-old male with chronic hepatitis B viral infection; both e antigen and e antibody weakly positive. Taking three types of herbal remedies. Flare of ALT, up to 3000. This could be seroconversion from eAg to eAb positive that is seen naturally with HBV infection, but biopsy shows cholestatic hepatitis with bridging collapse being more typical of a drug reaction.

of hepatotoxicity after enflurane or isoflurane is extremely rare with reviews identifying only a handful of instances [20].

Distinction between intrinsic toxicity and idiosyncrasy is less clear than was previously thought; e.g. in susceptible patients, some drugs previously considered allergens appear to damage cell membranes directly via toxic intermediate metabolites.

SUSCEPTIBILITY

There are various polymorphisms (common genetic variants) in the control of drug metabolism found within populations and wide individual variations in biotransformation pathways. The importance of this was first recognised in people who were 'slow acetylators', as they had an increased risk of hydralazine-induced systemic lupus erythematosus. Similarly, an increased risk of hepatotoxicity with the former anti-anginal agent perhexilene was identified in the 5–10% of Caucasians who are poor oxylators of debrisoquine; chronic injury with phospholipidosis and non-alcoholic steatohepatitis, some with development of cirrhosis, have been described in this at risk group after long-term ingestion. Despite the obvious importance of the p450s there has been little helpful data for identifying specific polymorphisms that could be predictive of liver injury; studies have tended to be small and retrospective and the findings have been contradictory [22]. There are also sizable questions to be addressed about the cost-effectiveness of genotyping for different polymorphisms before an individual can receive a prescribed drug.

In addition to these aspects of pharmocogenetics, other drugs, and also alcohol, affect the pharmacokinetics through enzyme induction. Age also has an affect, changes in p450 activity levels being most marked within the paediatric and elderly population. The elderly are at more risk for the majority of agents [6], [7], [23], [24] although some paediatric predisposition is seen with valproate [25] and aspirin, which was responsible for Reye's syndrome [6]. There appear to be some gender differences, females are more at risk of DILI, up to double the rate in patients over the age of 50 years [6], [7], although men appear more at risk of azathioprine toxicity (Fig. 11.2) [6]. The general nutritional status is also important; obesity may be a risk factor for the development of some steatohepatitic injury, while malnourishment can predispose to glutathione deficiency.

There are several examples where the frequency of drug hypersensitivity is increased in the presence of a viral infection, particularly in HIV infection [15]. This may reflect the role of the immune system in seeing a hapten, neoantigen, formed as a 'dangerous' molecule. The previous use of potential hepatotoxic agents and, possibly metastases, may also make the liver more susceptible to injury [26].

Multiple medications also seem to increase the risk of DILI [6], [27], and if the combination includes two potential hepatotoxic drugs, the risk may be increased 6-fold [8].

SPECTRUM OF CHANGES WITH DILI

PATTERNS OF INJURY

Although the morphological spectrum of disease is wide, the most common is an acute hepatitis, then a mixed hepatitic-cholestatic injury, followed by cholestasis [7], [10]. The degree of necrosis may vary from spotty, to confluent and bridging, or massive loss with multiacinar collapse. The cholestatic injuries may be complicated by a degree of duct damage that can lead to protracted jaundice or abnormal liver function tests [28]. Other relatively common manifestations are steatosis and granulomas, with some cases of steatohepatitis. More rare are the architectural and chronic changes – sinusoidal dilatation and peliosis,

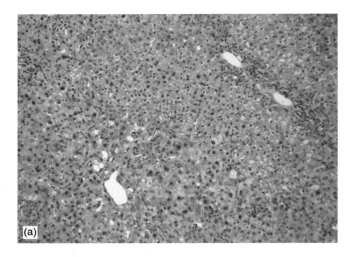

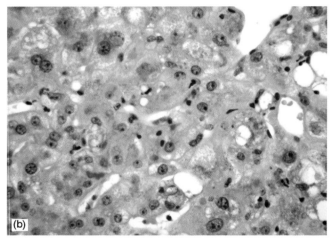

Fig. 11.2 A 75-year-old male on azathioprine and a statin, for 18 and 12 months respectively, with a diagnosis of cryptogenic fibrosing alveolitis; 2 weeks jaundice. A predominant bland cholestasis with Kupffer cell reaction. Although azathioprine can give a cholestatic picture this is usually seen within the first month. Direct questioning revealed a completed course of antibiotics for a chest infection 3 weeks prior to symptoms; this is the more likely candidate.

veno-occlusive disease, fibrosis, cirrhosis, and very rarely, mimickers of primary biliary cirrhosis, primary sclerosing cholangitis, autoimmune hepatitis and neoplasms.

ADAPTATION

Many drugs, including those capable of causing significant liver injury can be associated with transient, and apparently harmless, abnormalities.

DILI with isoniazid is estimated to be around 2%, being in the range of 0.5–4% depending on the age group [24] and a major cause of idiosyncratic induced acute liver failure [29]; however, a significant rise in alanine transaminase (ALT) is seen in nearly 20% of patients following initiation of therapy. Similarly, in the early trials of the novel anti-diabetogenic agent troglitazone (Rezalin), around 2% of recipients had ALT rises greater than three times the normal upper limit [30]. In the majority, this was harmless, as the subsequent incidence of symptomatic liver injury, after general marketing of the drug, was 0.1%. A range of histology was seen – hepatitis, steatosis, granulomas – but there were many cases of fatal severe hepatitis and, due to the large number of patients likely to receive it, this drug has now been withdrawn. Some 50% of recipients have shown an elevation in ALT during a trial with the cholinesterase inhibitor, tetrahydroaminoacridine (Tacrine), in the use of moderate dementia [6]. The drug was not stopped in all patients, partly as there appeared to be some cognitive improvements, and a return to normal ALT values was seen in the majority, regardless of whether the drug was stopped. Definite DILI has been described, however, with necrosis present on liver biopsy [31].

It would appear that some adaptive phenomenon is occurring with transient changes in up- and down-regulation of the responsible enzyme systems. This adaptation does appear to have a memory: re-exposure to Tacrine in patients with previously abnormal LFTs being associated with hardly a flicker of rise in the ALT.

This adaptive process leads to even further difficulty in the early stages of clinical trials, when potential toxicity is sought with monitoring of liver function tests. A recent review of serious hepatotoxicity from the now-withdrawn NSAID bromfenac, suggests that there are frequently constitutional, flu-like symptoms which, in conjunction with elevated ALTs, may predict serious DILI [32].

COMMONLY IMPLICATED DRUGS

In addition to the classic cases listed in Table 11.1 many other drugs have been implicated anecdotally and in single case reports.

SEVERITY OF INJURY

There has been a steady increase in the percentage of patients developing acute liver failure due to drugs. The combination of paracetamol toxicity (Fig. 11.3), both therapeutic misadventure and deliberate, with idiosyncratic drug reaction has now replaced viral hepatitis as the most frequent cause of acute liver failure within the United States [33]. Similarly, in the UK and Sweden paracetamol toxicity accounts for 50% of cases of acute liver failure [34], [35]. Idiosyncratic drug reactions, which are severe enough to lead to the full clinical manifestations of liver failure with encephalopathy, coagulopathy and jaundice have over an 85% mortality [36]. Lesser degrees of DILI but with jaundice and a high ALT may have a mortality as high as 10% [37]. Although over 4500 cases of fatal acute liver failure (ALF) with a drug as the implicated aetiology, have been reported through the World Health Organisation (WHO) over a 30-year period, just

Table 11.1 Drugs commonly implicated in DILI, derived from standard texts

Morphological picture	Implicated drug/toxin
Hepatitis-like	Carbon tetrachloride, chloroform, chloroalkanes (e.g. trichloroethylene), paracetamol (which affects zone 3 predominantly), allyl alcohol, phosphorus, ferrous sulphate (zone 1 first)
Necrosis − zonal	Isoniazid, ketoconazole, indomethacin, phenytoin, halothane, clozapine, diclofenac
Pure cholestasis	Antibiotics, especially flucloxacillin, oral contraceptives, anabolic steroids
Cholestatic hepatitis	Chlorpromazine, erythromycin, trimethoprim
Fibrosis/cirrhosis	Methotrexate, arsenic, chlorpromazine or nitrofurantoin, thorotrast, vinyl chloride, copper sulphate
Adenomas	Oral contraceptives
Vanishing bile duct syndrome (PBC-like)	Amoxicillin, amoxicillin−clavulanic acid, amitriptyline, carbamazepine, chlorpromazine, clindamycin, cyamemazine, cyproheptadine, erythromycin, flucloxacillin, glycyrrhizin, ibuprofen, sulpride, trimethoprim, sulfamethoxazole and troleandomycin
Granulomas	Phenytoin, carbamazepine, hydralazine, isoniazid, nitrofurantoin, sulphonamides, allopurinol, phenylbutazone
Steatosis	Corticosteroids, tamoxifen and estrogens, tetracycline, sodium valproate, salicylates
Steatohepatitis	Amiodarone, stilboestrol, nifedipine
Chronic hepatitis	Methyldopa, nitrofurantoin, minocycline (autoimmune like)
Veno-occlusive disease	Azothioprine, chemotherapy (especially post bone marrow transplant)
Peliosis hepatis	Anabolic and contraceptive steroids, azathioprine

20 drugs are responsible for the majority, each with over 50 well-substantiated cases [38]. The most common drug types found were analgesics, drugs against human immunodeficiency virus, anticonvulsants and antibacterial drugs.

MAKING THE DIAGNOSIS

This can be very difficult, as there are no specific markers of a drug injury and the diagnosis is often one of exclusion. Compounding factors include the presence of multiple drugs and also underlying disease, which may include liver disease (Fig. 11.4). Scoring systems have been devised to assess causality, e.g. Roussel Uclaf Causality Assessment Method [39] and Clinical Diagnostic Scale [40]. All have some limitations due to their complexity and user interpretation. A score is generated, using several categories, which suggests whether a DILI is highly probable to unlikely.

All systems take into account such factors as a positive history of drug ingestion with an appropriate temporal association; ingestion of a drug previously

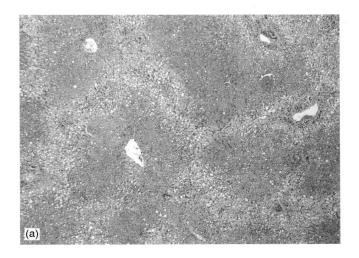

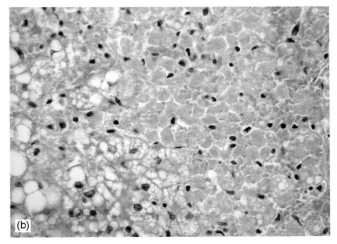

Fig. 11.3 A 44-year-old male, heavy alcohol consumption; 4 weeks of flu-like illness then diarrhoea and vomiting, abdominal pain, rectal bleeding and generalised bruising: bilirubin 120 μmol/l, alkaline phosphatase 150 U/L, ALT 6000 U/L. (a) Post-mortem liver showing zones 3 and 2 possible haemorrhage on low power; (b) shows coagulative necrosis of the all hepatocytes in these areas. This was unintentional paracetamaol toxicity; alcohol was probably acting as an enzyme inducer and he took several different medications containing paracetamol for his 'flu'.

reported to cause toxicity; the absence of factors to suggest a different aetiology. These factors include a lack of risk factors for alcohol abuse; or for contracting viral hepatitis, negative viral and autoimmune serology and normal biliary tract imaging (see Table 11.2). Further support comes from normalising of liver function tests (LFTs) after stopping the drug. The definitive test of a suspected drug is a rechallenge but this can be dangerous, especially in hypersensitivity reactions where there is increasingly severe liver damage with repeated exposure. An expert panel is perhaps the most suitable assessment, especially with the possibility of future litigation [41].

Table 11.2 Making the diagnosis

History of drug ingestion
Temporal association
Drug known to cause toxicity
No alcohol abuse
No viral hepatitis risk factors
Negative viral serology
Normal biliary tract imaging

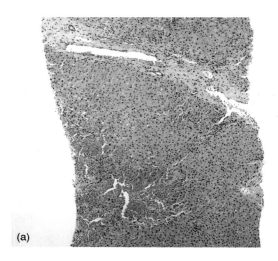

(a)

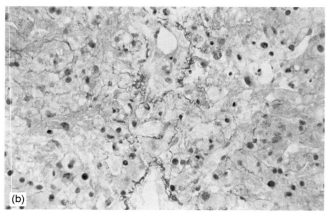

(b)

Fig. 11.4 A 43-year-old male transplanted for primary sclerosing cholangitis. 7 months later diagnosed with autoimmune hepatitis. Treated with azothioprine, mycophenalate, and prednisolone; abnormal LFTs and slight ascites at 9 months. (a) Zone 3 haemorrhage with little inflammation; (b) shows the architectural stain chromotrope alanine blue (CAB) with partial obliteration of a terminal hepatic venule. Azathioprine induced veno-occlusion, confirmed by wedge pressure measurement.

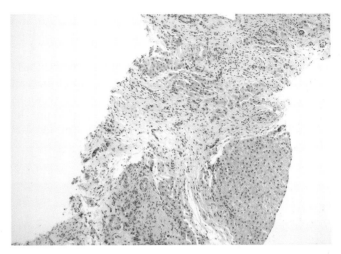

Fig. 11.5 A 10-year-old female with signs of portal hypertension and mildly abnormal LFTs two years after receiving chemotherapy for acute lymphoblastic leukemia. Massive fibrosis and distortion with sclerosed hepatic veins — an inactive cirrhosis. Probable veno-occlusion with 6-thioguanine.

A temporal association can be a useful pointer to the diagnosis, with most forms of liver injury occurring within 1–12 weeks of the exposure; although this may be more rapid if there is hypersensitivity and a repeat exposure. Other reactions involve chronic insidious injury (Fig. 11.5) and it may take many months of regular ingestion of a drug before liver injury becomes apparent, e.g. methotrexate fibrosis and oral contraceptive-induced adenomas.

There are numerous resources detailing drug hepatotoxicity including many textbooks (the most exhaustive being Zimmerman's *Hepatotoxicity* [24]) but also Medline and Internet sites. Resources include The UK Committee on Safety of Medicines, Yellow card reporting; monoclonal antibody studies which assess potential toxicity by seeing which cytochrome P450 enzymes are used to metabolise the drug; the MHRA, Medicines and Healthcare products Advisory Agency in the UK; Medwatch and the Adverse Events Reporting System (AERS), both run by the US Food and Drug administration. Local pharmacists and drug manufacturers themselves are often good sources.

ROLE OF LIVER BIOPSY

Although frequently considered the 'gold standard' in many aspects of liver pathology this is less true with histology in DILI, as frequently the changes seen may be relatively non-specific. However, the severity and type of injury in any individual are still important parameters to determine, as the same drug may show variable DILI changes in different patients. Biopsy also plays an important role in excluding other liver pathology and should have a role in assessing damage caused by drugs in trials. There may be some other risk factor for liver injury, e.g. in the alcoholic or with chronic viral infection, and a biopsy may help establish the relative degree of injury ascribable to these aetiologies.

Some clues from the biopsy are unusual patterns of injury, particularly mixed hepatitis or the presence of prominent eosinophils or granulomas. It may also be worth establishing the pattern of injury when multiple medications are being taken, to try and determine if there is a most likely candidate; the drugs being taken may be of considerable benefit in disease control and not easily replaceable.

PROBLEMS IN MAKING THE DIAGNOSIS OF DILI

NON-PRESCRIPTION DRUGS

Complementary and alternative medicines (CAM)

There is a booming industry and consumer confidence in complementary and alternative medicines, in particular herbal remedies. Over 40% of the general US population and over 75% of the German population regularly take some form of CAM [42], [43]. Meta-analyses of several randomised clinical trials have come to positive conclusions about the efficacy of herbal remedies, including palmetto in symptomatic prostatism, ginkgo biloba in slowing dementia, horse chestnut seed extracts for chronic venous insufficiency and St John's wort for depression [44]. The initial reports of the efficacy of St John's Wort use in mild and moderate depression [45], was followed by a 2800% increase in sales [44]. The seemingly active component, hyperforin, is a potent inducer of one of the cytochrome p450 enzymes (CYP 3A4) and has the potential for serious interactions with other drugs also metabolised by these enzymes [46]. Its effects can lead to a lowering in the serum level of the anti-rejection drug cyclosporine and, in the liver transplant setting, has been associated with acute rejection [47]. Of more widespread importance is its association with over a 40% reduction in the level of the active metabolite of some chemotherapeutic agents, and this effect can last for several weeks [48].

Toxic injury from CAM is more frequently seen in women; there is conflicting evidence as to whether females actually consume more of these products, particularly as several of the CAM side-effects have been associated with their use with the aim of weight reduction. But overall, this is in line with the greater susceptibility of females to drug-induced liver injury with conventional therapies.

Cumulative dosage seems important for some cases of liver injury. Although the elderly seem to also be at increased risk of ADRs, there have been cases of acute liver injury in children following use of a 'slimming agent', in which the problem offending agent was kava [49].

There is wide media reporting of available herbal remedies, raising expectation in areas where conventional medicines have little or no effect. There seems to be resistance and scepticism on the part of patients if they feel clinicians' attitude to be wholly negative towards CAM. Numerous studies have shown that the vast majority of patients either currently taking, or having previously taken CAM, would not mention this to a doctor who was trying to take a drug history [42], [50]. Perhaps rather contradictorily, people taking these CAMs, despite believing they have some potency in their actions, assume that, because they are 'natural' they are also 'safe'. Practitioners of CAM also emphasise the lack of side-effects; there were several upheld complaints to the advertising standards agency in the UK in 2005. However, there are numerous examples from conventional medicines of the potential toxicity of 'nature', e.g. digoxin from the foxglove, vincristine and morphine [44]. This assumption of safety can lead to problems when the initial symptoms of an ADR are not recognised and ingestion continues or, alternatively, when higher than recommended doses of such 'safe' products are consumed.

CAM agents are sold as 'food supplements' and are therefore not regulated for their safety and quality, as in the pharmaceutical industry. The quality control of some agents has been heavily criticised [44], [51]. One company has had over 1500 products withdrawn from circulation [52] after errors in manufacture had been identified; these included substitution of some products and an unacceptable range (of 0 to $\times$ 7) in the concentration of the indicated active compound. This action followed the identification of nearly 100 cases of adverse reaction to a travel sickness remedy, with 20% having a life-threatening reaction. Although this case involved an Australian firm, globalisation means that some of these products are available in the UK, and problems have also been seen with European manufacture [44].

Adulteration can be a problem with some products, either with orthodox drugs, pesticides or heavy metals [53], [44]. In the UK, the majority of herbal creams that were being marketed as suitable for cases of eczema illegally contained dexamethasone [54]. Other studies have shown the presence of paracetamol in herbal remedies [55]. Worse instances include the presence of known toxic agents; alacholic acid has been responsible for cases of nephrotoxicity in China and the UK [56] and subsequent development of urological malignancies [57].

There can be problems with identification of the exact herbs — and also what parts of the plant, roots, seeds, leaves, etc., contain the correct active ingredients [58]. There is also the scope for further herb—herb and herb—drug interaction; not least as the herb is given in its entirety, often taken as a tea mixture when hundreds of active chemicals may be present. Despite the centuries of knowledge in China of the use of herbs, there appear to be differences in manufacturing standards, and problems in the way information about their usage is crossing language and cultural barriers.

Traditional Chinese medicines, and also those from Japan, India and Africa, are usually a combination from several plants. Although the idea of isolating, and thereby purifying the active compound along Western pharmaceutical lines has a certain appeal, not least to the pharmaceutical companies, these isolates seem to be much weaker than the intact herbs as traditionally used [51].

And, of course there is still the potential for allergic and idiosyncratic reactions as with other xenobiotics.

Since 2004 the European Union has embarked upon a simple registration procedure for traditional medicines, and in the UK a Herbal Medicines

Advisory Committee has been established. There is a need to distinguish herbal therapies, of little effectiveness but with adverse reaction risks, from efficacious ones with an acceptable risk level [59].

OTHER AGENTS

There are other products, available without prescription, which may not be perceived as drugs, including tonics, slimming agents and vitamins. The use of the Japanese products Chaso and Onshido, as part of weight loss, may be associated with acute liver injury, including ALF. *N*-nitroso-fenfluramine, related to an appetite depressant, has been discovered in them, and this may be responsible for the hepatotoxicity [60].

Hypervitaminosis A can lead to acute and often rapidly fatal toxicity, through accidental consumption of bear or fish liver. More common is an insidious fibrosis which can lead to non-cirrhotic portal hypertension [25]. The risk seems proportional to the total cumulative dose. Self-medication, predominantly for skin and eye complaints, that has resulted in damage, has usually been many times higher than the normal daily recommended dose and taken over many years [61].

Some drugs may not have a license for use in the UK, but may be widely available in Europe and the rest of the world, and so become available for purchase over the Internet. Further, drugs limited to prescription in the UK may also be purchasable over the Internet. One such non-licensed drug is Pyritinol, which is marketed for improvement in brain function in dementia syndromes, but which is frequently taken by the healthy with a view to 'memory improvement'. Recent ADRs, with a severe and prolonged cholestatic hepatitis, requiring hospitialisation in nearly 70% of those affected has been described [62].

As the variety of herbal medicines available is large, so are the possible presentations of liver disease induced by them. Bush teas, used primarily in Jamaica and Africa, have long been associated with acute and chronic veno-occlusive disease. They contain pyrrolizidine alkaloids that can be found in many plants, e.g. *Heliotroprium*, *Senecio*, *Crotalaria*, *Symphytum* and t'u-san-chi'i (*Compositae*). A large epidemic of veno-occlusive disease has been seen following ingestion of wheat flour contaminated by heliotrope seeds [63].

Chaparral (*Larrea tridentata*) is marketed as a dietary and energy supplement and is used for a variety of conditions, mainly anti-infective but also for weight reduction. There is limited evidence of efficacy. It can cause a spectrum of liver injury, including acute hepatitis, subacute hepatic necrosis progressing to liver failure, and a cholestatic hepatitis that can progress to cirrhosis [64]. The mechanism of injury with such agents is very complex; although the cholestasis described is thought to be an oestrogen-like effect, due to the structural similarity of lignans, other potentially active substances include flavonoids, aminoacids and volatile oils.

Not all is doom and gloom and conflict in the worlds of CAM and hepatology: currently several CAMs, including Silymarin (milk thistle), Glycyrrhizin, *Plantago asiatica*, Sho-saiko-to and various other herbal mixtures are being

Table 11.3 Histological features of liver injury caused by complimentary medicines

Histological pattern of injury	Medicine	Refs
Massive hepatic necrosis	Ma huang	[79]
	Chaparral	[80]
	Greater celedine	[81]
	Jin bu huan	[82]
	Black cohosh	[83], [84]
	Kava	[85]
	Chaso, Onshido	[60]
Cholestatic hepatitis	Chaparral	[80], [64]
	Kava	[85]
Chronic hepatitis	Jin bu huan	[86]
	Greater celedine	[81]
Fibrosis and cirrhosis	Chaparral	[64]
	Vitamin A	[87], [88]
Autoimmune hepatitis	Black cohosh	[89]
	Syo-saiko-tu	[90]
Veno-occlusive disease	Pyrrolizidine alkaloids	[91], [92]
Microvesicular steatosis	Margaso oil	[93], [94]
Giant cell hepatitis	Isabgol	[95]

tried in acute and chronic liver disease in controlled clinical settings, although as yet, proof of efficacy is still awaited [42].

Table 11.3 lists some CAM agents which have been implicated in several cases of liver injury.

ILLICIT DRUG USE

Therapeutic use of anabolic steroids, along with the other C-17 alkylated steroids, has been associated with jaundice and, with more prolonged use, neoplasia. There has been an increase in their illicit use for body building and enhancement of sport performance, being possibly as high as 10% in regular gymnasium users [65].

Amphetamine derivatives are widely used in the UK and are known by a variety of names, the most common being 'Ecstasy' (3,4-methylenedioxymethyl-amphetamine). Fatalities have occurred with their use and in the late 1990s this led to massive media coverage, although the actual estimated fatal incidence is 0.0002%. A hyperthermia syndrome was responsible for some acute deaths; the majority had myocardial and cerebral changes and liver injury was universal [66]. Liver injury is predominantly hepatitic, involving zone 3, but with a variability from spotty necrosis to confluent and massive hepatic necrosis, leading to ALF with death or transplantation in a few cases. Chronic use has also been implicated in acute hepatitis and cholestasis [28].

Despite the chronic and widespread abuse of cocaine and its well-documented affects on the cardiovascular system and central nervous system, isolated hepatotoxicity is rare. Acute liver injury is seen, some probably related to systemic effects, particularly hypotension. There is also evidence for a direct liver effect with zonal microvesicular steatosis and zonal necrosis; interestingly, this can affect any of the zones, including periportal areas [67]–[69].

Overwhelmingly, the major risk of liver injury with intravenous drug use is the concomitant risk of chronic viral infections, in particular hepatitis C virus infection in the UK, due to the use of shared needles.

OVER-THE-COUNTER PREPARATIONS

The most important DILI associated with non-prescription agents is with paracetamol (referred to as acetaminophen in the USA). This is a widely used, and effective analgesic: it is estimated that over a quarter of the population will have self-medicated with it in any single month. There is a very rare incidence of toxicity but this carries a high medical burden: paracetamol toxicity is the leading cause of acute liver failure in both the UK and USA [33], [35]. However, there appear to be important differences in the patient populations: in the UK over 90% of patients have taken a supratherapeutic dose as a deliberate act of self-harm, usually well over the recommended maximum dose of 4 g/day [70], whereas in the USA over 50% of cases are considered unintentional, on average 7.5 g/day being taken over several weeks to days, the indication being chronic pain in the majority [33].

Nearly half of patients suffering from unintentional toxicity consumed more than one preparation containing paracetamol; this may be due to recklessness but also because of unawareness of the many different-sounding preparations that contain paracetamol. Nearly two thirds of patients were receiving prescription medications for pain, with paracetamol combined with a narcotic, but bought and consumed further over-the-counter paracetamol [33]. The aetiology is not always clear-cut; after all, paracetamol may have been taken for symptomatic relief for another illness, including a viral infection. There may even be dual pathology; paracetamol has been implicated as a co-factor with acute hepatitis B infection and with anti-tuberculosis therapy [71].

The majority of paracetamol is biotransformed by conjugation, with only around 5% being metabolised by p4502E1 to the potentially toxic electrophilic intermediate. This, in turn, is conjugated with glutathione and rendered nontoxic. Toxic levels accumulate when there is a large amount of substrate for metabolism, e.g. with an overdose; when there has been prior enzyme induction, e.g. with anti-epileptics, or when glutathione levels are depleted, e.g. with malnutrition or fasting.

High alcohol consumption also appears to be a risk factor for unintentional paracetamol toxicity [72]. Alcohol is an inducer of cytochrome p450 and is partly metabolised itself by p4502E1, although this induction disappears five days after cessation of alcohol consumption. Glutathione levels are also lower in the alcoholic, partly due to impaired synthesis and partly to general malnutrition.

The liver injury shows a striking zonality, with coagulative necrosis of hepatocytes with preservation of the architecture and little inflammatory cell infiltrate. The injury is within zone 3, but can extend into zone 2 and even 1 with greater levels of toxicity. Residual hepatocytes may show variable ballooning and steatosis.

OTHER AGENTS

Many household products can be injurious to the liver, the toxicity appearing to be a direct effect, with the formation of free radicals and massive change to proteins and cell structures leading to cell death, e.g. carbon tetrachloride, metallic salts, antifreeze and paraquat [24]. The use of childproof tops on the containers of such products minimises the risk of accidents, although unusual agents may still cause injury with deliberate abuse. Some naturally occurring hepatotoxins may be ingested in error, the classical example being the wild mushrooms *Amanita phylloides* and *A. lepiota* [28]. This has a more indirect toxic effect with selective interference with cell components or pathways, leading to mitochondrial dysfunction and microvesicular steatosis.

An important clue to this sort of liver injury, apart from the history, is a striking zonality of necrosis, with dead hepatocytes of similar age. Zone 3 is the most frequent site, due to the concentration of p450s in those hepatocytes, although zone 1 necrosis is also occasionally seen, e.g. with phosphorous and ferrous salts and with high concentrations of acetic acid [73]. With extreme toxicity complete haemorrhagic necrosis of hepatocytes may develop, e.g. with acute zinc toxicity from coin ingestion [74]. Rarely do such agents cause cholestasis, although paraquat does by direct damage to bile ducts. The other important pattern of severe toxic injury is microvesicular steatosis, e.g. mushroom poisoning, and Reye's syndrome.

PRESCRIPTION DRUGS

Although there may be a clear history of ingestion of prescription drugs, there may still be problems in making a positive diagnosis of DILI, and there may even be an extra level of complexity due to drug–drug interactions. Different trade names for the same drug can lead to confusion and inadvertent overdosing; as can alteration in the composition of a drug, e.g. to a slow-release preparation, which may have a different bioavailability and be less well-tolerated by a patient who had been tolerating the drug well for some years [28].

Due to the variable onset of symptoms of DILI, the patient may no longer be taking the injurious agent; the most obvious and frequent one being a previously completed course of antibiotics, some weeks before the development of jaundice (Fig. 11.6).

The lack of clear temporal association may cause difficulties in the diagnosis, with sometimes the onset of injury not being seen for many months. There may

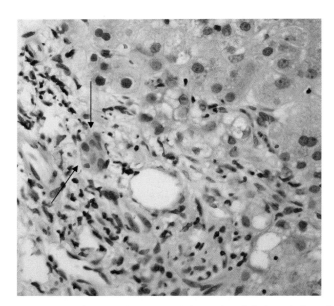

Fig. 11.6 A 79-year-old female with 2 months of cholestatic jaundice (alkaline phosphatase × 3 fold increase over normal levels, ALT × 3 fold increase); two courses of flucloxacllin in the month prior to onset. Predominantly cholestasis with some portal inflammation but very irregular bile ducts seen, a second biopsy showed loss of the inflammation with increased cholestasis but absence of bile ducts in several portal tracts. The bilirubin remains raised after 18 months of follow-up.

also be no previously recorded instances of DILI; particular attention should be paid to drugs that are in the first few years of general marketing, as this is when idiosyncratic reactions are most likely to be detected.

Seemingly of increasing importance is the assumption that abnormal LFTs are explicable due to some pre-existing condition, that the patient may be either known to have or be suspected of having. This is not infrequently seen in patients with high alcohol consumption. Initially malaise, jaundice and abnormalities in LFTs may be ascribed to chronic liver disease. A biopsy may be crucial in establishing the absence or limited presence of chronic injury with fibrosis.

A good example of the potential complexity and particular challenges of cases of possible DILI is in the assessment of abnormal LFTs in patients who are HIV-positive. Up to 50% of deaths in patients are now due to liver disease [75] and part of this is DILI. Patients with HIV are more susceptible to developing hepatotoxicity due to anti-tuberculosis medications or HAART (highly active antiretroviral therapy) [76]. HAART can result in hepatotoxicity through mitochondrial toxicity, lipodystrophy syndrome and steatohepatitis, whereas non-nucleoside reverse transcriptase inhibitors cause more hypersensitivity reactions [77].

Abnormalities of liver enzymes in patients with HIV may be due to a myriad of aetiologies, including viral hepatitis, opportunistic infections and drug toxicity. In HIV, elevation of transaminase levels may not be specific or clinically relevant (the majority are asymptomatic), since in most instances they resolve

Table 11.4 Clinical difficulties in making the diagnosis of DILI

Non-specific clinical presentation	
Non-specific histological appearance	
Unclear temporal association	Although some reactions occur within days or weeks of drug ingestion, others are insidious presenting months later
Drug not mentioned	Patients often do not consider over-the-counter or alternative therapies as drugs, and may hide illicit drug use
	They may have stopped taking the drug before onset of symptoms; particularly completed courses of antibiotics
Toxicity of drug not realised	No record of previous toxicity; most adverse effects are discovered after trials are completed, within the first two years of general release
Unintentional overdose	Use of several preparations with different names but which contain the same drug, e.g. numerous paracetamol preparations
Other liver disease known or suspected, which is believed to explain symptoms	Often patients with a history of high alcohol intake, but in whom chronic liver disease may not be present

despite continued drug therapy [76]. In addition, the diagnosis of DILI is more complicated by being one of exclusion and the presence of multiple medications.

All protease inhibitors and non-nucleoside reverse transcriptase inhibitors are substrates and potent inhibitors or inducers of the cytochrome p450 system. Other drugs can therefore potentially interact with antiretrovirals, including recreational drugs such as methylenedioxymethamphetamine (MDMA), gamma-hydroxybutuyrate (GHB), benzodiazepines and amphetamines.

Nucleoside analogues also have an expanding role in the treatment of other viruses, in particular the heptotropic viruses, and there have been some similar instances of toxicity. Severe toxicity was encountered in an early, phase II trial of fialuridine in the treatment of chronic HBV infection. Two-thirds of recipients developed hepatotoxicity, 50% with a severe and rapid deterioration in the third month of treatment. Despite withdrawal of fialuridine their condition worsened with lactic acidosis and death or the need for liver transplantation. Pancreatitis, myopathy and neuropathy were also identified. Histology of the liver revealed massive microvesicular and macrovesicular steatosis, suggesting abnormality of mitochondrial function [78]. The phase I trial had been performed on patients with symptomatic AIDS, and although several deaths were seen, they were originally thought due to progressive viral liver disease; some were probably missed fialuridine toxicity.

CONCLUSIONS

DILI is an important clinical problem. Although any pattern of damage may be seen, the most common is acute hepatocellular damage, followed by cholestasis. Important groups of drugs responsible are analgesics, anti-infectives and also antipsychotics.

Although the incidence of idiosyncratic injury is rare there is a high morbidity and mortality. Possible agents include prescribed drugs as well as complementary and alternative medicines.

Direct toxic injury is the most important cause of acute liver failure in the UK, due to paracetamol; in the USA many cases of unintentional toxicity are being recognised.

Table 11.4 gives a summary of the general problems encountered in making the diagnosis.

REFERENCES

1. Health and Social Care Information Centre. Prescription Cost Analysis: England 2004. (Department of Health, London, 2005).
2. Pirmohamed M, James S, Meakin S *et al*. Adverse drug reactions as cause of admission to hospital: prospective analysis of 18 820 patients. *BMJ* 2004; **329**: 15–19.
3. Pirmohamed M, Breckenridge AM, Kitteringham NR, Park BK. Adverse drug reactions. *BMJ* 1998; **316**: 1295–8.
4. Ebbesen J, Buajordet I, Erikssen J *et al*. Drug-related deaths in a department of internal medicine. *Arch Intern Med* 2001; **161**: 2317–23.
5. Bagheri H, Michel F, Lapeyre-Mestre M *et al*. Detection and incidence of drug-induced liver injuries in hospital: a prospective analysis from laboratory signals. *Br J Clin Pharmacol* 2000; **50**: 479–84.
6. Larrey D. Epidemiology and individual susceptibility to adverse drug reactions affecting the liver. *Semin Liver Dis* 2002; **22**: 145–55.
7. Sgro C, Clinard F, Ouazir K *et al*. Incidence of drug-induced hepatic injuries: a French population-based study. *Hepatology* 2002; **36**: 451–5.
8. de Abajo FJ, Montero D, Madurga M, Garcia Rodriguez LA. Acute and clinically relevant drug-induced liver injury: a population based case-control study. *Br J Clin Pharmacol* 2004; **58**: 71–80.
9. Bagheri H, Michel F, Lapeyre-Mestre M *et al*. Detection and incidence of drug-induced liver injuries in hospital: a prospective analysis from laboratory signals. *Br J Clin Pharmacol* 2000; **50**: 479–84.
10. Ibanez L, Perez E, Vidal X, Laporte JR. Prospective surveillance of acute serious liver disease unrelated to infectious, obstructive, or metabolic diseases: epidemiological and clinical features, and exposure to drugs. *J Hepatol* 2002; **37**: 592–600.
11. Farrell GC, Liddle C. Drugs and the liver updated, 2002. *Semin Liver Dis* 2002; **22**: 109–13.
12. Bohan A, Boyer JL. Mechanisms of hepatic transport of drugs: implications for cholestatic drug reactions. *Semin Liver Dis* 2002; **22**: 123–36.
13. Liddle C, Goodwin B. Regulation of hepatic drug metabolism: role of the nuclear receptors PXR and CAR. *Semin Liver Dis* 2002; **22**: 115–22.
14. Li AP. A review of the common properties of drugs with idiosyncratic hepatotoxicity and the "multiple determinant hypothesis" for the manifestation of idiosyncratic drug toxicity. *Chem Biol Interact* 2002; **142**: 7–23.
15. Pirmohamed M, Naisbitt DJ, Gordon F, Park BK. The danger hypothesis – potential role in idiosyncratic drug reactions. *Toxicology* 2002; **181–182**: 55–63.

16. Kontorinis N, Dieterich DT. Toxicity of non-nucleoside analogue reverse transcriptase inhibitors. *Semin Liver Dis* 2003; **23**: 173−82.
17. Kenna JG. Immunoallergic drug-induced hepatitis: lessons from halothane. *J Hepatol* 1997; **26**(Suppl 1): 5−12.
18. Mikatti NE, Healy TE. Hepatic injury associated with halogenated anaesthetics: cross-sensitization and its clinical implications. *Eur J Anaesthesiol* 1997; **14**: 7−14.
19. Christ DD, Kenna JG, Kammerer W *et al*. Enflurane metabolism produces covalently bound liver adducts recognized by antibodies from patients with halothane hepatitis. *Anesthesiology* 1988; **69**: 833−8.
20. Zimmerman H. Even isoflurane. *Hepatology* 1991; **13**: 1251−3.
21. Morgan MY, Reshef R, Shah RR *et al*. Impaired oxidation of debrisoquine in patients with perhexiline liver injury. *Gut* 1984; **25**: 1057−64.
22. Pirmohamed M, Park BK. Cytochrome P450 enzyme polymorphisms and adverse drug reactions. *Toxicology* 2003; **192**: 23−32.
23. Bjornsson E, Olsson R. Outcome and prognostic markers in severe drug-induced liver disease. *Hepatology* 2005; **42**: 481−9.
24. Zimmerman H. *Hepatotoxicity: the Adverse Effects of Drugs and Other Chemicals on the Liver*. (Liippincott Williams & Wilkins, Philadelphia, 1999).
25. Scheffner D, Konig S, Rauterberg-Ruland I *et al*. Fatal liver failure in 16 children with valproate therapy. *Epilepsia* 1988; **29**: 530−42.
26. Robinson K, Lambiase L, Li J *et al*. Fatal cholestatic liver failure associated with gemcitabine therapy. *Dig Dis Sci* 2003; **48**: 1804−8.
27. Perez GS, Garcia Rodriguez LA. The increased risk of hospitalizations for acute liver injury in a population with exposure to multiple drugs. *Epidemiology* 1993; **4**: 496−501.
28. Davies SE. Drugs and the liver. *Curr Diagnostic Pathol* 1997; **4**: 135−44.
29. Russo MW, Galanko JA, Shrestha R, Fried MW, Watkins P. Liver transplantation for acute liver failure from drug induced liver injury in the United States. *Liver Transpl* 2004; **10**: 1018−23.
30. Watkins PB, Whitcomb RW. Hepatic dysfunction associated with troglitazone. *N Engl J Med* 1998; **338**: 916−17.
31. Hammel P, Larrey D, Bernuau J *et al*. Acute hepatitis after tetrahydroaminoacridine administration for Alzheimer's disease. *J Clin Gastroenterol* 1990; **12**: 329−31.
32. Goldkind L, Laine L. A systematic review of NSAIDs withdrawn from the market due to hepatotoxicity: lessons learned from the bromfenac experience. *Pharmacoepidemiol Drug Saf* 2006; **15**: 213−20.
33. Ostapowicz G, Fontana RJ, Schiodt FV *et al*. Results of a prospective study of acute liver failure at 17 tertiary care centers in the United States. *Ann Intern Med* 2002; **137**: 947−54.
34. Bjornsson E, Jerlstad P, Bergqvist A, Olsson R. Fulminant drug-induced hepatic failure leading to death or liver transplantation in Sweden. *Scand J Gastroenterol* 2005; **40**: 1095−101.
35. O'Grady JG. Paracetamol-induced acute liver failure: prevention and management. *J Hepatol* 1997; **26**(Suppl 1): 41−6.
36. O'Grady JG, Alexander GJ, Hayllar KM, Williams R. Early indicators of prognosis in fulminant hepatic failure. *Gastroenterology* 1989; **97**: 439−45.
37. Reuben A. Hy's law. *Hepatology* 2004; **39**: 574−8.
38. Bjornsson E, Olsson R. Suspected drug-induced liver fatalities reported to the WHO database. *Dig Liver Dis* 2006; **38**: 33−8.
39. Danan G, Benichou C. Causality assessment of adverse reactions to drugs − I. A novel method based on the conclusions of international consensus meetings: application to drug-induced liver injuries. *J Clin Epidemiol* 1993; **46**: 1323−30.
40. Maria VA, Victorino RM. Development and validation of a clinical scale for the diagnosis of drug-induced hepatitis. *Hepatology* 1997; **26**: 664−9.
41. Macedo AF, Marques FB, Ribeiro CF, Teixeira F. Causality assessment of adverse drug reactions: comparison of the results obtained from published decisional algorithms and from the evaluations of an expert panel, according to different levels of imputability. *J Clin Pharm Ther* 2003; **28**: 137−43.
42. Seeff LB, Lindsay KL, Bacon BR, Kresina TF, Hoofnagle JH. Complementary and alternative medicine in chronic liver disease. *Hepatology* 2001; **34**: 595−603.

43. Tuffs A. Three out of four Germans have used complementary or natural remedies. *BMJ* 2002; **325**: 990.
44. Ernst E. Herbal medicines: where is the evidence? *BMJ* 2000; **321**: 395–6.
45. Linde K, Ramirez G, Mulrow CD *et al*. St John's wort for depression – an overview and meta-analysis of randomised clinical trials. *BMJ* 1996; **313**: 253–8.
46. Stedman C. Herbal hepatotoxicity. *Semin Liver Dis* 2002; **22**: 195–206.
47. Karliova M, Treichel U, Malago M *et al*. Interaction of *Hypericum perforatum* (St. John's wort) with cyclosporin A metabolism in a patient after liver transplantation. *J Hepatol* 2000; **33**: 853–5.
48. Mathijssen RH, Verweij J, de BP *et al*. Effects of St. John's wort on irinotecan metabolism. *J Natl Cancer Inst* 2002; **94**: 1247–9.
49. Risks of herbal therapies . . . and a caution about "skinny pill for kids". *Child Health Alert* 2003; **21**: 2.
50. Eisenberg DM, Kessler RC, Van Rompay MI *et al*. Perceptions about complementary therapies relative to conventional therapies among adults who use both: results from a national survey. *Ann Intern Med* 2001; **135**: 344–51.
51. Houghton P. UK needs greater expertise in TCM. *The Pharmaceutical Journal* 2004; 273.
52. Burton B. Complementary medicines industry in crisis after recall of 1546 products. *BMJ* 2003; **326**: 1001.
53. Espinoza EO, Mann MJ, Bleasdell B. Arsenic and mercury in traditional Chinese herbal balls. *N Engl J Med* 1995; **333**: 803–4.
54. Keane FM, Munn SE, du Vivier AW *et al*. Analysis of Chinese herbal creams prescribed for dermatological conditions. *BMJ* 1999; **318**: 563–4.
55. Huang WF, Wen KC, Hsiao ML. Adulteration by synthetic therapeutic substances of traditional Chinese medicines in Taiwan. *J Clin Pharmacol* 1997; **37**: 344–50.
56. Lord GM, Tagore R, Cook T *et al*. Nephropathy caused by Chinese herbs in the UK. *Lancet* 1999; **354**: 481–2.
57. Lord GM, Cook T, Arlt VM *et al*. Urothelial malignant disease and Chinese herbal nephropathy. *Lancet* 2001; **358**: 1515–16.
58. Atherton DJ, Rustin MH, Brostoff J. Need for correct identification of herbs in herbal poisoning. *Lancet* 1993; **341**: 637–8.
59. Ferner RE, Beard K. Regulating herbal medicines in the UK. *BMJ* 2005; **331**: 62–3.
60. Adachi M, Saito H, Kobayashi H *et al*. Hepatic injury in 12 patients taking the herbal weight loss aids Chaso or Onshido. *Ann Intern Med* 2003; **139**: 488–92.
61. Geubel AP, De GC, Alves N *et al*. Liver damage caused by therapeutic vitamin A administration: estimate of dose-related toxicity in 41 cases. *Gastroenterology* 1991; **100**: 1701–9.
62. Maria V, Albuquerque A, Loureiro A *et al*. Severe cholestatic hepatitis induced by pyritinol. *BMJ* 2004; **328**: 572–4.
63. Mohabbat O, Younos MS, Merzad AA *et al*. An outbreak of hepatic veno-occlusive disease in north-western Afghanistan. *Lancet* 1976; **2**: 269–71.
64. Sheikh NM, Philen RM, Love LA. Chaparral-associated hepatotoxicity. *Arch Intern Med* 1997; **157**: 913–19.
65. Korkia P, Stimson GV. Indications of prevalence, practice and effects of anabolic steroid use in Great Britain. *Int J Sports Med* 1997; **18**: 557–62.
66. Milroy CM, Clark JC, Forrest AR. Pathology of deaths associated with "ecstasy" and "eve" misuse. *J Clin Pathol* 1996; **49**: 149–53.
67. Freeman RW, Harbison RD. Hepatic periportal necrosis induced by chronic administration of cocaine. *Biochem Pharmacol* 1981; **30**: 777–83.
68. Wanless IR, Dore S, Gopinath N *et al*. Histopathology of cocaine hepatotoxicity. Report of four patients. *Gastroenterology* 1990; **98**: 497–501.
69. Kanel GC, Cassidy W, Shuster L, Reynolds TB. Cocaine-induced liver cell injury: comparison of morphological features in man and in experimental models. *Hepatology* 1990; **11**: 646–51.
70. Makin AJ, Wendon J, Williams R. A 7-year experience of severe acetaminophen-induced hepatotoxicity (1987–1993). *Gastroenterology* 1995; **109**: 1907–16.
71. O'Grady JG. Broadening the view of acetaminophen hepatotoxicity. *Hepatology* 2005; **42**: 1252–4.

72. Zimmerman HJ, Maddrey WC. Acetaminophen (paracetamol) hepatotoxicity with regular intake of alcohol: analysis of instances of therapeutic misadventure. *Hepatology* 1995; **22**: 767–73.

73. Kamijo Y, Soma K, Iwabuchi K, Ohwada T. Massive noninflammatory periportal liver necrosis following concentrated acetic acid ingestion. *Arch Pathol Lab Med* 2000; **124**: 127–9.

74. Bennett DR, Baird CJ, Chan KM *et al.* Zinc toxicity following massive coin ingestion. *Am J Forensic Med Pathol* 1997; **18**: 148–53.

75. Bica I, McGovern B, Dhar R *et al.* Increasing mortality due to end-stage liver disease in patients with human immunodeficiency virus infection. *Clin Infect Dis* 2001; **32**: 492–7.

76. Wit FW, Weverling GJ, Weel J *et al.* Incidence of and risk factors for severe hepatotoxicity associated with antiretroviral combination therapy. *J Infect Dis* 2002; **186**: 23–31.

77. Kontorinis N, Dieterich DT. Toxicity of non-nucleoside analogue reverse transcriptase inhibitors. *Semin Liver Dis* 2003; **23**: 173–82.

78. McKenzie R, Fried MW, Sallie R *et al.* Hepatic failure and lactic acidosis due to fialuridine (FIAU), an investigational nucleoside analogue for chronic hepatitis B. *N Engl J Med* 1995; **333**: 1099–105.

79. Skoulidis F, Alexander GJ, Davies SE. Ma huang associated acute liver failure requiring liver transplantation. *Eur J Gastroenterol Hepatol* 2005; **17**: 581–4.

80. Batchelor WB, Heathcote J, Wanless IR. Chaparral-induced hepatic injury. *Am J Gastroenterol* 1995; **90**: 831–3.

81. Benninger J, Schneider HT, Schuppan D *et al.* Acute hepatitis induced by greater celandine (*Chelidonium majus*). *Gastroenterology* 1999; **117**: 1234–7.

82. Woolf GM, Petrovic LM, Rojter SE *et al.* Acute hepatitis associated with the Chinese herbal product jin bu huan. *Ann Intern Med* 1994; **121**: 729–35.

83. Lontos S, Jones RM, Angus PW, Gow PJ. Acute liver failure associated with the use of herbal preparations containing black cohosh. *Med J Aust* 2003; **179**: 390–1.

84. Levitsky J, Alli TA, Wisecarver J, Sorrell MF. Fulminant liver failure associated with the use of black cohosh. *Dig Dis Sci* 2005; **50**: 538–9.

85. Stickel F, Baumuller HM, Seitz K *et al.* Hepatitis induced by Kava (*Piper methysticum rhizoma*). *J Hepatol* 2003; **39**: 62–7.

86. Picciotto A, Campo N, Brizzolara R *et al.* Chronic hepatitis induced by jin bu huan. *J Hepatol* 1998; **28**: 165–7.

87. Geubel AP, De GC, Alves N *et al.* Liver damage caused by therapeutic vitamin A administration: estimate of dose-related toxicity in 41 cases. *Gastroenterology* 1991; **100**: 1701–9.

88. Babb RR, Kieraldo JH. Cirrhosis due to hypervitaminosis A. *West J Med* 1978; **128**: 244–6.

89. Cohen SM, O'Connor AM, Hart J *et al.* Autoimmune hepatitis associated with the use of black cohosh: a case study. *Menopause* 2004; **11**: 575–7.

90. Kamiyama T, Nouchi T, Kojima S *et al.* Autoimmune hepatitis triggered by administration of an herbal medicine. *Am J Gastroenterol* 1997; **92**: 703–4.

91. Chitturi S, Farrell GC. Herbal hepatotoxicity: an expanding but poorly defined problem. *J Gastroenterol Hepatol* 2000; **15**: 1093–9.

92. McDermott WV, Ridker PM. The Budd–Chiari syndrome and hepatic veno-occlusive disease. Recognition and treatment. *Arch Surg* 1990; **125**: 525–7.

93. Zimmerman HJ. Drug-induced liver disease. *Clin Liver Dis* 2000; **4**: 73–96, vi.

94. Sinniah D, Baskaran G, Looi LM, Leong KL. Reye-like syndrome due to margosa oil poisoning: report of a case with postmortem findings. *Am J Gastroenterol* 1982; **77**: 158–61.

95. Fraquelli M, Colli A, Cocciolo M, Conte D. Adult syncytial giant cell chronic hepatitis due to herbal remedy. *J Hepatol* 2000; **33**: 505–8.

Index